Devin Starlanyl and her work are incredible resources to the Fibromyalgic community. She has tirelessly researched her subject and freely and lovingly shared it with those who have suffered pain and disability.

—Dr. Craig N. Anderson, D.C., past president of
the Vermont Chiropractic Association

Fibromyalgia & Chronic Myofascial Pain Syndrome

A SURVIVAL MANUAL

Devin Starlanyl, M.D.
Mary Ellen Copeland, M.S., M.A.

NEW HARBINGER PUBLICATIONS, INC

Figures 1-1, 7-8, and 8-7 were prepared by Tracy Marie Powell.

Except for the above figures, all figures have been previously published in *Myofascial Pain and Dysfunction: The Trigger Point Manual, Volumes I and II* by Janet G. Travell and David G. Simons, 1983 (Vol I), 1992 (Vol II), Williams and Wilkins, Baltimore, MD, and are reproduced here with permission of the copyright holder.

Copyright © 1996 Devin J. Starlanyl and Mary Ellen Copeland
New Harbinger Publications, Inc.
5674 Shattuck Avenue
Oakland, CA 94609

Text design by Tracy Marie Powell.

Distributed in the U.S.A. by Publishers Group West; in Canada by Raincoast Books; in Great Britain by Airlift Book Company, Ltd.; in South Africa by Real Books, Ltd.; in Australia by Boobook; and in New Zealand by Tandem Press.

Library of Congress Catalog Card Number: 95-72229

ISBN 1-57224-046-6

10 9 8 7 6 5

No Matter the Limits
by Rita Shaw (FMily member)

It is such a relief when you first find out
That the pain really does have a name,
And then you will ask (and everyone does),
"Just where can I place all the blame?"

No matter the limits, no matter the pain,
There's no evil, cruel "Master Plan."
It just simply happens. It just simply is.
You adapt, and you change what you can.

But even with knowing the best and the worst,
All the pitfalls the future could hold,
You still have a choice, you quit or you fight.
You determine the story that's told.

And every small step that we take, my dear friends,
Each battle that we slowly win,
Just credits the love and the caring we share
With the FMily that we call our friends.

To blaze any trail in science and medicine, no matter how small the trail, one must stand on the shoulders of giants. I am deeply grateful for Drs. Janet G. Travell and David G. Simons (and Sir William Osler who went before us) for holding me up so high, and for so long.

—Devin Starlanyl

Contents

Illustrations   **xi**

Preface   **xiii**

Acknowledgments   **xvii**

Introduction   **1**

PART I   COMING TO TERMS

Chapter 1   Fibromyalgia Syndrome: What It Is and Isn't   **7**

Chapter 2   The Myofascia   **17**

Chapter 3   Myofascial Trigger Points   **23**

Chapter 4   Chronic Myofascial Pain Syndrome   **29**

Chapter 5   FMS/MPS: The "Double Whammy"   **35**

Chapter 6   Coexisting Conditions   **41**

Chapter 7   Perpetuating Factors   **49**

PART II   COMMON SYMPTOMS AND WHY THEY OCCUR

Chapter 8   Questions and Answers About Common Symptoms   **67**

PART III   INTERNAL AFFAIRS

Chapter 9   Chronic Pain States: A Different Animal   107

Chapter 10   Sleep   113

Chapter 11   Irritable Bowel Syndrome   121

Chapter 12   Flare   127

Chapter 13   Pregnancy   133

PART IV   MIND OVER MATTERS

Chapter 14   The Body-Mind Connection   139

Chapter 15   Taking Control   143

Chapter 16   Coping Day to Day   155

Chapter 17   Keeping a Journal   163

Chapter 18   Fibrofog and other Absurdities   171

Chapter 19   Positive Change   179

PART V   HEALING TOOLS

Chapter 20   Meditation and Mindfulness   191

Chapter 21   Fibromyalgia/Myofascial Pain Syndrome Medications   201

Chapter 22   Enhancing Your Medications   209

Chapter 23   Guaifenesin   219

Chapter 24   Nutrition: Keep It Natural   227

Chapter 25   Bodywork: Helping Your Body Work   237

Chapter 26   Bodyworkers   243

Chapter 27   Bodywork You Can Do Yourself   253

Chapter 28   Alternatives: Other Cultures, Other Ways   267

PART VI   LIFE ISSUES

Chapter 29   Advocating for Yourself   279

Chapter 30   The Home Front   285

Chapter 31   Building Your Support Structure   305

Chapter 32   Past Issues   315

Chapter 33   The Workplace   **321**

Chapter 34   Disability: There Oughtta Be a Law   **333**

Chapter 35   Travel   **345**

Chapter 36   Children with FMS or FMS/MPS Complex   **351**

Chapter 37   Finding Your Primary Care Physician   **355**

Appendix A   Resources   **365**

Appendix B   Additional Reading List   **371**

Appendix C   Suppliers of Health Care Items   **377**

              Bibliography   **381**

              Subject Index   **391**

              Name Index   **403**

Illustrations

Figure 1-1: Location of tender points (2 views)   **11**

Figure 3-1: Location of trigger points in the right scalene   **26**

Figure 3-2: Sternocleidomastoid (SCM) trigger points   **27**

Figure 6-1: Trigger points in the right subcapularis   **42**

Figure 7-1: Trigger points along the iliopsoas   **54**

Figure 7-2: Trigger points in the right piriformus   **55**

Figure 7-3: Trigger points in the gluteus maximus   **55**

Figure 7-4: Trigger points in the peroneals   **59**

Figure 7-5: Trigger points in the intrinsic foot muscles   **60**

Figure 7-6: Morton's foot   **60**

Figure 7-7: Morton's foot callus pattern   **61**

Figure 7-8: Typical FMS/MPS foot and callus pattern   **61**

Figure 7-9: Shoe insert designed by Janet Travell   **61**

Figure 8-1: Trigger points in the right digastric   **77**

Figure 8-2: Trigger points in the left medial pterygoid   **78**

Figure 8-3: Trigger points in the masseter   **78**

Figure 8-4: Trigger points in the platysma   **79**

Figure 8-5: Trigger points in the upper trapezius   80

Figure 8-6: Trigger points in the temporalis   80

Figure 8-7: Extrinsic eye muscles   81

Figure 8-8: Trigger points in the upper and lower splenius cervici   82

Figure 8-9: Trigger point in the orbicularis oculi   82

Figure 8-10: Trigger points in the posterior cervicals   83

Figure 8-11: Trigger points in the right levator scapulae   83

Figure 8-12: Trigger point in the splenius capitus   84

Figure 8-13: Trigger points in the right brachioradialis   84

Figure 8-14: Trigger point in the adductor pollicis and in the opponens pollicis   85

Figure 8-15: Trigger points for the external oblique (heartburn), lower quadrant   87
              oblique, "belch button," and abdominals

Figure 8-16: Trigger points in the serratus anterior   88

Figure 8-17: Trigger points in the left pectoralis   89

Figure 8-18: Trigger points in the left sternalis   90

Figure 8-19: Trigger points in the right infraspinatus   90

Figure 8-20: Trigger points in the multifidi   93

Figure 8-21: Trigger points in the iliocostalis and longissimus   94

Figure 8-22: McBurney's point   95

Figure 8-23: Trigger points in the gluteus minimus   96

Figure 8-24: Trigger points in the hamstrings   97

Figure 8-25: Trigger points in the peroneals   97

Figure 8-26: Trigger points in the tibialis   98

Figure 8-27: Trigger points in the sartorius   99

Figure 8-28: Trigger points in the gastrocnemius   99

Figure 8-29: Trigger points in the soleus   100

Figure 8-30: Trigger points in the vastus medialis and quadriceps   101

Figure 8-31: Trigger points in the adductor longus   101

Figure 8-32: Trigger points in the quadriceps femoris   102

Preface

Devin's Story

I knew of the need for a book such as this long before I began this project. In vain, I tried to talk others into writing it. I felt I had already reached my own limits, even working very part-time (less than 60 hours a year, in short sessions). Eventually, even this became too much. By then, I was holding my own, as long as I didn't work outside my home.

One day I went to a support group in Keene, NH, with the hope of learning something, but fate intervened: the facilitator had run into an emergency and couldn't be there. I wound up giving an impromptu two-hour talk on fibromyalgia syndrome (FMS) and myofascial pain syndrome (MPS). I met many wonderful people at this talk. One of them, Pat, changed my life.

Pat came to see me several weeks after my talk, and I held my first FMS/MPS counseling session. Because of my condition, I hadn't renewed my license, so the meeting was very informal. (All I have learned about MPS and FMS was acquired after my formal schooling was long over—after I got my "FMS/MPS degree.")

We were just two people sitting at a kitchen table, listening and talking to each other. But Pat urged me to start a Brattleboro Support Group. Previously, Pat had met the Vermont Arthritis Foundation Community Relations Representative, and she urged me to arrange a meeting with the Brattleboro Memorial Hospital community liaison, Barbara Gentry (whom I knew), and Lue McWilliams of the Arthritis Foundation. Pat said that she would be there, too, because I was concerned about my ability to facilitate such a group, since both my FMS and MPS are severe, and I tend to turn into a pumpkin by 6 p.m.

We met, and a little more than two weeks later, we held the first support group meeting. I wanted to supply information, but could find little written material. The people who attended asked many questions, and I promised to write up some answers for the next meeting. Participating in this local group led to my participation and current role in the Internet fibrom-l support group.

That was over two and a half years ago. Since then, I've seen more than 400 people with FMS/MPS, and I've written a lot of handouts. I've listened a lot, observed a lot, and done some research. Because of my medical constraints, I did this a little at a time. I've learned a lot, and one of the things I've learned is that people with FMS and/or MPS are very special. They have been through the fire and survived.

Back then, I already knew that FMS and MPS are two separate conditions, even though they often occur together. When the two syndromes form what I call the FMS/MPS Complex, their combined symptoms are more than compounded. The then-current treatments produced very poor results. Since then, I've found some effective medications and treatments for FMS/MPS Complex, which are described in this book.

Last year, one of the people I met was an extraordinary woman named Mary Ellen Copeland. She also has FMS/MPS Complex, compounded with other conditions. In spite of her medical condition, she has written and published two excellent books. She convinced me to collaborate with her on this book, because trying to manage individual consultations was proving impossible, and was ruining my health.

Working on this book, even two hours a day with frequent breaks, became an endurance test. What kept me going was the knowledge that there are so many people out there hurting, misdiagnosed or undiagnosed, who could be greatly helped by the information in this book. I passed the endurance test because of such people.

If you are one of them, there is much for you to learn. I hope the rewards that will result from learning the information contained within will make a careful reading worth your while. All I ask is that you inform others with similar symptoms—and there are many—that there may be answers to their anguished questions and relief for their pain.

Mary Ellen's Story

I awaken after a fitful night's sleep to find my foot in a severe, excruciatingly painful cramp. The day has begun without any reprieve.

I work to release the cramp by massaging my foot with my hand. That doesn't work. I clamber out of bed to try and walk it out. After a while, the cramp subsides, replaced by a dull, aching persistent pain. My whole body feels stiff and sore. The walk to get the paper is a nightmare. Now the irritable bowel is starting to kick up and I have to make a fast dash for the bathroom. Another day in my life with fibromyalgia.

Sometimes when I first awaken, when I am still relaxed and groggy from sleep, before I move, before I am aware how radically my life has changed in the last 18 months, I briefly feel that all is well. I treasure such infrequent moments before I stretch or turn, when I feel no pain.

About eight years ago, strange things began to happen to the lower end of my digestive system. Various gastroenterologists told me it was irritable bowel syndrome and that I should learn to live with it. They also intimated that if I could learn to relax, it would go away.

Various parts of my body began to tingle or to go numb. My doctor said it was arthritis of the neck, common to people my age—nothing to worry about. I didn't buy the arthritis-of-the-neck diagnosis. The numbness and tingling was all over my body and worsening each day.

I went back to the doctor. He said if it would relieve my anxiety, he would refer me to a neurologist. When I walked into the neurologist's office, it was clear he had been coached by my doctor. After the most perfunctory examination, he confirmed my doctor's diagnosis. Arthritis of the neck. Take some anti-inflammatories. Two weeks later I got a bill for $270. The symptoms worsened.

The next few months were a haze of doctors' offices, big machines that made loud noises, and well-meaning physicians telling me that there was nothing wrong with me. I wish they could have walked a mile in my shoes.

Then, one evening a friend dropped in with a well-worn copy of the *Merck Manual*. He opened it to a page he had marked and said, "This is what you have." I thought, "Hmm. Your local friendly amateur diagnostician." It was the same disease I had seen described in an article in our local newspaper about a doctor named Devin Starlanyl, who had fibromyalgia.

Several days later, I had my annual check-up with my gynecologist. She asked me how I'd been. I said "horrific" and then I blurted out some of my symptoms. I said, "You know, I think I have fibromyalgia." She said, "Of course you do," and then she gave me Devin Starlanyl's phone number on a piece of paper.

Eight months later, after working intensively with Devin and other supportive health care professionals, I am beginning to feel some hope that I may be able to pick up some of the shattered pieces of my life and go on; that I may be able to play with a grandchild without wincing in pain; and that I may view the world from the top of a mountain, again.

An Invitation

Both of us have firsthand knowledge of the consequences of having severe FMS/MPS Complex and know full well the losses and challenges that you face every day of your life. We give you this book to help you reclaim a measure of control over your life. Having climbed our own Matterhorns and set down our flags, we have built some warm, snug cabins and laid out a nourishing feast. This is an invitation for you to join us. The road is a little steep and it certainly can be rocky in places, but nothing can beat the view.

Acknowledgments

To my coauthor, Mary Ellen Copeland, I am grateful that she talked me into this project, and for her help and encouragement. I also have a deep appreciation for the work of Dusty Bernard and Kayla Sussell, our editors. They took a wealth of data and formed it into a cohesive and understandable book, usable to the lay reader. I am especially thankful for the encouragement and companionship I received from Kayla, as I struggled to finish the book before it finished me.

This book has been greatly enriched by the gracious guidance and help of David G. Simons. The work he did with Janet G. Travell is the foundation of much of the book. I am grateful for his help in securing the marvelous illustrations by Barbara D. Cummings, from the *Trigger Point Manuals*.

I give thanks to Craig Anderson, who first told me about Janet Travell. As my physician and chiropractor, he not only worked at keeping me healthy, but he helped to write the sections on chiropractic and electronic stimulation, and was a fount of information. I thank the rest of my medical team: Martha Wilmot, massage therapist; Tina Wyman, hospital physical therapist; Drs. Bob and David Fagelson, and Carolyn Taylor-Olson who supplied the needed extra care and support that enabled me to write. I thank Jeffrey Wallace, Arti Carrasquillo, and Cheri Brodhurst for insight into the special needs of their patients.

This book is the greater for information supplied by Margo McCaffery from the book she wrote with Alexandra Beebe on pain. I thank R. Paul St. Amand for his work on guaifenesin, and for sharing his wisdom and time with me. Thanks go to Sharon Butler, Lynne August, Lonny Brown, Wayne London, Camilla Cracciola, and David Nye for their additions to this book.

I am truly grateful for Brattleboro Memorial Hospital and Barbara Gentry for providing a home for our local FMS/MPS support group, for the hospital library and librarian, Marty Finn, and for Pat Remick who gave me the courage to start the group.

I thank my friend Miryam Williamson, who helped me get onto the Internet and the fibrom-l listserv, and Susan Fuller who first read the manuscript.

Kudos go to the amazing and ever-patient librarians at Brooks Memorial Library in Brattleboro, VT, who came up with obscure literature and exact information when I needed it.

I would also like to thank my fibrom-l FMily, especially Rita Shaw, who's poem graces this book, and for the cyberdocs and others who kindly sent me so much information, and for my local FMily who gave me so much support, insight, and data. I love them all.

My last thanks goes to those who supported me from the first, throughout this endurance trial, with love and encouragement. To my husband Rick, my sister Peggy, Mom and Dad Lawrence, Aunt Peg, and Elliot, Jenni, Trib and Ian, and to our Creator, thank you very much.

Fibromyalgia & Chronic Myofascial Pain Syndrome

A S U R V I V A L M A N U A L

Introduction

Most people love a mystery. They search for clues and eventually find out "who done it." When the "who done it" turns out to be fibromyalgia and/or myofascial pain syndrome, the real mystery remains: What can you do about all your mysterious symptoms, many of which are frightening, not to mention disabling?

Think of the solution to that mystery as buried treasure. To find it, you need a map. In the realm of diagnosis and treatment, the maps are sometimes obscure and written in a dialect that most people don't readily understand. Fortunately, when it comes to fibromyalgia syndrome (FMS) and myofascial pain syndrome (MPS), the maps are already there. This book will guide you through them.

In the case of MPS, the map leading to diagnosis and treatment is specific and accurate, thanks to the *Trigger Point Manuals* by Drs. Janet G. Travell and David G. Simons. This book refers to them often. Unfortunately, though, many members of the medical profession have not read them. For this lapse in medical education, their patients pay. With your help, this book can lead them to these invaluable manuals.

What's in This Book

You are about to embark on a journey of discovery. You will learn how to tell whether you have myofascial pain trigger points, FMS, MPS, or the FMS/MPS Complex, and you will discover many, many steps you can take to manage your symptoms successfully.

In Part I, Coming to Terms, you'll find out what FMS and MPS are. These conditions can exist separately or together, and identifying which of your symptoms result from which condition is crucial in treating them. An important element of Part I is its discussion of trigger points, complete with illustrations; if you have MPS either with or without FMS, you'll find you—and your doctor—can't do without this information. You'll also learn about coexisting conditions and perpetuating factors that must be taken into account for diagnosis and treatment.

Part II, Defining Your Limits, contains only one chapter, but you'll be referring to it often. Whatever symptoms you may be experiencing from FMS and/or MPS—including symptoms that may well have been misdiagnosed as caused by other illnesses—you're likely to find them described and explained here, along with cross-references to more detailed discussions in other parts of the book.

Part III, Internal Affairs, addresses the issue of chronic pain, which is often the overriding symptom in FMS and MPS. It also examines the sleep factor and other internal happenings, including irritable bowel syndrome (IBS), flare (significant increase in intensity, frequency, and number of symptoms), and, in case you're expecting a child or planning to have one, pregnancy.

In Part IV, Mind over Matters, you'll learn about the power of the mind to counteract physical symptoms—and what to do when your otherwise useful mind is befuddled by "fibrofog." Perhaps you will choose to meditate, to keep a journal, or to find peace of mind by taking long walks. Perhaps you will use a judicious mix of these and other mental disciplines. Whatever techniques you decide to use, you'll find that by holding on to a positive attitude and applying it daily to the many challenges you face, you can make a significant, lasting difference in the quality of your life.

Part V, Healing Tools, starts by examining the medications available for treating your symptoms and the steps you can take to enhance their effects. An entire chapter is devoted to guaifenesin—an over-the-counter medication that is just now emerging as a possibly effective treatment for FMS. In addition, you'll find out how to use bodywork, by yourself and with professional practitioners, and how to optimize your diet. Part V ends with a description of less commonly known treatments, often from other cultures, that have been effective in treating the symptoms of FMS and MPS.

Part VI, Life Issues, gives you a chance to pinpoint and improve conditions in specific areas of your life, including your home and family, your workplace, and travel situations, and shows you how to build a support structure that works. You'll find out how to examine past issues that may be affecting how you feel now. You'll learn about your rights as a person with a disability, and take a look at the special challenges faced by children with FMS and/or MPS. The final chapter in Part VI describes the procedures to follow to find the best primary care physician you can.

The Bibliography provides the specific references used as source material in the text. Appendix A offers the names of agencies to contact for further information and assistance. In Appendix B, you'll find suggestions for further reading, and Appendix C provides a list of suppliers of useful health care items that have been mentioned in the text. If you don't find a reference in the Bibliography it will be in Appendix B, the Additional Reading List.

The illustrations in this book are very special. That's because in addition to trigger points (TrPs) causing pain where they are located, they refer pain to other parts in the body from the point of origin. They refer pain in specific patterns that are replicated from patient to patient.

To use the illustrations, find the pain pattern that reminds you of the area of pain that you experience. The worst of the pain pattern is marked by solid areas. The stippled (dotted) areas show other locations where the pain is referred to—where it is less severe. Then you want to look for the "x." That is the actual site of the trigger point (TrP), and that is where you need to focus your attention. Note that, sometimes, the referred pain pattern is in the front of the body and the TrP is in the back. You will learn more about this in the book.

At times, you may very well want to bring this book with you to your doctor's office. Most doctors are not trained to diagnose and treat FMS or MPS at all. Many doctors don't "believe" in these medical conditions, although they are quite common and have been recognized by official medical authorities and organizations. Armed with this book, you may be able to educate these physicians and help them to change their minds.

Ideally, this book will already be on your doctor's bookshelf. If it is not, with your own copy in hand, you can point to the description of a symptom and exclaim, "I told you I wasn't imagining it!" You can say, "There's a lot of detailed information in here about trigger points, and I don't understand it all. I'd appreciate it if you would take a look and help me out." You can ask, "Have you ever heard of this treatment (or symptom)? Will you help me find out more about it?"

Use this book as a positive force—a survival manual. When you've finished reading it, you will know exactly what you're up against and the tools you will need to manage the many issues that arise with FMS, MPS, and FMS/MPS Complex. With these tools you can significantly improve the quality of your life—as well as the lives of those around you.

PART I

COMING TO TERMS

CHAPTER 1

Fibromyalgia Syndrome: What It Is and Isn't

Before you read this chapter, a word of warning: Having fibromyalgia syndrome (FMS) is no fun. You know that already. But reading about it shouldn't depress you. Fibromyalgia is neither progressive nor deadly. There are many things you can do to improve the quality of your life and you'll learn about them in this book. We both have FMS and we've learned how to take control of our lives; as we hope to teach you how to take control of yours. Whatever your previous experience with FMS has been, you are no longer alone.

The best place to start is to describe what you may be experiencing in your body and mind.

What's in a Name

Fibromyalgia Syndrome (FMS) is pronounced "fie-bro-my-al-jia sind-rome." The word "fibromyalgia" is a combination of the Latin roots "fibro" (connective tissue fibers), "my" (muscle), "al" (pain), and "gia" (condition of). The word syndrome simply means a group of signs and symptoms that occur together which characterize a particular abnormality.

FMS is not a new syndrome. It was first described by William Balfour, a surgeon at the University of Edinburgh, in 1816 (van Why 1994), but for many years the medical profession called it many different names, including chronic rheumatism, myalgia, pressure point syndrome, and fibrositis, and the condition was also thought to be psychological by some physicians. (Note that FMS is not the same as myofascial pain syndrome (MPS), which is discussed in Chapters 3, 4, and 5.) In other words, the prevailing belief was that "It was all in your head" or "It was your own fault that you were sick."

In 1987, the American Medical Association (AMA) recognized FMS as a true illness and a major cause of disability. Now, nearly ten years later, it is still, unfortunately, too often dismissed as the "newest fad disease," and most physicians still lack the diagnostic skills needed to differentiate it from other chronic pain conditions. In fact, until recently, it was rare to find a doctor who had even heard of FMS as a "real" condition, and very few doctors have received any substantial training in treating the syndrome.

Many physicians are defensive about their lack of training in this field and there are some who still refuse to acknowledge that FMS (and MPS) really exist. You may have encountered such practitioners. Fortunately, this attitude is becoming less common.

Aiming for a Diagnosis

The average FMS patient suffers for five years and spends thousands of dollars on medical bills before receiving an accurate diagnosis. As a result of misdiagnosis, more than half of all patients undergo unnecessary surgery.

It isn't unusual for those who are fibromyalgia patients to feel a profound sense of relief when they learn they have a recognized illness and they come to understand that it isn't progressive.

If this has been your experience, you may cry with relief at not having to doubt yourself any longer. At last, someone believes you and believes in you. You really *do* have these symptoms, and you are no longer fighting the world alone. Debilitating self-doubt can be replaced with appropriate self-care.

Admittedly, if your doctor has no specific training in FMS, his or her initial diagnosis can be extremely difficult. Patients come in with very different symptoms every visit, which often do not appear to be related to each other. These can run the gamut from sleep problems, blurred vision, falling, itching, and pelvic pain, to hearing loss, and soft tissue aches and pains. The list sometimes seems endless.

Many patients don't even tell their doctors *all* of their symptoms because they sense the doctor's disbelief. Our culture expects its physicians to know all and see all, which is a recipe for trouble for both doctor and patient when the illness presents as complicated a diagnosis as FMS does.

With FMS, the standard medical tests can come back negative, and the doctor can become very frustrated. The patient may look fine but he or she has constant, unsubstantiated complaints. To make things even more confusing, the signs and symptoms can, and frequently do, fluctuate from hour to hour and day to day.

> I coined the word "FMily" to describe the special bond those of us who have fibromyalgia all share. We often have more in common with our fellow fibromites (another newly coined word you'll find in this book) than we do with members of our family.
>
> D.J.S.

In desperation, many doctors often send their patients to physical therapy or for psychological counseling. Yet, most often, every treatment a person with FMS tries only aggravates the symptoms further.

It is important to understand that FMS is not a catch-all, "wastebasket" diagnosis. "FMS is a specific, chronic non-degenerative, non-progressive, non-inflammatory, truly systemic pain condition—a true syndrome"(van Why 1994). Very recently, however, the National Institutes of Health have reclassified it as a true disease, but most authorities today still say that, technically, FMS is not a disease. *Diseases* have known causes and well-understood mechanisms for producing symptoms. Instead, FMS is called a *syndrome,* which means it is a specific set of signs and symptoms that occur together.

Don't let this categorization fool you into thinking that fibromyalgia is any less serious or potentially disabling than a "disease." Rheumatoid arthritis, lupus, and other serious afflictions are also classified as syndromes.

The essential symptom of FMS is pain (see Chapter 9, Chronic Pain) except in the case of elderly patients. Older patients are more troubled by fatigue and depression. In younger people, discomfort after minimal exercise, low-grade fever or below-normal temperature, and skin sensitivity are also common.

Laboratory Tests

Laboratory tests for fibromyalgia are valid only to rule out other conditions. As this book goes to press, there is still no blood test that can accurately identify fibromyalgia.

Unfortunately, although some doctors claim to have a blood test for it, thousands of dollars worth of blood tests later, their patients still have received no diagnosis. Then, these doctors often send their patients to see psychiatrists, because "nothing showed up in the blood test, so therefore nothing can be wrong." Unfortunately, until physicians learn to ask the right questions, they will be unable to provide the right answers.

An "Official" Diagnosis

The official definition of fibromyalgia came about as a result of the Copenhagen Declaration (see Bibliography), which established fibromyalgia as an officially recognized syndrome on January 1, 1993, for the World Health Organization. This definition was presented at the Second World Congress on Myofascial Pain and Fibromyalgia, which was held in Copenhagen in 1992.

The Copenhagen Declaration defines FMS as a painful, but not articular (not present in the joints), condition predominantly involving muscles, and as the *most common cause of chronic, widespread musculoskeletal pain.*

The diagnostic fine points of FMS had been defined (van Why 1994) by the American College of Rheumatology (ACR) in 1990. The World Health Organization considered the ACR definition as "suitable for research purposes" and added the following symptoms to the syndrome. (Note that these are often overlooked):

". . . . the presence of unexplained widespread pain or aching, persistent fatigue, generalized morning stiffness, non-refreshing sleep, and multiple tender points. *Most* patients with these symptoms have 11 or more tender points. But a variable proportion of otherwise typical patients may have less than 11 tender points at the time of the examination." (See the next section for a discussion of tender points.)

In addition, the Copenhagen Declaration states that fibromyalgia syndrome is "part of a wider syndrome encompassing headaches, irritable bladder, dysmenorrhea, cold sensitivity, Raynaud's phenomenon, restless legs, atypical patterns of numbness and tingling, exercise intolerance and complaints of weakness."

Note: Here the document appears to be referring to the FMS/MPS Complex, which consists of fibromyalgia complicated with Myofascial Pain Syndrome (MPS). MPS will be explained and discussed in Chapters 4 and 5.

The Copenhagen Declaration goes on to state that the psychological state of FMS patients, which is often one of depression and anxiety, could well be *caused* by the physical conditions. Chronic pain, especially pain of undiagnosed origin, is a frequent source of depression and anxiety.

Lately, there have been some educational articles about FMS in the popular press. This has alerted many patients to the true nature of their problem. For example, one member of a local support group (you'll find out more about support groups in Chapter 31) had been seeing a specialist for some time, without receiving a diagnosis. She took one of these articles to her doctor and told him, "This is what I have. It's fibromyalgia." His response was, "I've known that for two years. I didn't tell you, because there's nothing you can do about it anyway." This physician's attitude has no place in the practice of medicine—nor anywhere else. There are effective treatments for FMS, and he owed it to his patient to inform her of her correct diagnosis. Anything short of that is unethical.

Tender Points

The Copenhagen official Fibromyalgia Syndrome definition states that you must have at least 11 of the 18 specified *tender points* to be diagnosed with FMS. Tender points hurt where pressed, but they do not refer pain elsewhere—that is, pressing a tender point does not cause pain in some other part of the body. (Note that when examining yourself for tender points, you must use enough pressure to whiten the thumbnail.)

The official definition further requires that tender points must be present in all four quadrants of the body—that is, the upper right and left and lower right and left parts of your body. (See Figure 1-1.) Furthermore, you must have had widespread, more-or-less continuous pain for at least three months. Because tender points can fluctuate and vary from day to day, if you don't have "11 out of the 18" on a given day, your doctor may diagnose "possible FMS" and may need to count the tender points again on future visits.

As Figure 1-1 shows, tender points occur in pairs on various parts of the body. Because they occur in pairs, the pain is usually distributed equally on both sides of the body.

On the back of your body, tender points are present in the following places:

- along the spine in the neck, where the head and neck meet;

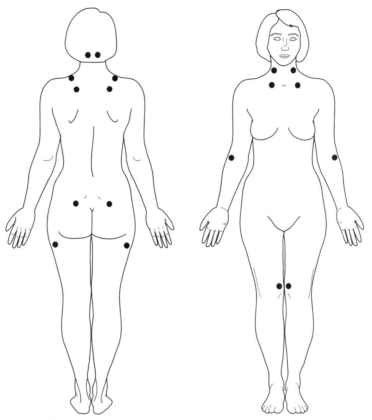

Figure 1-1: Location of tender points

- On the upper line of the shoulder, a little less than halfway from the shoulder to the neck;

- Three finger widths, on a diagonal, inward from the last points;

- On the back fairly close to the "dimples" above the buttocks, a little less than halfway in toward the spine;

- Below the buttocks, very close to the outside edge of the thigh, about three finger widths.

On the front of your body, tender points are present in the following places:

- On the neck, just above inner edge of the collarbone;

- Still on the neck, a little further out from the last points, about four finger widths down;

- On the inner (palm) side of the lower arm, about three finger widths below the elbow crease;

- On the inner side of the knee, in the "fat pad."

Note, however, that the tender point locations shown in this diagram are not "written in stone." They can vary from person to person, which can cause further problems with diagnosis. In *traumatic FMS*, for example, tender points are often clustered around an injury instead of, or in addition to, the 18 "official" points. These clusters can also occur around a repetitive strain or a degenerative and/or inflammatory problem, such as arthritis.

Looking at the Facts

Knowledge, as they say, is power. This is especially true with fibromyalgia syndrome. The more you know about it, the better able you will be to deal with it.

FMS can occur at any age. Most patients, when questioned carefully, reveal that their symptoms began at an early age. Often the first sign is "growing pains."

Pain is frequently the most prominent symptom of FMS, but there are many others. For example, your eyes may often be too dry, but at other times they will water. Your thermal regulatory system is out of whack. You may notice this thermal fluctuation when you get out of bed (often due to bladder irritability) during the night. You may have to wait for your temperature to cool down after getting back in bed, before you can pull the bedcover up again.

Another symptom of FMS is spasticity (tightness) which can constrict the peripheral blood vessels—those close to the skin. This symptom, especially in the winter, makes certain parts of our bodies—most often the buttocks and thighs—feel like cold slabs of meat.

You may experience skin mottling, and nail ridges. Fingernails can break off, often in crescent-shaped pieces. If nails do grow, they sometimes start to curve under.

Often FMS is found coexisting with one or more other disorders (see Chapter 6, Coexisting Conditions), and FMS may also amplify the symptoms of another disorder.

FMS adds stress to everything we do. Many fibromites cannot sit still or maintain any other position for longer than 20 minutes without becoming stiff. Morning stiffness can take an hour or more to wear off.

The course of FMS can be mild, moderate, or severe. In some cases there are remissions (van Why 1944). Nearly everyone with FMS exhibits reduced coordination skills and decreased endurance abilities. FMS can be as disabling as rheumatoid arthritis. Approximately 30 percent of FMS patients cannot hold down their jobs due to their chronic, unrelenting symptoms (Wolfe 1989). It often creeps up, one symptom at a time. The person with FMS learns to live with those symptoms until his or her quality of life becomes seriously compromised.

The Inheritance Factor

It appears that the tendency to develop FMS is inherited.

The bad news is that a study by Pellegrino, Waylonis, and Sommer (1989a) at Ohio State found that FMS is inherited on an "autosomal dominant basis." This means that approximately half of the children of an FMS parent will eventually develop FMS.

If the person with FMS *is* a child, his or her needs are different from those of adults with the same condition. Chapter 36 deals with this issue.

Sensitivity Amplification

FMS is a sensitivity-amplification syndrome. Because of this it has been called the "Irritable Everything Syndrome." This means that fibromites are sensitive to smells, sounds, lights, and vibrations. The *noise* emitted by fluorescent lights can drive them crazy.

FMS sensitizes nerve endings, which means that the ends of the nerve receptors have changed shape. Because of this, for example, your body might interpret "touch, light, or sound" as "pain." Your brain knows pain is a danger signal—an indication that something is wrong and needs attention—so it mobilizes its defenses. For example, adrenaline starts pumping and your muscles tense, ready for "fight or flight" action. Your heart speeds up. Blood flow slows to areas that are not immediately needed for action, such as your digestive tract, but blood flow to your muscles increases. Then, when those defenses aren't used (or when no action is taken) the body/mind system becomes anxious.

Frequently, for fibromites, the pain does *not* indicate a dangerous situation. But our bodies are getting the wrong signals. Pain itself causes stress and depression, which may cause further contraction and then more pain. The pain signal is an indication that it's time to do something about the problem. (See Chapter 9, Chronic Pain.)

Sleep

Sleep plays a crucial role in FMS. Perhaps you aren't getting enough sleep, or the right *kind* of sleep. You may have insomnia, or a host of other sleep-related problems. See Chapter 10, Sleep, for information about sleep disorders and what you can do about them.

Muscle Communication

Much of our mental and physical sense of continuity and security as fibromites depends upon our ability to repeat appropriate and predictable actions, but this ability is disrupted in FMS. *Neurotransmitters,* which are the biochemical substances that transmit nerve impulses across synapses, normally inform our muscles constantly about what they're doing so that their actions can be modified. For fibromites, much of our muscle tension function is improperly controlled by these neurotransmitters.

Healthy people think nothing of picking up a glass of water and bringing it to their lips. They know just how tightly their hand has to maintain a grip, how heavy the glass of water feels, and how much speed is appropriate to accomplish this act smoothly. Fibromites, however, lack proper sensory feedback. Their thumbs grasp with too little pressure, and their wrist muscles let go when flexed. The economy of effort is not there. To enable us to sit, walk, and stand, the entire musculature must be able to feel its own activity accurately.

Triggering Events

In FMS, a triggering event often activates biochemical changes, causing a cascade of symptoms. For example, unremitting grief of six months or longer can trigger FMS. It's sort of like "Survivors Syndrome." Cumulative trauma, protracted labor in pregnancy, open-heart surgery, even inguinal hernia repair have all been triggering events for FMS. Life stressors can overwhelm the body's balancing act, turning life itself into an endurance contest.

Note, however, that only about 20 percent of FMS cases have a known triggering event that initiates the first obvious *flare*. During a flare, current symptoms become more intense, and new symptoms frequently develop.

> About 25 percent of the FMS patients I see are men. This ratio differs from most sources in the literature. I think that this is due to FMS being underdiagnosed in males. Some doctors even refuse to believe that men can contract FMS. I've talked with a few physicians I know who can diagnose FMS with accuracy, such as Paul St. Amand in California (who has FMS). They are also finding that about 25 percent of their patients with FMS are male.
>
> D.J.S.

Debunking the Myths

There are some myths about FMS that must be silenced. The following list is adapted from Richard van Why's work. Van Why is a nurse and massage therapist, who gives excellent weekend courses on fibromyalgia for massage therapists. (See Bibliography.) Doctors and patients are invited to attend his seminars. He's one of our FMily, and a fountain of knowledge.

- **FMS is a controversial condition.**

   This implies that it may not really exist. The American College of Rheumatology, American Medical Association, World Health Organization, and the National Institutes of Health have all accepted FMS as a legitimate clinical entity. There is no excuse for doctors "not believing" in its reality. It's real.

- **FMS is benign, meaning nonmalignant.**

   True, it isn't malignant. But "benign" is often wrongly translated as "harmless and easy to live with." FMS is neither.

- **FMS is psychogenic, meaning it is a physical sign of mental illness.**

   Studies have shown that the incidence of mental problems is no higher with FMS patients than with any other type of chronic pain syndrome.

- **FMS is curable.**

   Not yet, although there are a lot of researchers working on it. On a more positive note, there are ways to achieve a remission of symptoms.

Dealing with Other People

As an FMS patient, you have probably been burdened with a long history of undiagnosed illness. Because your condition is more or less invisible, friends and family may not believe you when you say you hurt, so you may also be suffering from a loss of self-esteem. In other words, you may be deprived of the normal support network that forms around a chronically ill person because "you look just fine." And without the support of family and friends, you may well withdraw from others to conserve what little self-esteem and energy you have left. Chapter 31, Building Your Support Structure, provides a number of techniques to help you pull yourself out of this box.

The difficulties you may encounter when dealing with government and insurance services to receive the support you need can further contribute to your loss of self-esteem and can complicate work and economic issues. Chapter 34, Disability, covers this subject in detail.

Then there's also the issue of dealing with the furnishings and people in your workplace. A lot of how you are accommodated there is up to you. Chapter 33, The Workplace, explains what you can do to make your workplace less stressful.

In Conclusion

In this chapter we've taken a brief look at the basic components of FMS and have touched on some of the difficulties that having FMS creates in our lives. The good news is that this book describes many of the tools that are available to help you create your own personal health care system and to improve the quality of your life. These include support groups, exercises, medications, bodywork, relaxation techniques, and organizational skills.

So, it's time for an attitude adjustment. True, you have a high maintenance body. But so do expensive sports cars, and there is no question that they are valuable and coveted!

CHAPTER 2

The Myofascia

When we were in grade school, we learned about the various systems of the body: the digestive system, the reproductive system, the respiratory system, and so forth. At that time, we were led to believe that we'd learned a bit about every part of the body. However, one "part" that was never mentioned in any of the elementary overviews of the body that we studied is the myofascia.

Myofascia, a thin almost translucent film that wraps around muscle tissue, is the tissue that holds all the other parts together. It gives shape to and supports all of the body's musculature.

For people with fibromyalgia syndrome (FMS) and / or myofascial pain syndrome (MPS), the myofascia takes on a new importance. You've already learned a bit about FMS in Chapter 1 and MPS is discussed in Chapters 4 and 5. To fully understand these syndromes, however, you will need some information about the myofascia.

Myofascia and the Fight or Flight Response

Half a century ago, Hans Selye, the "Father of Stress Theory," studied the effects of stress on the human organism. He found that when the body experiences a "stressor," that stressor may trigger the "fight or flight" response. That is, when responding to stress, the body undergoes certain complex physiological changes that will enable it either to fight the stressor or to flee from it.

When some of Dr. Selye's patients responded to *repeated* stressors with the fight or flight response again and again, he saw something he called *calciphylaxis* occurring in their tissues. He defined calciphylaxis as "an induced hypersensitivity in which tissues respond to various challenging agents with a sudden calcification" (Selye 1975). It didn't matter whether the stressor was chronic illness, severe emotional trauma, or multiple injuries, repeated experience of the fight or flight response caused tissue changes.

It appears that this "calcification" or tightening in the myofascia occurs in many cases of FMS and/or MPS. If both of these conditions are present, this tightening causes more than double the trouble. When the myofascial tissues become thickened and lose their elasticity, the neurotransmitters' ability to send and receive messages between the mind and body is damaged, and the communication between the mind and body is disrupted. Myofascia, then, may well be the *key* to what is wrong with people with FMS/MPS.

Neurotransmitters

Neurotransmitters are electro-biochemical agents that transmit information across nerve synapses. They are the vehicles that carry information back and forth between your body and mind. One might say that neurotransmitters are the "information superhighway" between the body and mind.

Ground Substance

In the myofascia there is a material called *ground substance*. This material can exist in a solid, semi-solid, or fluid state, sort of like the character Odo on "Deep Space Nine." (Odo can change from humanoid form to a gelatinous liquid and then back to humanoid again.) When ground substance changes from a liquid to a gel, and then changes into its more solid form, the myofascia tightens, and it is difficult to get it to reverse to a liquid state again without intervention.

Myofascia from the Inside Out

You can see myofascia when you cut up a fresh chicken: It is the thin, sticky, somewhat filmy material that wraps around the muscle tissue. We are going to look inside a muscle. Start with an image of thin, nearly transparent, stretchy gauze with the strength of Lycra™.

Muscles are made up of fibers. We'll start at the smallest level and work our way up. Sharon Butler described the changes that can take place in the myofascia as follows:

"Inside a muscle, the tiniest muscle fiber is wrapped with fascia. Then, bundles of those fibers are wrapped with fascia, then the whole muscle is wrapped with it. Can you see the three-dimensionality of it all?

At some point in the anatomy of the muscle, the muscle fibers end. But, here is the kicker . . . the fascia *continues* until it joins, attaches to, and blends into the bone. This band of fascia that used to be permeating through the muscle now becomes a tendon. The same fascia that was spread in many layers, running lengthwise through the muscle, now joins together because there are no more muscle fibers holding the planes of fascia apart.

Muscle fibers are what contract to make movement happen. Muscles are not attached to bone. The tendons are. So when a muscle contracts, it creates a shortening in the planes of the fascia wrapping its sections, and it is the tendon (made up of fascia) attaching to bone that actually causes the bone to move.

When you bend your elbow, your biceps (upper front arm) muscle shortens, but the triceps (upper back arm) muscle has to lengthen. If there is imbalance in the amount that each muscle can move in relation to the other, then one muscle will have to work harder, making it feel fatigued.

The fascia that forms ligaments has a slightly different job. While tendons connect muscle to bone, ligaments attach muscle to muscle and bone to bone. Some ligaments are soft and filmy, like the ones that suspend organs in place, and other ligaments are tough and fibrous. When ligaments are missing or cut, as in surgery, then the organized structure of the body suffers.

Try to imagine the fascia running in three-dimensional planes throughout the body, connecting everything to everything else. Now, when fascia is strained, it has the truly unique characteristic of being able to chemically change in order to protect the body. When it goes through this change, the collagen fibers that make up the fascia bunch together, forming a sort of thickened or denser bunch of fascia. The body creates this so that the overworked muscles can have some support and protection.

Now, remember that this thickened bunch of fascia is somewhere in the middle of a muscle, or is a tendon or a ligament. If the body creates enough sites where the fascia has changed, then this restriction begins to affect the quality of movement, making one muscle work harder to pull against the restriction present in the opposite muscle. This causes more strain in the muscle and affects more of the fascia in the area. That fascia, in turn, changes chemically and becomes thicker and more restricted, and the downward spiral continues." (Butler 1995)

Note: Sharon Butler's book, *Conquering Carpal Tunnel Syndrome and Other Repetitive Strain Injuries*, deals with upper body self-myofascial release. It is a helpful tool for anyone with a myofascial problem.

The Results of Myofascial Changes

The fascial changes that Butler describes are the cause of the lumps and taut bands called *trigger points* (TrPs), which are described more completely in Chapter 3. Fascia changed in this way can entrap nerves, constrict blood vessels, and tighten around lymph vessels. By now, you can probably see why TrPs can cause so many different kinds of symptoms.

Fascia also forms adhesions and scar tissue. People with FMS seem to have a lot of thickened tissues. Once fascia changes, it needs help to return to its previous form. This is where bodywork is particularly helpful. (See Chapters 24, 25, and 26.)

Note that the majority of connective tissue consists of fluids and fibers. Because of this, it is not uncommon for bodywork to cause nausea or headaches from the large amounts of toxins and wastes that are moved out of the intercellular fluids and into the blood stream. This movement is necessary for the body to rid itself of toxins and wastes (Juhan 1987).

Travell and Simons (1992) also found that the medication Potaba™ loosened tight myofascia. (See Chapters 21 and 22 for information regarding medications.)

> The myofascia also helps to regulate circulation. I believe that tight myofascia results in "spider veins" in legs. I also believe it holds the explanation for the mysterious "livido reticularis" areas (see Chapter 8, Questions and Answers About Common Symptoms) of hypersensitive skin overlain by a network of veins and capillaries that are sometimes seen in FMS/MPS Complex patients.
>
> D.J.S.

In some people, increasingly restricted capillaries need higher than usual blood pressure so that the blood can adequately supply the extremities and skin areas. When a sufficient number of capillaries is compressed, this results in "cold spots" on the skin, and/or cold feet and hands. When an individual cellular area becomes stagnant and toxic to an extreme, the accumulated waste can kill the cell. The dead cell is then filled in by scar tissue. This kind of scarring is nearly impossible to reverse.

The Impact of Muscle Function

Normal muscle action is the patterned response of groups of muscles. This means that no muscle works alone. For every muscle that stretches, another one must contract. Muscle function depends on groups of muscles working together to create an effect.

Muscles must stay active to remain healthy and responsive. Activity helps to ensure that the fluids in the body keep moving. Anything that interferes with muscle activity—such as FMS/ MPS—interferes with muscle health.

Muscles and Wastes

The products of the body's cellular factories and all the wastes from its cellular processing must pass through the connective tissue to reach the lymph and blood vessels. When the myofascia is "gunked up" and sticks together, neurotransmitters, those biochemical messengers that run the body, can't work properly. When wastes accumulate, muscles receive insufficient fuel and oxygen. This can result in confused sensations, foggy thoughts, numbness in some areas, and hypersensitivity in others. (See Chapter 8, Questions and Answers.)

When wastes back up in the tightened muscle, local nerve endings become irritated. The irritated nerves tell the brain to activate its arousal system, so the body knows something is going wrong. This is a stress signal and the ground substance becomes more solid because the "fight-or-flight" response is activated when the entire body mobilizes to rid itself of the irritation (Juhan 1987).

Myofascia and Nerves

When a muscle contracts, the fascia becomes compressed or squeezed. When myofascia is squeezed in this way, blood and lymph vessels, as well as the nerves that pass through the myofascia, are also squeezed. When the body is on constant alert, the myofascia forms taut bands, or ropes, that tighten throughout the muscle, called *contractures*. When a nerve passes through a muscle between taut bands, or between taut bands and muscle or bone, the unrelenting pressure on the nerve causes the loss of nerve conduction. This is called *neuropraxia*. Neuropraxia produces aching pains, numbness, tingling, or hypersensitivity.

Contractures appear to be beyond mental control. The muscle becomes increasingly firm and tight, so that muscle definition and mobility are lost and the muscle appears to be cast in concrete. This tightness, called *spasticity*, becomes painful in itself. The pain, in turn, causes more tightness, which, yet again, causes more pain.

When you voluntarily relax your muscles, you can reduce the number of nerve signals transmitted by that muscle. If the muscle is only tense, it will be able to relax. If the muscle is contractured, it will stay contractured until it is treated. A contracture may loosen up when you stretch or instinctively massage the problem muscles, but specific therapy (see Part V, Healing Tools) is the only way out for anyone with multiple contractures.

In Conclusion

You now have some understanding of the interaction between the muscles and the myofascia. You also have some information on how trigger points are formed. The next chapter will give you a crash course in trigger points, those instigators of pain.

CHAPTER 3

Myofascial Trigger Points

Chapter 2 introduced the term *trigger points* (*TrPs*), which are extremely sore points that can occur as ropy bands throughout the body. They can also be felt as painful lumps of hardened fascia (see Chapter 2, Myofascia). Trigger points can be present as single points, multiple trigger points, as a part of chronic MPS, or as a part of the FMS/MPS Complex. People diagnosed with FMS, who actually have a lot of their pain caused by MPS, recognize the pain patterns.

Unlike tender points (see Chapter 1), trigger points can and do refer pain to other parts of the body. Note that trigger points are *not* part of FMS. This chapter deals with individual TrPs, which can, but do not always, go on to become chronic MPS, which can, but does not always, become FMS/MPS Complex. This chapter provides some basic information about TrPs to help you and your doctor pinpoint your problems.

Note: The brief sketches and explanations offered in this book are by no means meant to serve as a complete diagnostic trigger point manual for the doctor. There are two very large medical texts, loaded with wonderful diagrams and details, by Drs. Travell and Simons, for that. (See Bibliography.) Most of the information in this chapter comes from Travell and Simons. All of the illustrations of trigger points in this book were also adapted from those manuals. Your doctor should be familiar Travell and Simons' work. What this chapter will show you is just how important it is to have a doctor who knows those texts. We have tried to simplify the explanations, but the locations of the TrPs are meant to be used just as guidelines. Remember, every patient is different.

What Causes Trigger Points?

Trigger points can occur in the myofascia, skin, ligaments, bone lining, and other tissues. In this book we are primarily concerned with TrPs in the myofascia. Although you may never have heard of TrPs before, they are actually quite common.

Note: It's been said that practitioners in the medical community take approximately ten years to catch up with research. In the case of trigger points and myofascial pain syndrome, that rule of thumb has been far too optimistic.

The Stress Response

Trigger points can form throughout life as a stress response to many things that happen to your body, including overuse, repetitive motion trauma, bruises, strains, joint problems, surgery, and so on. Acute pain creates a neuromuscular response, and the muscle around the pain site tightens, "guarding" the hurt area.

When muscles are in a state of sustained tension, they are working, even if you're not. A working muscle needs more nutrition and oxygen, and produces more waste, than a muscle at rest. This creates an area in the myofascia starved for food and oxygen and loaded with toxic waste. Such an area is a trigger point.

Physical stress isn't the only thing that can cause TrPs. They can also occur as a result of emotional stress. These are not the psychological results of tension; they can be the physiological effects in the body resulting from long-term emotional abuse or mental trauma. If you are constantly holding your muscles tight in a fight-or-flight stress response, this changes your body's musculature patterns. (See Chapter 2 for a brief discussion of the fight or flight stress response.)

Coexisting Conditions

Trigger points also often form as a result of other medical conditions. For example, a case of arthritis may be otherwise well managed, but the accompanying TrPs could be overlooked. The pain load of such a patient could be substantially lessened if the associated TrPs were treated successfully. (See Chapter 6 for a further discussion of coexisting conditions.)

In addition, many of the aches and pains thought to be due to "old age" could be from TrPs resulting from the wear and tear of life. Treating them would not restore the vigor of youth, but it might enable senior citizens to cut down on medication and improve the quality of their lives.

Perpetuating Factors

Often, one stress activates a TrP and another stress may cause it to continue. (See Chapter 7 for a complete discussion of perpetuating factors.) It is vitally important that doctors identify their patients' perpetuating factors. For example, symptoms such as unequal leg length or another kind of musculoskeletal imbalance may not even be noticed until something else activates a trigger point in that area. Then, the unequal legs become a perpetuating factor of that trigger point.

Latent Trigger Points

The trigger point is an exquisitely sore point that not only hurts where it is pressed, like an FMS tender point, but it also "triggers" a referred pain pattern to somewhere else in the body. A *latent* type of TrP also occurs. The latent TrP doesn't hurt at all, unless it is being pressed. You might not even know it's there, but your body does. It restricts movement, and weakens and prevents full lengthening of the affected muscle. If you press on the latent TrP, it does refer pain in its characteristic pattern. A latent TrP may be activated by overstretching, overuse, or chilling the muscle. People who rarely exercise have a much greater chance of developing latent TrPs.

Trigger Point Symptoms

Often, TrPs can be felt as painful lumps of hardened fascia, possibly due to the constriction of blood and other fluids, as discussed in Chapter 2. The ropy bands are often easier to feel along the arms and legs. If you stretch (extend) your muscle about two thirds of the way out, you might be able to feel them. Sometimes the muscles get so tight that you can't feel the lumps, or even the tight, ropy bands. Your muscle simply feels like hardened concrete.

When TrPs are present, muscle strength becomes unreliable. For example, if you have arm and hand TrPs, your grip is weakened so that things may drop unexpectedly from your hand. That's because the pain is translated by the brain as damage—so your body won't allow you to complete acts that cause pain. Your tightest grip just isn't what it used to be.

When a nerve passes through a muscle between the ropy bands, or when a nerve lies between the band and bone, the pressure on the nerve can produce numbness, but only in the area of compression. That's called TrP *nerve entrapment.* You may have noticed that if one part of your body rests over another part while you are sleeping, the part being compressed goes numb. For example, if you fling one arm over the other arm, the compressed arm will go numb. If you want to be able to distinguish between a TrP with an entrapped nerve and one without such entrapment the following simple test will help. If ice makes it feel better, that is a sign of nerve entrapment; but if heat relieves the pain and ice makes it worse, then there is no nerve entrapment.

Where trigger points are involved, no two patients' problems are exactly alike. TrPs also can vary in irritability from hour to hour and day to day. The amount of stress needed to activate a latent TrP depends on the conditioning of the muscle, and that also varies. If you have stubborn chronic pain, you should expect multiple causes and perpetuating factors.

Some trigger points refer pain only in close proximity to the TrP itself. Others, such as those in the scaleni muscles, refer symptoms in a very large pattern. (See Figure 3-1.)

This pain pattern is *similar* from patient to patient, which is a great aid in diagnosis.

A *satellite* TrP develops in a muscle because that muscle is in the primary TrP's referred pain area. A *secondary* TrP develops in a muscle that is overloaded because it is compensating or substituting for a muscle that contains the primary TrP. These are important concepts, because

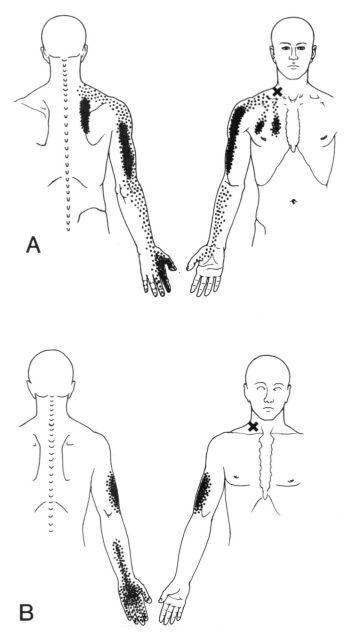

Figure 3-1: Location of trigger points in the right scalene (A) Scalenus anterior (B) Scalenus posterior

they explain how TrPs seem to "spread." It has given rise to the mistaken impression that FMS and/or MPS are "progressive." There is a large difference between a condition "worsening" and a "progressive" illness. The difference being that a progressive condition cannot be reversed whereas trigger points definitely can be.

Often these trigger points produce other symptoms, usually in a referred pain zone. Such a TrP hurts whenever you use the involved muscle.

The fact that the referred pain patterns are very similar from patient to patient with TrPs really helps the physician to make a diagnosis—*if* that physician is familiar with the patterns as described by Travell and Simons. That's why familiarity with TrPs and an ability to take a good medical history are so important. An educated doctor will know *where* to look for TrPs before the physical exam begins.

Note: There has been some confusion about nomenclature in recent medical literature. A muscle group with many TrPs is often called MPS. The term *MPS* should refer to chronic, body-wide Myofascial Pain Syndrome.

Pain from trigger points is usually steady, dull, deep, and aching. However, the intensity can range from mild discomfort to incapacitating torture. If a nerve is trapped, the pain can be burning, sharp, and lightning-like. Trigger point pain, unlike the tender point pain of FMS, is rarely distributed equally on both sides of the body.

The effects of low-back pain of myofascial origin can be as bad as or worse than low-back pain from a herniated disc (Cassisi, et al. 1993). If you have a bad back, be sure your doctor is familiar with and understands trigger points. Needless surgery can be avoided, and you will get much better treatment and results.

Chapter 9 delves further into the subject of chronic pain in FMS/MPS and offers various ways to deal with it.

Sternocleidomastoid TrPs

Now, let's take a look at what are called the Sternocleidomastoid (SCM) trigger points to give you a better idea of how important trigger points can be. See Figure 3-2.

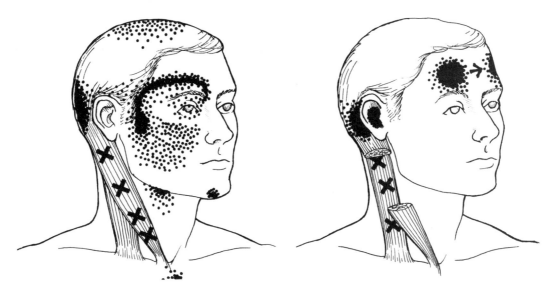

Figure 3-2: Sternocleidomastoid (SCM) trigger points

Dr. Janet Travell, in her autobiography, *Office Hours Day and Night* (1968), explains how dizziness, ringing of the ears, loss of balance, and other symptoms can all be caused by SCM trigger points. The sternocleidomastoid group has a great many functions, one of which is to hold up the head. Receptors in the SCM muscle complex transmit nerve impulses that inform the brain of the position of the head and body in the surrounding space. When trigger points are present, the receptors lie. What they tell the brain is not what the eyes tell the brain. If there are TrPs in the muscles surrounding the eyes, the eyes also send incorrect data to the brain—*different* incorrect data than the receptors in the neck do.

When head movement changes the SCM message, for example, when you turn your head to look around or you look up from changing the kitty litter, you get dizzy. This, coupled with poor balance, can make it seem as though the walls are tilting. In fact, a common symptom of SCM trigger points is called the "drunken" walk, because it causes you to bump into doorways and walls.

People with SCM TrPs often have trouble glancing downward; doing so can cause them to fall forward. They can become so disoriented that they can get nauseated and may even vomit.

When you take corners while driving, you get the impression that you're "banking" the turn at a steep angle, as if you were tilted on a motorcycle. This kind of altered perception can occur when you stop the car and you feel as if it were still moving. This can be frightening. These perceptual changes can be very hard to explain to your doctor.

Chronic dry cough, pain deep in the ear canal, pain in the throat and back of the tongue, and pain to a small round area at the tip of the chin also can be part of the SCM trigger point package. Localized sweating and vasoconstriction can be a problem, as well as pain in the "skull cap" area of the head. (What SCM TrPs don't cause is a pain in the neck, although they figuratively become one due to their wide-ranging symptoms.)

Note that cold drafts alone can bring on neck TrPs.

Where, Oh Where Are Those Trigger Points?

Travell and Simons warn against thinking of published TrP sites as the only places that trigger points can occur. These published sites are only guides; places to start looking. TrP sites in a given muscle may vary from person to person and many muscle groups may hold multiple TrP locations. Multiple TrPs may create overlapping and differing pain patterns.

To add to the diagnostic confusion, TrPs often can overlay FMS tender points. Diagnosis becomes really challenging when FMS and MPS occur together. The hunt for TrPs can seem like a search for lost treasure. Thanks to Drs. Travell and Simons, we have the treasure map.

CHAPTER 4

Chronic Myofascial Pain Syndrome

In Chapter 3, you learned some basic information about trigger points (TrPs). In this chapter TrPs are discussed in somewhat greater detail.

- The good news is that if TrPs are treated immediately and vigorously, and perpetuating factors (conditions that aggravate and perpetuate the TrPs, as described in Chapter 7), are avoided or remedied, the TrPs can be eliminated.

- Unfortunately, if TrPs are left untreated, or are inappropriately treated, the TrP will remain active. If muscle action is restricted to avoid pain, the TrPs will become latent.

- If the muscle is pushed to work in spite of the pain, especially if perpetuating factors exist, active TrPs may develop secondary and satellite TrPs.

Secondary and Satellite Trigger Points

Secondary trigger points develop when a muscle is subject to stress because another muscle with a trigger point isn't doing its job. Another muscle compensates for the muscle that is not working and the overworked muscle can develop a secondary TrP as a result. Note that a TrP located on a muscle on one side of the body can cause secondary TrPS on the other side of the body in this manner. *Satellite trigger points* develop when a muscle is in a referred pain zone of another TrP. Without proper intervention and with perpetuating factors, the TrPs can lead to severe and widespread chronic Myofascial Pain Syndrome (MPS).

Developing secondary and satellite TrPs can give the false impression that MPS is a condition that will steadily worsen with time—that it is what is called *progressive*. However, MPS

I believe that one reason why "traumatic" FMS is more severe than nontraumatic FMS is that trauma often produces TrPs. When FMS is accompanied by trigger points, it frequently goes on to develop MPS. I know that is true in my case. Every patient I've ever seen with a tentative diagnosis of "traumatic fibromyalgia" actually had either chronic MPS or FMS/MPS Complex. Some people think that FMS is a progressive condition because such FMS begins in one area and slowly spreads throughout the body. Often this "spreading" consists of the developing of myofascial trigger points.

D.J.S.

is *not* progressive. With proper intervention, which you will learn about throughout this book, these trigger points can be broken up and eliminated.

Post-Traumatic Hyperirritability Syndrome

There is a severe form of MPS called *post-traumatic hyperirritability syndrome* (PTHS). It begins with some kind of trauma sufficient to injure the sensory moderating system of the brain. This is the system that translates impulses from different receptors in the body to the brain.

With PTHS, the sensory moderating system has been modified to register extreme sensitivity to any kind of stimulus. Noise translates as pain. Touch translates as pain. Vibration, light, all these sensory signals reach the brain screaming "pain!" People with this condition must avoid all types of strong sensory stimuli. They are a challenge to their health care team: they often can't do any exercise and frequently can't tolerate ice or heat.

Note: In this book, chronic MPS is defined as a condition of multiple TrPs present in all four quadrants of the body for at least six months—that is, the upper and lower left side and upper and lower right side of the body all must have had TrPs for at least six months.

An Example: Neck Congestion and TrPs

Some patients can trace the start of their troubles to a severe illness or to a fall or an auto accident. The illness or accident often exhibited neck congestion as a common factor. Such neck congestion can activate TrPs. That's because normal fluid passages become constricted with muscle tightening. Fluids back up in the sinuses and there is a constant post-nasal drip, although the nasal passages themselves may be dry and bleeding—especially in the winter.

When people with this condition are asleep, the nose stuffiness moves from side to side as they toss and turn. Gravity pulls the stuffiness to the downward side—that is the side of the head on the pillow if you are sleeping on your side. Post-nasal drip irritates the back of the throat all night. This happens either on the down side if you are on your side, or in the back of the throat if you lie on your back. As a result, throat and neck TrPs develop—especially in the sternocleidomastoid (SCM), a group of muscles located at the side of the neck. (See Figure 3-1.)

As the muscles tighten, the area becomes more constricted. More fluid backs up. The constant drip into ever-more-restricted vessels ultimately can result in a sinus infection, because viruses and bacteria will take advantage of the moist, constricted areas. Trigger points cascade down the arm, and the neck and shoulders lose some mobility.

A trigger point *cascade* results when a primary TrP develops satellite and secondary TrPs, which then develop satellite and secondary TrPs of their own. For example, sternocleidomastoid (SCM) TrPs can result in TrPs developing in other neck muscles, in the chest and shoulders, and in the head and face. The chest and shoulder TrPs can then result in arm/hand/finger and belly/back/hip TrPs, and so forth. Eventually, you can have TrPs from the top of your head to the tips of your toes. A true "cascade" effect.

Note: A similar cascade of TrPs often takes place in the lower body. For example, painful menses, childbirth, a hysterectomy, or a hernia can activate TrP activity (hips to thighs to knee to lower leg to foot to toe).

Differences Between FMS and MPS

FMS and MPS are different syndromes. However, the vast majority of physicians tend to lump them together because they see many patients with the FMS/MPS Complex (or at least FMS and individual TrPs). Unless doctors have a thorough knowledge of and familiarity with individual TrPs, they don't stand a chance of sorting out the symptoms. The works of Travell and Simons explain the differences in great detail and supply supporting data. (See Bibliography.)

One interesting difference between the two syndromes is that more women than men have FMS, but MPS affects men and women in equal numbers.

Another difference is that muscles in locations that are some distance from the trigger points of MPS have normal sensitivity. In fibromyalgia, there is a generalized sensitivity. This means there is a bodywide, diffuse achiness with FMS, whereas with MPS there are specific pains in specific areas. In MPS, the areas not affected with TrPs do not hurt; whereas in FMS, the areas outside the tender points still ache (Travell and Simons 1983 and 1992).

Remember that FMS is, among other things, a *systemic neurotransmitter dysregulation, with many biochemical causes.* Since neurotransmitters are the means by which the body and brain speak to each other, a systemic dysregulation causes communication breakdowns and failures.

This process somewhat resembles a familiar game that children sometimes play in school. They line up, and whisper a sentence, child to child, down to the end of the line. By the time the last child in the line hears the sentence, its meaning has been garbled. In very simplistic terms, this is similar to what happens in FMS. There are other problems as well, but they are all systemic in nature, such as the alpha-delta sleep anomaly described in Chapter 10, Sleep.

Fibromyalgia is a *biochemical* disorder. It occurs as part of a biochemical imbalance, and we are far from understanding the "whys" of it. We just know that a number of biochemical balances in the body are in disarray. This is part of the reason why FMS is so complex. There are many neurotransmitters, and they can be disrupted in many ways. Some of these ways influence how other biochemicals, including medications, are metabolized.

Myofascial Pain Syndrome, however, is a *neuromuscular* condition. MPS happens because of mechanical failures—the mechanics of physics, not biochemistry. Due to the nature of trigger points, some of the symptoms may *seem* to be systemic, but they are not. Initiating events, such as repetitive motion injury, trauma, and illness, can start a cascade of TrPs.

One of the most damaging misconceptions concerning chronic pain syndromes made the medical rounds during the time when FMS was just beginning to be accepted as a "real" syndrome. Doctors were advised, when testing patients for fibromyalgia tender points, to try pressing areas other than the designated 18 sites. If patients complained of pain, they were to be branded as malingerers. This patently false (and dangerous) "test" made its ugly way into print. (Patients are still suffering because of it.)

Today, we know that traumatic FMS—that is, FMS caused by an auto accident, repetitive motion, degenerating discs, and so forth—often exhibits tender points at areas clustered around the damaged area in addition to or instead of the "18 standard points" (Pelligrino 1993). In addition, we now know that the MPS patient has trigger points *all* over his or her body.

Diagnosing MPS

Unfortunately, most pain management clinics spend a lot of time helping people to learn to live with their pain when, often, some of the pain can be eliminated. Once identified, trigger points —those lumps of fascia and waste materials—can be broken up, or at least minimized.

Myofascial Pain Syndrome isn't easy to diagnose, and neither is FMS. There are often multiple interacting factors. (MPS is a great mimic of other conditions.) No matter how much doctors might enjoy a mystery, they have little time to play Sherlock Holmes; and no two patients are alike. But the Travell and Simons *Trigger Point Manuals* are invaluable tools in making a diagnosis.

A chronic pain state causes many problems. To diagnose such a condition correctly, your physician must keep looking for the *source* of the pain. With chronic MPS, your doctor should take the following steps, one at a time.

1. Identify active and latent trigger points and perpetuating factors.

2. Estimate TrP importance in the pain/symptom load. Those TrPs that interfere with vital functions (breathing, sleeping) and those that cause the most debilitating effects (migraines, dizziness, and so on) should be the first treated. Note that many TrP-referenced pain zones may overlap.

3. Develop a treatment plan for the major TrPs, using an order and combination that respects their interaction.

What You, the Patient, Can Do

It is important for you as a patient to learn about the relationship between TrPs and MPS. Then, you can demand that your medical care team become at least as well-informed as you are.

At one time, my physical therapist mapped the worst TrPs I had. On a scale of one to ten, one being noticeable pain and ten being barely tolerable pain, we only mapped those off scale. If I started exhibiting shock symptoms because the pain was so bad, we considered it "off scale." It was pain that my body could not take. I had studied meditation and various mind-control techniques for many years, but this was the only time I have come close to "levitating."

We stopped mapping at about 100. I had over 100 TrPs that could not be pressed hard without having me develop shock-like symptoms. I have never seen anyone with a case as bad as I had. At the time, I had no idea what was wrong, neither the FMS nor the MPS had yet been diagnosed.

Although an examination to discover the trigger points can be very painful, a lot of the pain can be minimized if a very careful medical history is taken by the physician.

D.J.S.

It is true that many people have emotional problems, and these can worsen the physical symptoms of MPS. Nonetheless, make sure your medical care team understands that the constant effort of dealing with your "untreatable pain" has reduced your physical activity, limited your social activity, impaired your sleep, caused loss or change of your family role, and perhaps been responsible for loss or change of your job.

Janet Travell says, "Above all, clinicians must believe that their patients hurt as much and in the way that they say they do." She speaks of the "mystery of history," and says that to take a good history, the physician must first be willing to believe the patient.

Your doctor may need your help in finding the perpetuating factors—those factors that reinforce, aggravate, and continue the conditions that sustain the TrPs (see Chapter 7). (Note that FMS is one of the most common perpetuating factors of MPS.) Your doctor and/or physical therapist can uncover such factors as skeletal defects, but you can help by becoming more aware of how you move through your life.

You should provide your physician with specific data concerning your daily routines, including sleep positions, work conditions, and family dynamics. You may observe that certain repetitive motions give rise to strain and stress on certain muscles, which can result in specific TrPs, so you should probably make a careful evaluation of your movements, postures, and so on. Ask your health team for assistance in observing your body. They can tell you what to look for.

If you're like most people, you want to understand your medical condition and will do everything within your power to get as well as possible. You don't want to be sick. With MPS, you may need to develop a willingness to limit your activities to avoid pushing yourself too hard and then suffering later from the "good sport" syndrome.

In Conclusion

It's easy to understand why trigger points can give the impression of a spreading disease. It's a relief when you understand what is happening and learn that this "spread" can be reversed once you find out what is perpetuating the TrPs.

Now that you know something about the pain caused by MPS alone, you can imagine the problems that arise when it occurs with a pain-amplification syndrome such as fibromyalgia. In the next two chapters we will look at what is called the FMS/MPS Complex.

CHAPTER 5

FMS/MPS: The "Double Whammy"

People with the FMS/MPS Complex face more than just the two sets of symptoms of both conditions. Today, a few researchers are realizing that FMS and MPS not only occur together, they reinforce each other. Therefore, physical therapy and all other forms of treatment must proceed carefully. Any treatment tried will be both more complicated and less successful than if the patient had only one of the two conditions.

Many studies have confirmed that Myofascial Pain Syndrome (MPS) pain is restricted to trigger point (TrP) referred pain areas, whereas fibromyalgia (FMS) causes a generalized pain amplification in the tested tissues (*Fibromyalgia Network Newsletter* October 1995). In FMS/MPS, a *chronic* pain condition exists, with many different symptoms and the trigger points of MPS, which are all magnified by the pain amplification aspect of fibromyalgia (FMS). Furthermore, some of the treatments normally prescribed for FMS patients can cause damage to MPS patients, and the reverse is also true.

In some people, the chronic pain of MPS seems to lead to FMS. And in those who have a genetic tendency toward contracting FMS, chronic pain changes the chemistry of their bodies in many ways (Russell 1994).

Making a diagnosis of FMS/MPS can be extremely complicated. As stated previously, the symptoms of each person can vary in many ways. From the MPS point of view, not only is there a wide variety of combinations of trigger points, there are also many different kinds of nerves entrapped (see Chapter 2). There are also many kinds of perpetuating factors (see Chapter 7) and many different kinds of initiating events.

In the context of the fibromyalgia syndrome, many different neurotransmitters are affected, and FMS can affect them in many different combinations. Also, different combinations interact in different ways, and other biochemicals in the body are affected to different degrees.

Various biochemicals may be involved. Histamine, for example, a neurotransmitter, is often an important factor when there are many allergic manifestations; but the possible combinations are endless.

The FMS/MPS Connection: Some Theories

To understand the FMS/MPS complex, we need to look at the big picture. Most of the body's processes rely on the unobstructed movement of fluids through the system.

- Blood circulates, carrying food, fuel, oxygen, and other materials. It also carries away wastes.

- Lymph circulates, carrying fats, salts, proteins, white blood cells, and other substances.

- On a microscopic level, every cell in the body depends on the motion of liquids from outside to inside the cell, and back. In one "Star Trek" episode, an alien called human beings "bags of dirty water." The description, while unsavory, is quite correct. Your body depends on the motion of this "dirty water" in and out of its cells.

Neurotransmitter activity determines the elasticity of the tissues, but in FMS/MPS, connective tissues become stiffened, shortened, and tightened. That means that the fluid exchange is disrupted as well. This often starts with simple FMS.

In FMS, muscles in the area of the tender points that characterize FMS "guard" the painful area. The myofascia forms a sort of splint, trying to minimize the pain. The body reacts to pain immediately, because pain signifies damage. So the body goes into a self-protective stress mode.

The muscles around the tender points are in a state of sustained tension—and they become tight and hard. This means they are working all the time, even when you are resting. When muscles are working, their need for nutrition is greater than when they are at rest, and they produce more wastes. But in FMS, the sustained contraction hampers the delivery of fuel and oxygen and the removal of waste. In a relatively short time, the tender point can become a toxic waste dump—what we call a myofascial trigger point.

FMS perpetuates MPS and the reverse is also true. This is a true "catch-22" situation. You can't get rid of the MPS until you successfully treat the FMS and you can't successfully treat the FMS until you get rid of the MPS. They each perpetuate the other. Then, too, chronic pain, all by itself, causes stress, which can create TrPs. That's another reason why so many cases of FMS are accompanied by MPS.

The spiral of pain/contraction/pain/contraction continues until it is interrupted by an outside force, or by relief in some form. But don't despair. A lot can be done to relieve MPS and to lighten the pain load. And there are many things that work for FMS as well. Part IV discusses these matters in depth.

Some Definitions

To aid in your understanding of the FMS/MPS Complex, here are definitions of some basic terms:

- A *fibroblast* is a cell that develops into connective tissue, such as myofascia.

- *Mast cells* are types of connective tissue cells that contain histamine (a neurotransmitter) and heparin (an important substance that helps blood clotting and cell repair).

- *Ground substance* is the material in the myofascia that can change its form from liquid to solid and back to liquid. (See Chapter 1.)

- *Collagen fibers* are a type of protein found in connective tissues.

These all affect the thickening and tightening of the myofascia in FMS/MPS Complex.

Growth Hormone

Growth hormone is significant in wound healing, where rapid production of collagen fibers by many fibroblasts is necessary for repair. It's an important neurotransmitter and has a powerful effect on the myofascia. It stimulates the production of fibroblasts and mast cells, ground substance, and collagen fibers.

But growth hormone is released only during delta-level sleep. People with fibromyalgia have the alpha-delta sleep anomaly. This means that fibromites never stay in delta-level sleep. As the delta level is reached, alpha waves intrude and disrupt slumber. They either jolt the sleeper totally awake, or cause a shallower (lighter) slumber.

People with FMS have very low levels of growth hormone, so the body has problems with cellular repair itself. Not only is the myofascia a major information highway and repair mechanism of the body, its chemistry also monitors inflammatory response, and its fluids deliver antibodies and white blood cells to fight infection. All of these functions of the myofascia are disrupted in FMS/MPS Complex. Killer cells from the immune system are present in the normal amounts, but most don't function.

Serotonin

The body uses tryptophan to form *serotonin*. Serotonin is an important neurotransmitter that, among other things, regulates and affects sleep, mood, and sensory perception. Serotonin is regulated in delta-level sleep, which, as stated above, is constantly disrupted in FMS, so serotonin levels in people with FMS are very low.

But tryptophan does not always cross the blood-brain barrier in FMS/MPS. The *blood-brain barrier* is a membrane that separates the circulating blood and the brain. Its job is to filter out damaging substances before they reach the brain. Unfortunately, in FMS, it also filters out needed substances, as well.

The "Deconditioning" Myth

One of the cruelest misunderstandings about FMS/MPS is that it is caused by deconditioning. *Deconditioning* means that the muscles have become flabby from disuse. It isn't unusual for a doctor to examine a patient with FMS/MPS and say, "It looks like fat to me." People come to the medical system for help, expecting at the very least understanding and compassion. When the doctor fails to meet these minimum expectations, they feel betrayed.

It appears that deconditioning often occurs as a *result*, not as a cause, of FMS/MPS Complex. There are ways to prevent deconditioning from happening, however, if you know what you're dealing with. Just remember, you are also dealing with that aspect of FMS that amplifies pain. This means decreased endurance as well as muscles that don't repair themselves very well. Be gentle with yourself.

What You, the Patient, Can Do

For the person with MPS/FMS the body and mind is a war zone, but they are frantically trying to work together! It's important for people with this combination of syndromes to take on the responsibility of managing their own treatment. It isn't easy, and it takes concentrated focus to change the habits of a lifetime. Getting as well as possible—optimizing your quality of life—takes commitment. What is done to or for you can help a lot, but getting better is also a function of what *you* do. (See Chapter 15, Taking Control.)

If you have the FMS/MPS Complex right now, you might feel as though it has put you in the bottom of a deep, dark hole. Throughout this book, we will shine some light in the darkness for you, and then try to help you find the footholds to climb out of that dark hole. *The first thing you must do to get out of the hole is to stop digging it!* Smoking, alcohol, junk food and other bad habits, including negative thoughts, add to the depth of the hole.

Changing the habits of a lifetime is hard. Keep this thought in mind:

The night is long, it is not endless—there will be a dawn.

The pain is now, but not forever—there will be a healing.

The path is hard, yet there is hope—you do not walk alone.

As just about anyone knows, emergency room work in a major city hospital is not a job for those who lean toward a couch-potato existence. Neither is being the Technical Director of a pharmaceutical plant. I've done both, and also played goalie on an ice hockey team during the same time period. Before I contracted FMS/MPS, I was exceedingly active and usually weighed about 105 pounds. I was very healthy (coping well with what I now know was FMS and episodic TrPs) until, after an auto accident, I developed severe FMS/MPS Complex. So much for deconditioning.

D.J.S.

Why Treat MFS/MPS Complex Differently?

In Part IV of this book you will learn many ways to help ease the burden of FMS/MPS Complex. For the time being, be aware that this condition doesn't respond to any treatment as either of its two components do.

Consider trigger point (TrP) injections, for example. This treatment often works on TrPs after other methods fail, and is a treatment of last resort. Injection consists of procaine in an isotonic saline *without epinephrine*. For those allergic to procaine, saline solution provides some local analgesic relief (Simons 1988(b)).

But if you have FMS/MPS Complex, the injections don't work as well. You are not as likely to experience any pain relief from them. Some people get pain relief for a few weeks. Some get no relief at all. If you do receive some relief, often you may have more severe post-injection soreness. And any relief you get from the pain doesn't last as long (Hong 1995). It's a whole new game, and your doctor needs to understand both FMS and MPS as distinct entities, as well as FMS/MPS Complex before you can be helped.

In Conclusion

So far, you've read about myofascia, fibromyalgia, individual trigger points, myofascial pain syndrome, and the FMS/MPS Complex. That's a lot of information to absorb. Don't be concerned if you don't understand all the concepts right now. You have the jigsaw puzzle frame in place, and the picture will become clearer as we help you fit in more of the individual pieces.

Soon we will be talking not only about basic survival techniques, but also about restoring creativity, dignity, self-esteem, and identity. Before we leave Part I, however, Chapter 6 takes a look at some conditions that may coexist with FMS/MPS.

CHAPTER 6

Coexisting Conditions

Fibromyalgia (FMS) and Myofascial Pain Syndrome (MPS) are great mimics of other medical conditions. Because the myofascia is everywhere and touches on or interacts with so many other parts of the body, someone may seem to have many different medical problems, and yet they could all turn out to be part of the FMS/MPS Complex. Of course, that isn't always the case. For example, one study found FMS in 51 percent of osteoarthritis patients, 55 percent of lupus patients, and 32 percent of rheumatoid patients (*Fibromyalgia Network Newsletter* January 1993).

As a rule, if you are jogging in the park and hear hoofbeats, you expect to see a horse—not a giraffe or a zebra. True, a horse would be most likely, but a zoo or circus truck could have broken down, and there is always a possibility that the hoofbeats are those of a zebra or giraffe. If you have most of the symptoms, you probably have the FMS/MPS Complex. But the Complex may mimic other disorders and you could have some other condition or conditions *in addition* to FMS/MPS. In fact, the FMS/MPS Complex often appears in conjunction with another disorder and then amplifies symptoms of that disorder. We tend

One woman I had been seeing for FMS consultations became very ill. She had been treated by an alternative-treatment doctor who specialized in Vietnamese medicine. She had been taking herbal packs, brewed as tea, and was experiencing some relief from her symptoms.

Sometime later, though, her partner called me because she was running a very high fever. She had stopped the herbal "tea" packs, and her doctor was very angry at her. He said fevers were a common result of these herbs. I advised her that she should be checked out immediately by an M.D. She did. A few weeks later, I got a call from her; she had just recovered from *pneumonia* and had just been released from the hospital.

These kinds of things do happen. A proper diagnosis is essential.

D.J.S.

to shrug off our symptoms and blame everything on FMS/MPS, but this attitude can be dangerous. If in doubt, check it out.

Possible Coexisting Conditions

The following sections describe some of the most common medical conditions that may coexist with FMS/MPS Complex. Be sure to talk with your primary physician if you suspect you have any of these conditions. The chances are, you've already been tested for them. But if you have a confirmed diagnosis of FMS and/or MPS, have not been responding to treatment, and have eliminated perpetuating factors (see Chapter 7), you should have a thorough medical evaluation to detect coexisting conditions.

Carpal-Tunnel Syndrome

The symptoms of carpal-tunnel syndrome are wrist pain, and soreness and weakness of the thumb caused by pressure on the median nerve. Be aware, though, that other conditions, such as the subscapularis trigger points mimic carpal-tunnel syndrome. See Figure 6-1. If you are considering surgery for carpal-tunnel syndrome, make sure your doctor first checks

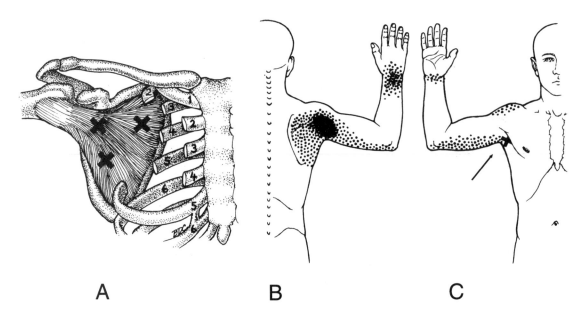

A   B   C

Figure 6-1: (A) The X's show trigger points in the right subscapularis. (B) and (C) show the trigger points and the referred pain zones emanating from those trigger points.

for subscapularis and scaleni TrPs. (If your arm hurts whenever you try to keep it raised for any length of time, such as for hanging curtains or painting, check for this TrP. True carpal-tunnel syndrome can occur in conjunction with FMS and/or MPS, and often results in TrPs.)

Cerebral Palsy

Cerebral palsy (CP) is a paralysis that doesn't worsen. It is usually the result of birth defects or birth trauma. It occurs symmetrically on both sides of the body and muscle imbalances from the paralysis can result in trigger points.

Chronic Fatigue Syndrome

Chronic fatigue syndrome (CFS) is characterized by a history of extreme exhaustion lasting at least six months, as well as biochemical abnormalities. This exhaustion can be brought on by the slightest effort. Often, the patient wants to sleep all the time, even when insomnia is present. Usually, aches and fever, sore throat and an inability to concentrate are part of CFS. Some patients meet the requirements for both fibromyalgia and chronic fatigue.

Depression

There are several kinds of depression. Some symptoms of depression include feeling very sad most of the time, an inability to experience pleasure, lethargy, confusion, poor memory, sleep problems, and appetite changes. Also, it is natural to grieve when you have a chronic pain problem, but those feelings are not the same as a clinical depression. (For information about coping with depression, see Chapter 16, Coping Day to Day.)

HIV

FMS/MPS may occur in those who are infected with the human immunodeficiency virus, HIV, which causes AIDS. A recent study found probable or definite FMS in 41 percent of HIV patients with musculoskeletal pain and in 11 percent of *all* HIV infected patients (Boston City Hospital Clinical AIDS Team 1992).

> Some publications and some doctors make the assumption that FMS and CFS are the same. Although I am not an authority on CFS, I do not believe this is true. I think they may be related, in a family of neurotransmitter dysfunctions. FMS has many subsets, depending on which neurotransmitters are affected. Some of these subsets are similar to CFS. People with well-managed FMS may have little or no fatigue at all. Many people diagnosed with CFS actually have FMS, and the alpha-delta sleep anomaly is causing the fatigue. CFS more often shows abnormalities in blood tests. FMS does not.
>
> D.J.S.

> In all the AIDS patients I've seen who have probable FMS, MPS has been present as well.
>
> D.J.S.

Hypoglycemia

Hypoglycemia is generally defined as a deficiency of sugar in the blood. Many women have hypoglycemia just prior to their menstrual period. Stress can also trigger hypoglycemia. A type of hypoglycemia called "reactive hypoglycemia" occurs in FMS when there is an insufficient amount of *usable* sugar in the blood (see Chapter 24, on nutrition).

Hypometabolism

Hypometabolism is a low or low-normal thyroid deficiency that makes people more susceptible to the development of trigger points. Thyroid hormones influence growth, energy production, and energy consumption.

Low-normal thyroid often escapes detection because doctors don't consider it serious. However, many of the symptoms are the same as some of the symptoms of FMS/MPS: Hypometabolism patients are usually cold most of the time, especially in the hands and feet. Some are intolerant of heat, as well, and don't sweat normally. Stiffness and achiness all through the body are common.

Hypermobility Syndrome

Hypermobility syndrome is characterized by joint relaxation that allows muscles to stretch beyond their normal range of motion. With this problem, stretching techniques should be avoided. Often trigger points appear in muscles that cross hypermobile joints. Hypermobility syndrome perpetuates TrPs.

Lupus

Lupus is a chronic, progressive auto-immune syndrome. There are two types of lupus. *Lupus myositis,* or *discoid lupus,* is a disorder confined to the skin. There is a scaling red, pink, or brown rash, often in the shape of a butterfly over the face, although it is not limited to that area. This rash is very photosensitive, and patients with this condition must avoid the sun.

Systemic lupus erythematosus occurs in connective tissue. It can also cause a butterfly rash, but *all* of the connective tissue can be involved, not just the skin. There may be involvement with any or many organ systems, producing a host of symptoms. As with FMS, MPS, or FMS/MPS Complex, symptoms may fluctuate. Fatigue, sun sensitivity, Raynaud's phenomenon, stiffness, muscle aches, swollen glands, low-grade temperature, hair loss, nausea and vomiting, lack of appetite can all occur. Other symptoms, too, may appear just as they can in FMS and/or MPS.

Mitral Valve Prolapse

This heart valve is made of connective tissue and doesn't flex as it should when it loses elasticity. This can cause the valve to change shape, and it no longer functions normally. Myofascia is connective tissue. This condition often occurs in conjunction with FMS and MPS.

Multiple Chemical Sensitivities

At the onset of multiple chemical sensitivities, a person may become sensitized to one chemical, such as formaldehyde from insulation or hair spray, after an exposure. Then, other environmental irritants, previously tolerated, begin to provoke allergic or sensitivity reactions.

The signs and symptoms are many and varied. They include fatigue, headaches, muscle aches, coughing, watery eyes, and tremors. Multiple chemical sensitivities are often present in people with FMS, which can make medication difficult. (See "Leaky Gut Syndrome.")

Multiple Sclerosis

Multiple sclerosis (MS) is caused by the breakdown of certain central nervous system (CNS) tissues that occur in multiple, random sites. Myelin is the fatty sheath surrounding some of the nerves (see Chapter 25, Bodywork—Helping Your Body Work). In MS, this sheath is damaged and neurotransmitter information is diminished or lost. There is cellular overgrowth at the damage sites, and areas of *sclerosis* (hardening) result.

Many patients with FMS/MPS Complex fear that they have MS, as there is often an overlap of symptoms. Loss of balance, muscular incoordination, and the weakness of the FMS/MPS Complex have lead to misdiagnoses. There are tests for MS. Some people do have both MS and the FMS/MPS Complex.

Osteoarthritis

Almost all people have osteoarthritis (OA) changes in their weight-bearing joints by the time they reach age 40. The cartilage of the joint begins to deteriorate, roughening and finally wearing away, and the bone changes. The joints become stiff. This later becomes pain when the joints are used. Inflammation is minimal, but range of motion is limited. MPS is often misdiagnosed as OA. Trigger points often develop due to arthritic changes.

Parkinson's Disease

Parkinson's Disease is a chronic nerve disease that causes a slowly spreading tremor and muscular weakness. The muscle tightness, twitching, nocturnal drooling, and postural instability of FMS/MPS Complex often lead patients to believe they are coming down with Parkinson's. In Parkinson's, the neurotransmitter dopamine is depleted. This can often happen in FMS as well. Some people have both Parkinson's and FMS/MPS Complex.

Post-Polio Syndrome

Post-polio syndrome (PPS), also called post-polio muscular atrophy (PPMA), occurs many years after recovery from an initial episode of polio. PPMA causes muscle weakness and recurrent paralysis, which can lead to respiratory paralysis, with slowly progressive muscle wasting.

Early PPS is often mistaken for FMS. Due to the possibility of PPS respiratory paralysis, FMS/MPS Complex patients who have had polio should be carefully monitored. It is not unusual for people to have FMS/MPS and PPS.

Raynaud's Phenomenon

Raynaud's Phenomenon is a condition in which fingers and/or toes turn white, then blue, and then red. This can occur during periods of cold or emotional stress. Numbness, tingling and burning may also be present at these times.

Reflex Sympathetic Dystrophy Syndrome

Reflex Sympathetic Dystrophy Syndrome (RSDS) (also called causalgia) is a disorder of the sympathetic nervous system. It causes irregular blood supply to the affected area: hand, foot, knee, hip, shoulder, and so on. It causes severe pain, often burning in nature. It often follows an injury (including surgery). In 30 percent of cases, there is no apparent cause. FMS/MPS is often misdiagnosed as RSDS.

Rheumatoid Arthritis

Rheumatoid arthritis (RA) is a chronic, systemic (biochemical) inflammatory condition that results in crippling deformities of the bone. RA almost always causes myofascial TrPs. RA patients should be checked for the presence of TrPs. Although the RA will continue to act as a TrP perpetuator, periodic TrP treatments can greatly lessen the patient's pain load.

Temporomandibular Joint Syndrome

Temporomandibular joint syndrome (TMJ) often occurs due to the presence of trigger points, although it can occur for other reasons. It is difficult for the dentist to deal with TMJ caused by TrPs, since the contraction of muscles due to TrPs can change so drastically. Often, as soon as the bite is corrected, it changes.

Severe pain is felt in the area of the jaw joint, with a clicking, crunching noise made by the jaw during chewing. Often, this is accompanied by ringing and/or itching of the ears. Sometimes there is some hearing loss.

Yeast Infections

Chronic yeast infections throughout the body often occur with FMS/MPS Complex. These perpetuate TrPs, as do all infections. Much of the body's defenses are tied up, fighting the infection. This is particularly true in the large subset of people with FMS/MPS Complex who also have reactive hypoglycemia, another FMS/MPS Complex perpetuating factor that also perpetuates yeast.

Yeast overgrowth can be responsible for at least part of the bloating, "fibrofog," abdominal upsets, and muscle aches in this subset of FMS/MPS Complex. Treatment with a systemic anti-yeast agent such as Diflucan™ (which crosses the blood-brain barrier) can result in dramatic symptom improvement. Note that it can also result in dramatic symptom *increase*.

This latter is due to the "yeast die-off" phenomenon. The dead and dying yeast can create all sorts of havoc, in the form of toxins and waste. Patients with long-term systemic yeast problems usually have developed yeast antibodies, and often are also allergic or sensitive to molds. This allergy or sensitivity will also perpetuate FMS/MPS Complex.

In Conclusion

The symptoms of FMS/MPS are widespread and varied. In some cases, though, those symptoms have other causes. Identifying other causes of your symptoms and treating them appropriately is as important as dealing with the symptoms that *are* due to FMS/MPS Complex. (When in doubt, check it out.)

CHAPTER 7

Perpetuating Factors

Perpetuating factors are conditions or stressors that cause a trigger point (TrP) to remain in place, in spite of attempts to break it up. Perpetuating factors may occur alone or with others. They may be behavioral, such as posture. They may be biochemical, such as nutritional inadequacy. They also may be mechanical, such as poorly fitting shoes. Frequently, one factor creates a TrP and another perpetuates it.

This chapter examines the most common perpetuating factors.

Behavioral Factors

Certain behaviors, that is, particular things that you do, whether voluntarily or involuntarily, can be perpetuating factors.

Facial Trigger Points

Grinding the teeth, clenching the jaw, late thumb sucking, chewing gum, loss of back teeth, and mouth breathing are often perpetuating factors in facial TrPs. The muscles you use for these activities are also the first to contract in situations of extreme emotional tension, desperation, and/or determination.

Smoking

Smoking is a terrible abuse of your body, and it is especially bad for people with FMS/MPS Complex. Nicotine causes the blood vessels to constrict and decreases blood flow. If you smoke, your body has to work harder to get adequate amounts of oxygen and nutrients to your muscles, and this added work increases tension and pain.

Carbon monoxide in a smoker's blood binds to hemoglobin, which is the oxygen-carrying workhorse of the body. This then blocks oxygen availability to the muscles. Sometimes when people with FMS/MPS quit smoking, they experience a sharp decrease in pain.

Air Pollution

Air pollution can add to the problems brought about by smoking. If you live in Mexico City, for example, just breathing the air is the equivalent of smoking 40 cigarettes a day! (What have we done to our environment, when breathing—the foundation of life itself—has become hazardous to our health?) We all must learn that we are part of the environment, and as it sickens, so do we.

Good Sport Syndrome

"Good sport syndrome" is one that probably all fibromites will find familiar. Perhaps it's a family outing, or relatives are coming and the house needs a super cleaning. Maybe your sister is moving and she needs help. You don't want to be thought of as a hypochondriac. And you *look* just fine. So you pretend you are fine, and go ahead with whatever. And you pay. And pay. And pay. (See Chapter 30, The Home Front, for some relatively graceful ways out of this situation.)

Non-Restorative Sleep

Lack of sleep perpetuates both FMS and MPS. Sleep problems can be activated by physical and emotional stress, maladaptive behaviors, postural abnormalities, caffeine beverages or alcohol before bed, menopausal hot flashes, or disturbances from children, noisy neighbors, or pets. (For more information, see Chapter 10, Sleep.)

Obesity

Obesity puts stress, both physical and emotional, on anybody. Unfortunately, as with many problems associated with FMS/MPS Complex, there are built-in self-perpetuators, such as altered carbohydrate metabolism and chocolate craving. (For more information, see Chapter 24, on nutrition.)

Depression/Anxiety

Depression and anxiety can occur for many reasons. Among them is the chronic pain of FMS/MPS; furthermore, if you start out feeling depressed or anxious, your physical symptoms can worsen. If you experience high levels of anxiety, you may express this in the form of tighter muscles. (For techniques to help you deal with depression and anxiety, see Chapter 16, Coping Day to Day.)

Muscle Abuse

If you aren't very careful, you can abuse your muscles. Perhaps you overuse them by pushing yourself too hard, or your boss pushes you too hard by requiring mandatory overtime, or you use muscles that you haven't warmed up properly.

The failure to listen to your body is another form of abuse. Pain, fatigue, weakness, tingling, numbness, heaviness, clumsiness, stiffness, and lack of control are all signs that something is wrong. Listen. You get only one body in this life. Take care of it.

Poor Posture

You may be contributing to poor posture by sleeping on two pillows, sleeping without adequate neck support (such as a well-fitting cervical pillow), protracted neck extension (watching a tennis match, or bird-watching), reading in bed with a light to one side, or rolling over in bed by lifting your head and "leading with it."

Try this. Lie down on your bed. Now, roll over, paying attention to which muscles you use, and how you use them. Do you lift your head? (Your head should remain flat when you turn. Otherwise you are placing stress on any TrPs in your neck.) Try rolling with your head flat. Does that feel odd? This motion may be one reason why you have sternocleidomastoid trigger points (SCM TrPs). (See Figure 3-2.) For more information about posture, see Chapter 27, Bodywork You Can Do Yourself.

Repetitive Motion

Repetitive motion is one of the most common perpetuators of TrPs. For example, if you start an exercise program, such as weight training or work hardening, before you have treated your TrPs, the repetitive motion training can become a perpetuating factor.

The subscapularis TrP (see Figure 6-1) severely restricts the rotating movement of the arm at shoulder level. Hanging curtains, folding sheets, throwing a ball overhand, keeping an arm raised at school, ironing, or almost any repetitive motion in this area will perpetuate this TrP.

> I have seen more people with active TrPs become disabled by repetitive motion exercises and inappropriate physical therapy than from anything else.
>
> D.J.S.

Treating One Side But Not the Other

Another common failing is stretching or otherwise treating one side of your body and not the other. Often, the non-symptomatic side, if there is one, is full of latent TrPs.

Compression

You may be compressing part of your body by wearing a tight collar, necktie, bra, belt, socks, or some other piece of clothing, or by grinding your teeth, among other things. You may tend to swell. For example, a bra that feels comfortable in the morning can become unbearably tight just hours later. Tight clothing can really aggravate TrPs, causing constriction of blood vessels, which, in turn, can amplify pain that is referred from TrPs.

Habitual Frowning or Squinting

If you are in the habit of frowning or squinting, perhaps you have astigmatism or light sensitivity. Repetitive motions can perpetuate TrPs around the eyes.

Biochemical Factors

Many biochemical factors can be the culprits in perpetuating TrPs. Some of the most common ones are discussed below.

Vitamin Inadequacy and Other Nutritional Factors

Vitamin inadequacy and other nutritional factors are extremely common perpetuating factors of FMS and MPS (Simons 1989). Other common biochemical perpetuators are low levels of electrolytes, especially ionized calcium and potassium. You need these minerals to run the body. Unfortunately, in FMS/MPS, either the body doesn't get enough of them or it can't use those it does get efficiently.

Sometimes, there's a catch-22 situation. For example, your body may need electrolytic balance, but it can't absorb the minerals that adjust the balance until its electrolytes are in balance. This can cause trouble.

Nutritional inadequacies such as very low levels of B complex and vitamin C are the rule for those who smoke, have mineral deficiencies, or metabolic and endocrine inadequacies. Hypometabolism due to low thyroid function, hypoglycemia, and other coexisting conditions are also important perpetuators of TrPs and fibromyalgia syndrome (FMS).

In FMS, often there are low blood serum levels of essential amino acids, including *tryptophan*, which contributes to sleep regulation, pain control, and immune system function. The result can be lack of sleep, pain, or frequent infection. These are all perpetuating factors.

The activity of TrPs tends to increase during any systemic viral, bacterial, yeast, or protozoal illness. Vulnerability to TrPs may start a few days before symptoms from infection worsen, and may last for several weeks after the infection. (Absorption of toxic products also makes the development of active TrPs more likely.)

Note that specific TrP therapy won't produce a lasting effect while a chronic infection, such as an upper respiratory infection, vaginal infection, or a parasitic infection such as tapeworm, is present. (For more information about nutritional factors, see Chapter 24, on nutrition.)

Impaired Muscle Metabolism

Certain conditions, including anemia and apoxia (people with FMS/MPS often have to relearn to breathe correctly), can contribute to impaired muscle metabolism.

Low Thyroid

People with low thyroid function, or even "low normal" thyroid, have what is called *hypometabolism.* This means they feel exhausted most of the time. They are also "weather reactors"; they don't need to watch the local weather broadcasts, because they always know when a storm is coming. (The National Weather Service could save big bucks if they just had a phone tree of fibromites with low thyroid function.)

People with hypometabolism often have skin that is rough and dry in places. They may carry excess weight, which seems impossible to lose. The standard thyroid tests don't give an accurate picture of people with FMS/MPS Complex. What is needed is a series of tests called the BT2 panel. This consists of Total T4, Free T4, Total T3, and TSH (London 1994).

Allergic Conditions

Illnesses such as asthma and hay fever are perpetuators of TrPs and FMS. The neurotransmitter, histamine, seems to be at least one of the culprits.

Hypoglycemia

Coexisting hypoglycemia makes treatment of FMS/MPS Complex extremely difficult. Myofascial TrP activity is so aggravated by it that it doesn't make sense to treat specific TrPs unless the hypoglycemia is also treated (Simons 1989).

Some initial symptoms of hypoglycemia are sweating, trembling, and shakiness before meals; rapid heart rate; and a feeling of anxiety. Sternocleidomastoid (SCM) TrPs may add headaches and dizziness. If the brain is not getting adequate oxygen, visual disturbances, restlessness, impaired speech and thinking, and sometimes fainting also occur.

Reactive hypoglycemia is a condition that shows up two to three hours after a meal rich in carbohydrates. It is this kind of hypoglycemia that is more common in FMS patients. There is a problem with carbohydrate metabolism in a subset of FMS patients that overstimulates the release of insulin. (See Chapter 24, on nutrition.)

> One of the most painful episodes I ever had was when Hurricane David, which came in with an incredibly low pressure area, was barreling in on the south Florida coast. We lived in the Fort Lauderdale area then, and I was busy trying to secure the house. I spent a lot of time meditating, trying to control the incredible feeling of "implosion." It felt as though every cell in my body was trying to collapse in on itself.
>
> D.J.S.

Coexisting Conditions

As you learned in the previous chapter, irritable bowel syndrome and yeast *are* possible coexisting conditions. Cancer and other internal illnesses can produce and perpetuate TrPs. Other common conditions that can act as perpetuating factors include Crohn's Disease, interstitial cystitis, painful menstrual periods (or just the periods themselves), ovulation, an irritated iliocaecal valve from constipation, and even uncorrected vision problems. When the problem is removed, the TrPs become latent—which, as you know, can reactivate and become the source of further problems.

It is wise to open the pelvic constriction by trigger point-tennis ball acupressure (see Chapter 27, Bodywork You Can Do Yourself) before menses, thus decreasing water retention and bloating. Eye exercises for those whose vision is impaired or for people who spend most of the day looking downward will help to remedy TrPs around the eyes.

Iliopsoas TrPs (see Figure 7-1) can worsen constipation, which, in turn, can perpetuate TrPs. This usually sets up piriformis TrPs and gluteus minimus TrPs. When it comes to TrPs, misery loves company.

Symptoms include pain in the front of the thigh, in the back close to the vertebrae, and in the front, on the iliac crest. These symptoms often occur as the result of a failed low-back surgery (Travell 1992). In this case pain can extend as high as the shoulder blade. Not just the surgery itself, but its analogs—immobility in bed, constipation, and so forth—are also perpetuators.

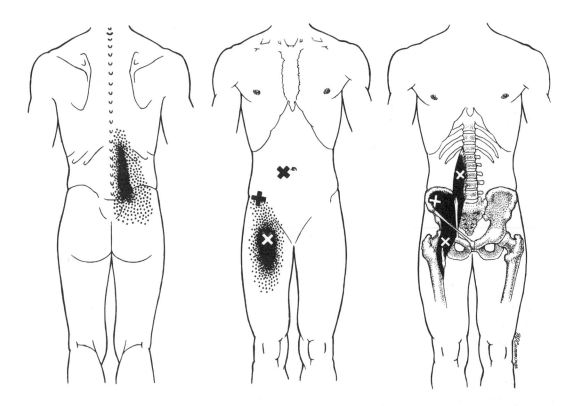

Figure 7-1: Trigger points along the iliopsoas and referred pain patterns

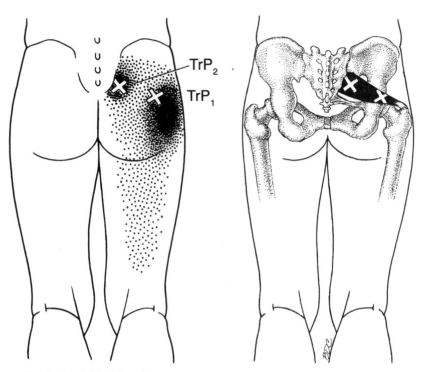

Figure 7-2: Trigger points in the right piriformis

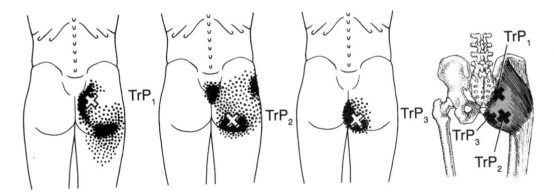

Figure 7-3: Trigger points in the gluteus maximus

The ileocaecal valve is located between the small and large intestines. Think of it as something like the valve between the kitchen refueling area and the garbage dumpster. This valve prevents the garbage from returning to the small intestine.

The last portion of the small intestine is called the *ilium.* This is where nutrient-laden moisture is absorbed. When it becomes irritated, with constipation or from an irritable bowel, one of the first consequences is a right iliopsoas TrP (see Figure 7-1). A cool gel pack on the area and proper treatment of the constipation will take care of the TrP. When it is latent, trigger point-tennis ball acupressure (see Chapter 27) will help to banish the TrP.

Chronic hemorrhoids can aggravate symptoms in related muscles, and TrPs can add to the problems that caused the hemorrhoids in the first place.

Mechanical Factors

People who develop FMS/MPS Complex often have mechanical irregularities that go unnoticed until something goes wrong. When that something is FMS and/or MPS, it tends to go wrong in a big way.

Body Asymmetry

To determine whether body asymmetry is an issue for you, take an inventory of your body, which is something we rarely do.

From the front, your shoulder blades, shoulders, nipples, and the space between your arms and your ribs should match on your right and left sides. The points of your hips should match, as should your knees and ankles.

From the back, your shoulders should be even and level. Your shoulder blades should match and not protrude. Your elbows and hip points should match, as should the backs of your knees, your ankles, and your heels.

When you stand straight, your feet should touch each other from the big toe to the heel. If you stand with your back against the wall and with your heels about three inches away from the wall, your head should feel comfortable against the wall.

If there is an internal rotation of your knees, shoulders, and/or hips, it creates a tightness of the musculature. This can create many deformities and inequalities. Some types of hypermobility are often due to this rotation. Muscles resist correction, and they resist change.

Your *diaphragm,* the big flat muscle that separates the chest cavity from the abdominal cavity, also may be warped and stiff, affecting your breathing.

Each elbow should reach the crest of the ilium, which is the outside top "point" of your hip. The corner of your mouth should be in line with the corner of your eye, and the sides should be symmetrical. If one shoulder is low, you may be tipping the other even lower to compensate.

If you wear glasses, you will know whether your ears are different heights. This can affect your vision, so be sure to mention it to your eye doctor.

If you have one leg longer than the other, the gluteals will often respond by developing TrPs. The abnormal weight distribution usually causes pronation (toeing out).

Note: Always check both sides of your body for TrPs. Active ones on one side are usually matched by latent ones on the other side, especially in the case of the scaleni and sternocleidomastoid TrPs. (See Figures 3-1 and 3-2.)

Hypermobility

You may have what are termed *hypermobile* joints—that is, they move beyond the normal range of motion. In this situation, physical therapists must be *very* careful not to overstretch your muscles, and exercise must be aimed at strengthening, not lengthening, the muscles. For hypermobile patients, it is essential to inactivate their TrPs by using techniques that do not extend their muscles to maximum length.

Sensory Changes

Sensory changes include such things as the change to and from daylight saving time, weather changes such as barometric shifts, and dampness and drafts.

Many fibromites are especially sensitive to temperature. (A hyperactive nervous system can increase any kind of hypersensitivity.) If this is the case for you, dress defensively in cool environments, and be especially careful of drafts; cold plus wind equals TrPs. Heat can also be a perpetuator, especially when accompanied by high humidity.

Ill-Fitting, Poorly Designed Furniture

Janet Travell is an amazing woman. This brilliant physician was not content simply to find out what was happening with FMS/MPS Complex; she also needed to know why. (And how to prevent it.) Thus, she spent some of her valuable time designing chairs, so that we might be more comfortable.

She says in her excellent video series (see Appendix C, Suppliers of Health Care Items) that chairs were originally designed as thrones to raise a king above his subjects. They were not designed for comfort. This is doubly true for those of us with short upper arms and/or short lower legs.

Ill-fitting pillows and beds also perpetuate TrPs.

Typewriter or Computer Use

When using a typewriter or computer keyboard, long fingernails can perpetuate TrPs, so keep your fingernails trimmed. You should be able to strike the keyboard with the point of the finger. Otherwise, there will be too much stress on too many muscle groups. Improper lighting and awkward areas in your workspace can also perpetuate TrPs.

Traveling

Traveling can really stress your body and mind, especially when you are driving. Then, you are relatively immobile, and many of your muscles are in shortened positions. Because of this, your circulation is often greatly impaired in the lower body. (For more information, see Chapter 35, Travel.)

Immobility

FMS/MPS stiffness is most apparent after immobility. Any kind of muscle immobility causes static electrical loading of the muscles. Casts, even walking casts, can produce TrPs. After being immobile for a time, you must be careful when you do move. Determining how to move, where to move, and for how long are critical issues in the world of FMS/MPS.

Running, Climbing, Jumping, Jogging

Running, climbing, jumping, or jogging on uneven ground can cause and perpetuate TrPs. Climbing uphill can also injure your legs. This makes FMS/MPS Complex especially tough for people who live in hilly and/or mountainous areas.

Prolonged Sitting

Prolonged sitting perpetuates TrPs in several ways. Circulation can be impaired if you do not have adequate clearance under your hamstrings when you sit. When much of your leg length is in the upper part of your legs, your feet don't touch the ground when you sit. This compresses the hamstrings and perpetuates TrPs.

Crossing your legs when you sit is also a perpetuating factor. This can be a problem for people with FMS and MPS, who often cross their legs to achieve better balance and support. The use of a gently sloping triangular footrest, to keep the foot in an ankle-down and toes-high position, is a great benefit. Some of the catalogs listed at the end of this book even offer portable, collapsible footrests. A large 3-ring binder works also well as a footrest.

Prolonged Bed Rest

Muscles must function to remain functional. They receive inadequate amounts of oxygen and nutrients when you stay in bed. Unless it absolutely cannot be avoided, prolonged bed rest is not a good idea for people with FMS/MPS.

Ill-Fitting Shoes (and Socks)

Shoe designers must really think very little of women. Finding shoes that fit can be a real challenge. How many women do you know who have a foot with a wide heel, and a narrow pointy toe, who walk around on their toes all day?

A shoe with a tight upper layer, and little room between shoe and foot, encourages the formation of TrPs. If you are using a shoe insert, take it to the store when trying on shoes. Orthotics, which are specially made shoe inserts, are usually unnecessary unless there is a foot deformity. The need is for soft-cushioning, not hard orthotics, which may perpetuate TrPs (Travell 1992). Shoes with extensive wear on the heels and soles may also perpetuate a foot problem.

Socks with tight elastic aggravate the peroneus TrPs. (See Figure 7-4.) It isn't unusual for people with FMS/MPS to retain indentations on their legs from their socks for a whole day or longer. Janet Travell recommends ironing the top of the sock with a hot iron. This may ease the elastic enough to avoid restriction of blood flow.

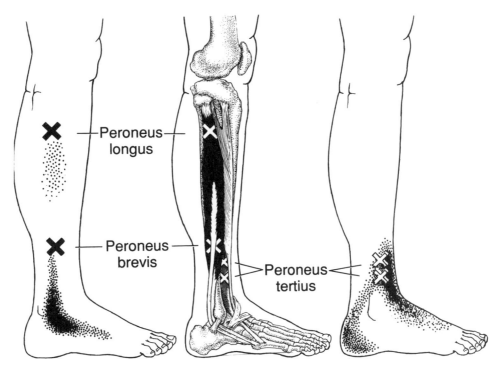

Figure 7-4: Trigger points in the peroneals

You may need to wear warm, loose socks at night during the winter months. (This can be a problem for those of us who need to stick their feet out from under the bedclothes at times during the night, to help equalize the temperature.)

Shoes with rigid soles that allow only ankle and no toe movement can perpetuate TrPs in the leg as well as in the foot. Selecting the right sole is important for other reasons, too. Wearing shoes with smooth soles on a hard slippery surface can perpetuate TrPs, as can chilling of the feet. It helps your feet and legs if you soak them in a tub of warm water and then do some gentle stretching.

Intrinsic Foot TrPs

Deep intrinsic foot TrPs can cause pain under the heel, an intolerance to orthotics, a staggering walk, and thickened calluses. Intrinsic foot TrPs can also cause a strange fluffy feeling of numbness, a sense of the skin swelling over the region of the metatarsal heads (these are the joints in the toes like the knuckles in the fingers), and a tingling of the great toe (see Figure 7-5).

Active or latent TrPs in the dorsal interosseous muscles can be associated with hammer toes, and any foot deformity will perpetuate TrPs. Note that deformations of the toes may disappear after correction of TrPs.

Foot Structure

Some common varieties of foot structure create additional hazards for the person with FMS/MPS. They are discussed below.

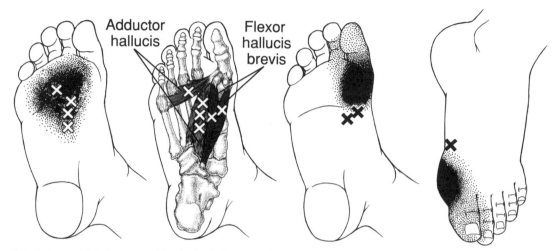

Figure 7-5: Trigger points in some of the intrinsic foot muscles

Fallen Arches

People with "fallen arches" often try specially made shoe orthotics without success. The undersurface of the foot near the middle continues to be painful, and the expensive inserts lie in the closet, unused.

Morton's Foot

The name of Dudley J. Morton, M.D. is forever linked with variations on the normal foot structure. One type of variation is hypermobility of the first metatarsal.

The second variation is the foot with a relatively short "big toe" metatarsal and longer second toe metatarsal, with a wide web between the second and third toes These variations are common. In a person with a tendency to develop TrPs, they result in a muscle imbalance stress situation of the whole leg. The peroneus and foot muscles are directly affected. The vastus medialis, gluteus medius, and gluteus mimimus TrPs are perpetuated due to the attempts these muscles make to compensate for the peroneus and foot dysfunction. There is a common callus pattern with this condition that aids diagnosis. (See Figure 7-7.)

The "FMS/MPS Foot"

There appears to be no technical term for what I call the FMS/MPS foot. This foot has a broad front, a narrow heel, and a high arch. There is usually a large space between the big toe and the second toe. There is also a typical callus pattern. The callus may wear a hole in your socks about the size of a dime right under the second metatarsal. The big toe is often slanted towards the little toe. All of these are perpetuating factors of foot and leg TrPs.

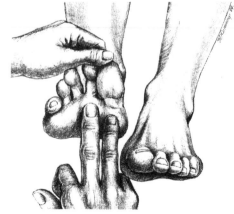

Figure 7-6: Morton's foot

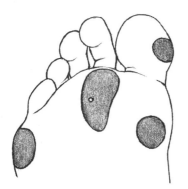

Figure 7-7: Morton's foot callus pattern

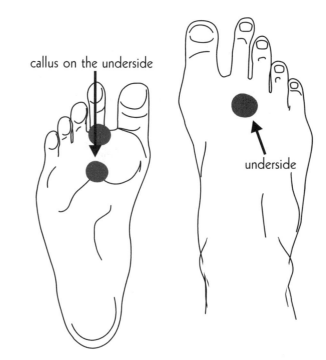

callus on the underside

underside

Figure 7-8: Typical FMS/MPS foot and callus pattern

Numbness and tingling can be caused by entrapment of the common peroneal nerve on the top of the foot in the triangle between first and second toes. Both of these types of structural foot problems can be remedied to some extent.

Janet Travell did some research for the best kind of shoe for people with MPS. (See Figure 7-9.) She found that pointed toes and any kind of heel are not good. The shoe should be flat. The sole of the shoe must be flexible at the metatarsal bend. There must be adequate room for the toes, and the heels must fit snugly. The shoe heel should be firm and fit well, to avoid sliding. That's because sliding irritates the Achilles tendon and can cause heel calluses. If the heel does not fit properly, the foot will "roll," causing heavy callus formation on the sides and back of the heels. A thick foam or felt pad inside the shoe can prevent the rolling

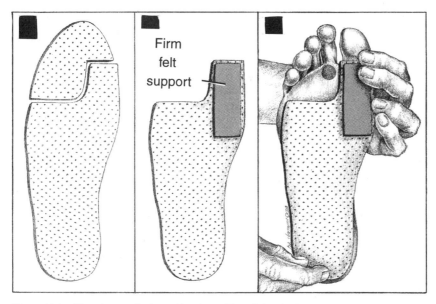

Firm felt support

Figure 7-9: Shoe insert designed by Janet Travell for the Morton foot.

and the calluses, and subsequent Achilles tendon irritation. The arch of your foot needs good support as well.

Morton's Neuroma

Morton's neuroma occurs as a result of entrapment of the nerve between the toes. At the base of the toe, where it joins the foot, there are bones called *metatarsals*. Nerve branching occurs in this same area. If the metatarsals are crowding the nerves or if the myofascia is tightly wrapped around these nerve branches and the musculature, a neuroma can result.

A *neuroma* is a swelling of the nerve, with scarring and constriction in the surrounding area. If you have this condition, it feels as though you always have a pebble in your shoe. Your foot hurts whenever you put pressure on it. Gradually this develops into shooting pains that feel like electric shocks originating from the toes. Eventually, your foot hurts all the time, and walking becomes torture.

By this point, conservative measures are often not enough. People with FMS/MPS and Morton's neuromas are in severe pain.

> I needed hospitalization for surgical removal of neuromas. The involved toes are always numb now, but the numbness beats the pain. There is nothing like having Morton's neuromas, Morton's foot, and FMS/MPS foot, to make shoe comfort a challenge.
>
> D.J.S.

Sacroiliac (SI) Joint Dysfunction

The sacroiliac is one of three joints in the body for which movement can neither be caused by nor opposed by muscles. Abnormal muscle tension from any cause can help to hold this joint in an abnormal, displaced position. It can become locked in place—which is a place that it should not be. For proper functioning, the joint must be mobilized.

The onset of sacroiliac (SI) TrPs can be a simple motion of bending forward while tilting the pelvis and twisting. This is common when making a golf swing or while shoveling snow, while stooping and reaching, after a slight fall, or in pregnancy.

What You, the Patient, Can Do

As you are learning more about your body, there are steps you can take to eliminate or lessen the effects of perpetuating factors. You will learn more as you continue reading this book. Because TrPs are at the heart of FMS/MPS Complex, however, it's important that you always try to prevent more TrPs from developing. You can do so in the following ways:

- Treat injuries aggressively

- Seek crisis intervention when appropriate

- Build proper and sufficient exercise and sleep into your program

- Use your body properly

- Control psychological trauma and stress load

- Make lifestyle modifications

You will find tips for accomplishing these goals throughout this book. These tips involve things you can do for yourself and ways in which other people can help you.

In Conclusion

Perpetuating factors have a tremendous impact on people with FMS/MPS. As you are beginning to learn, identifying these factors and treating them appropriately are essential elements of your treatment.

PART II

COMMON SYMPTOMS AND WHY THEY OCCUR

CHAPTER 8

Questions and Answers About
Common Symptoms

If there is a specific trigger point (TrP) causing a symptom, it is MPS-related. Otherwise, it is due to fibromyalgia (FMS). Some symptoms can have both FMS and MPS components. Symptoms can be caused by the biochemical changes of FMS, or by the mechanical effects of MPS trigger points. Some of these symptoms can also be worsened by the biochemical changes brought about by chronic pain. Any of these symptoms can occur in FMS/MPS Complex.

If you've read Part I, you know that the symptoms of FMS/MPS Complex are many and varied. This chapter consists of questions to ask yourself about your symptoms, as well as explanations of what these symptoms mean. You may be surprised to learn how many symptoms you experience are associated with FMS/MPS Complex. In some cases we've provided suggestions for eliminating or lessening a particular symptom, and in others we've included cross-references to other chapters, where you will find more detailed information on a particular symptom.

To make this long chapter more easily manageable, we have divided it into four sections. The dividing lines may seem a little fuzzy, but that's because they are. Everything in the body is connected and dividing lines are often arbitrary.

Some of the information in this chapter is still in the theoretical stage, and we have indicated that where appropriate. We have tried to draw logical connections whenever we could, but we are still trailblazing. We do feel sure that you will know more about your condition when you finish this chapter, and that information will give you a greater measure of control over your life.

Note: In the descriptions in this chapter, we have included the medical names of many of the specific TrPs that cause problems. Don't let these names scare you. You can refer to these figures throughout your reading for a better understanding of particular trigger points. The more you know, the more you can help your doctor to make a correct diagnosis. (This information will also help the efficiency of physical therapy and other treatments.)

Section I: No Bones About It

1. Did you have "growing pains" and chronic aches as a child?

Many people with FMS and/or MPS believe that their problems started fairly recently. When closely questioned, however, they often remember "growing pains," especially in the hips (Travell and Simons 1992 vol. II, p. 440).

> I have found that growing pains are often the first warning sign of a genetic predisposition toward FMS/MPS. A TrP in the gluteus maximus often causes pain in a rapidly growing child (see Figure 7-3).
>
> D.J.S.

2. Do you attract blackflies and mosquitoes?

For some reason, blackflies and mosquitoes seem to love people with FMS. There's something about their biochemistry that attracts these insects. (Perhaps you should hire yourself out for lawn parties. It might help pay your medical bills.) Northern New England blackflies prefer the taste of people with FMS. So do Alaskan blackflies. The attraction may have something to do with abnormal carbohydrate metabolism. It may be electromagnetic. In any case, blackfly bites swell into huge, hard lumps that take forever to go away and often leave scars. This symptom does seem to be diminished by guaifenesin therapy, however. (See Chapter 23, Guaifenesin.)

Mosquitoes are attracted to children, people with higher-than-normal body temperatures, anyone wearing bright clothes and scented products, and people with FMS. The best advice is to keep cool and unscented, and to wear white.

> I've been on guaifenesin now for a year and a half (as well as on diet modification for reactive hypoglycemia), and this summer, for the first time in years, I didn't swell with blackfly bites. Actually, this may be because there is less constriction now in my myofascia. My improved circulation carries the blackfly toxin away more efficiently, and the blackfly toxin is diluted. Unfortunately, I am still high on their flavor-favorite list.
>
> D.J.S.

3. Do you have bodywide achiness?

Several studies have confirmed the presence of three times the amount of substance P in the spinal fluid of patients with FMS (Russell 1994, pp. 101-115). *Substance P* is a neurotransmitter that can produce a nerve-generated response that leads to the dilation of the blood vessels. It can also cause fluid and proteins to migrate from inside the cells to outside the cells. This may be responsible for some of the aches, as well as some of the swollen feeling that FMS patients report.

4. Do you have allergies?

Allergies seem to be part of the FMS/MPS Complex's bag of tricks, and there are many reasons for this, but the chief one may just be that people with FMS/MPS have sensitized nervous systems. Histamine, a familiar name to allergy sufferers, is a neurotransmitter that is regulated in delta-level sleep. Multiple chemical sensitivities and sensitivity to odors are also common with FMS.

You may be hypersensitive to molds and yeasts. You may also have the "itchies." (See the answer to Question No. 12 below, and see Section II, Question No. 15, about itchy ears.) Add the post-nasal drip common to those with FMS, some TrPs, and the already mechanically irritated throat, and you have a perfect set up for allergies. Note, also, that people with FMS/MPS don't always react normally to allergy tests. Skin tests are not reliable due to altered biochemical responses. Many of our "allergies" are often really sensitivities without immune components. (See the discussion about the the leaky gut syndrome in Chapter 24 on nutrition.)

5. Do you experience extreme fatigue?

Fatigue and lack of endurance may be part of the disrupted hypothalamic-pituitary-adrenal (HPA) axis found in FMS. The hypothalamus, pituitary, and adrenal glands are tied together in many ways, each affecting the other as well as many other regulatory systems in the body. This interaction of the three glands is called the "HPA axis." (See Chapter 14 for an explanation of the HPA axis in some detail.)

If, for some reason, the hypothalamus stops functioning, then the ability to adjust rapidly to environmental change is damaged or lost. (Does that sound familiar?) The hypothalamus also integrates cardiovascular regulation, food intake, and body temperature regulation (including sweating). The gland receives its

---

The discoloration on my skin first began to be noticeable on my forearms. They became brown in rectangular patches. The color faded slightly with the winter and then darkened again in the sunlight. After a few years, the blotches turned an angry red and itched when they were exposed to the sun, although sunblock did prevent this symptom from occurring. I visited a dermatologist, who had no answers, except to rule out infection.

The clue for me came when I inadvertently left some salt gel residue from a muscle electrostimulator electrode on my forearm. I soon developed a brown mottled semicircle on my arm. It became obvious to me that the electrolytes—the "salts"—in the gel had reacted with something in the sunlight to cause the brownish mark on my arm. Observing my movements in the garden, I noticed that I often wiped my forehead on my arms. The photoreaction of the gel salts with sunlight and the salts in my sweat and, perhaps, unusual FMS biochemical components produced the mottling. I still have the mottling on my arms two years later, but, since I began wearing headbands while gardening, and frequently washing off any sweat accumulation, the mottling has not increased.

D.J.S.

Hair loss isn't as common in FMS/MPS Complex as the other symptoms described in the answer to Question 10, but I had clumps of hair fall out when I was young. I had bald patches all over my body. Hair loss seems to accompany some cases of FMS.

D.J.S.

control signals from (you guessed it) neurotransmitters.

Fatigue is also exacerbated by sleep deprivation and the constant barrage of disrupted neurotransmitters, which causes an overabundance of mixed messages and sensory overload. Your adrenals, which help to regulate your energy, are often overworked because of the adrenaline surges you get—often when you are longing to go to sleep. You may be very tired, "bone weary" even, yet your adrenaline starts pumping and suddenly you are wide awake. Naturally, this is exhausting. The toxic wastes resulting from the constriction of your myofascia also contribute to the energy drain on your resources. Is it any wonder you sometimes feel as if you've been tangling with a vampire?

6. Do you have mottled or blotchy skin?

Light activates the hypothalamus, which activates the pituitary. The pituitary is also responsible for secreting melanocyte-stimulating hormone. This influences the mottling on the skin.

7. Do you have loose ("double-jointed"or hypermobile) joints?

Hypermobility (or loose joints) is often due to rotation of internal musculature. Travell and Simons (1992) say that up to 5 percent of *all* adults have this problem. Overstretching hypermobile joints can seriously overextend the muscles, thus perpetuating the TrPs.

8. Do you crave carbohydrates or sweets?

Craving for chocolate stems at least partially from a lack of the neurotransmitter, serotonin, which can leave you agitated and distressed (Xenakis 1993). Chocolate causes the brain to produce more insulin, which enhances serotonin production. Serotonin is one of the main neurotransmitters in short supply in FMS.

Lack of serotonin can also cause a craving for carbohydrates (pasta, bread, and so on). On the other hand, craving salty things can mean fluctuating hormones, which indicate neurotransmitter dysregulation.

9. Do you have frequent yeast infections, itchiness on the roof of your mouth when you eat tangy cheese, or bloating if you drink beer?

If you have these symptoms, you may have a yeast problem. Many people with FMS/MPS do. And there is a good indication that at least some of the cognitive difficulties you may be experiencing are due to water retention from yeast overgrowth.

Often foods that are high in yeast, such as citrus fruits, peanut butter, and cashews, cause bloating or roof-of-the-mouth itch. There is a blood test for the candida (a common yeast) antibody. This test doesn't measure the candida yeast, but it looks for antibodies that we would form in response to recurring yeast infections. You may also find that allergy shots for molds are very helpful. (For more information on the "yeast beast," see Chapter 18, Fibrofog and Other Absurdities.)

10. Do you have overgrowing connective tissue—nail ridges or beads, nails that curve under, ingrown hairs—and do you scar easily?

Nail ridges or beads and/or nails that curve under; ingrown hairs; adhesions; easy scarring; cuticles that thicken and split painfully resulting in sore hangnails; cysts and fibroids; pierced ears that overgrow—all of these symptoms may be related. It appears that people with FMS/MPS frequently have overgrowing connective tissue. Also, fibrocystic breasts and fibroid tumors may be related, as they indicate an overgrowth and possible encapsulation of certain types of tissues. Hair loss may also be related, because hair tissue is similar to fingernail tissue.

> I considered the possibility of allergies when my arms started mottling and itching. The cortisone cream the dermatologist recommended did nothing. Both he and I failed to account for the sensory itch effect, which is where at least some of the itch originates.
>
> D.J.S.

11. Do you have sleep apnea?

Sleep apnea—temporary cessation of breathing while sleeping—is a very dangerous condition that often accompanies snoring. It is common in FMS, especially in men. For more information, see Chapter 10, Sleep.

12. Do you have generalized itchiness?

There are many types of itch. Often, when people itch, they look for an allergic reaction as the culprit, but allergies are not always the problem. The skin is the largest organ in the body. Too often it is regarded simply as a passive cover, but your skin is actually your first line of defense against a frequently hostile outer world. It is the main contact between your inside "world" and the outer world. However, as most science fiction fans know, problems do tend to occur when two worlds try to communicate.

There are pressure plate receptors in the outer skin layer called Merkel's discs (Xenakis 1993). They translate the tactile messages received by the skin to the brain. The brain then responds appropriately to the sensory input. For example, if you touch a thorn, your brain signals "sharp" and you move away. When the receptors don't know what message to send, they initiate a default mechanism. Unfamiliar pressures are translated and sent to the brain as "itch" signals. It may be that because of the dysregulation of neurotransmitters (in FMS) and/or the mechanical constriction of fluids around the Merkel's discs (in MPS), that people with FMS/MPS Complex itch more than most folks. Sometimes, it is enough to drive them to distraction and it often disrupts their meager amounts of sleep.

Cold helps to control the itch by numbing the pressure plate receptors. Dryness, which enhances pressure reception by the discs, makes the itch worse. (We hope to interest a dermatologist to do some research on this.)

> You can't imagine how many times I've finished huge blocks of this chapter and then accidentally deleted them. It even took me three tries to write the word "frustration." That kind of frustrating effort is sometimes typical for people with FMS/MPS Complex.
>
> D.J.S.

13. Do you experience frequent frustration?

Those of us with FMS and/or MPS must learn how to cope with chronic frustration in order to survive. On the Internet group (fibrom-l listserv), one correspondent commented on how many times she had written a heartfelt reply to someone, only to accidentally delete it instead of sending it. So it goes.

14. Do you experience unusual reactions to medications?

Sometimes just a small portion of a normal dose of medication will have very strong effects on you as a fibromite. Other times you can take whopping doses of the same medication and feel no effects at all. This phenomenon may be connected with altered metabolism.

15. Do you have thick mucus secretions?

A lot of people with FMS/MPS Complex experience thick mucus secretions. There may be times when you have to take off your eyeglasses before you can blow your nose, because the mucus from your nose can gunk up the lenses, and it's hard to remove from your eyeglasses. Guaifenesin ends this problem, and the way it thins secretions may be a part of why it is so effective. (See Chapter 23, Guaifenesin.)

16. Do you have an inability to sweat or extreme night/ morning sweats?

These symptoms seem to come in a specific order. First, there is a period when you hardly sweat at all. This can last for years. Then, later, you may have times when you can become drenched in sweat, even during sleep. Any exertion, even a walk to the mailbox, can cause extreme sweating. Sometimes, this is accompanied by a continual feeling of nerves firing up and down the legs, chest, and arms, although this is not as common as just sweating.

It is likely that the body is trying to eliminate toxins and built-up metabolic waste products in the sweat. Many fibromites have reported that their sweat often smells bad, as does their urine. Additionally, they report having less skin symptomology if they wash off the sweat as soon as possible. Some medications cause sweating as well.

17. Do you have patches of skin with a painful network of fine veins and capillaries?

This is the mysterious "livido reticularis" that is sometimes seen in FMS/MPS Complex patients, usually in the legs, but it also can occur in the arms. Areas of hypersensitive skin are overlain by a visible blue and red network of veins and capillaries.

18. Do you have dermographia (writing with a fingernail on your skin leaves red welts)?

One phenomenon that occurs in FMS/MPS Complex is called the "flare response." Richard van Why describes this in his book (1994). The flare response is part of a reaction to the neurotransmitter histamine, and to mast cell release at the trigger points and other trauma sites.

One Internet FMily member reported that red welts occurred with acupuncture. This can happen with any kind of trigger point therapy. It is a *neurogenic* (generated by the nerves) flare in response to even mild touch (such as writing on your skin), heat, or chemical contact.

Some people with FMS/MPS also experience a profound change in their ability to tolerate heat and cold and an increase in *skinfold* tenderness. (This is the sensitivity that results when you pinch the upper layer of skin, lifting it off the underlying tissues.) These people respond to touch with what is called "tactile defensiveness," or muscle tension. For many of us, this means that some types of deep-muscle work, such as Heller-work or Rolfing, can worsen our condition.

19. Do you have night-driving problems?

Many people with FMS/MPS Complex often have a problem driving at night. The lights of the oncoming cars really distress us. Beta-carotene seems to help this somewhat. The effectiveness of beta-carotene depends on how deficient you are at the beginning of supplementation.

20. Do you have an extreme susceptibility to infection?

This symptom can occur in a cycle of immune changes. You may go through a cycle when you don't catch any colds or any other types of germs that may be going around. Later on, the reverse is often true, and your immune system has no success attacking infections at all. At those times, you have to put antibiotic ointment on every scratch to prevent it from becoming infected. Both responses can be signs of immune dysfunction.

The *Fibromyalgia Network Newsletter* (April 1992) reported two studies that found decreased immune natural killer (NK) cell activity in FMS. These cells are our frontline warriors against outside attack. It seems that they are present in normal amounts in people with FMS, but they do little or nothing. So what gives?

Immune natural killer cells require serotonin to activate them. And serotonin is a nerve transmitter regulated in delta sleep, which is in short supply for people with FMS/MPS. When confronted by an "alien invader," our fibromite NK cells respond with "It's not my job."

> The thymus is a glandular structure that functions in the development of the immune system. I have found that if I take a thymus extract, which comes in pill form, it makes an important difference in my immune system's ability. Without the extract, I can expect at least one cold a month. With it, I may get one or two colds a year. The extract can be purchased at many health food stores.
>
> D.J.S.

21. Do you have delayed reactions when you are too active physically?

It is a common occurrence in FMS that when you overdo things, the reaction hits hardest the next day or even the day after that.

22. Do you get the shakes?

Perhaps you get the shakes when you are hungry, and they subside as soon as you eat. There is a certain type of hypoglycemia, or low blood sugar, that accompanies many cases of FMS. (See Chapter 24, on nutrition.) For some reason, fibromites don't show positive on the normal glucose tolerance test, which, for us, is useful only for ruling out diabetes (London 1994). If the blood sugar is low, normally the brain receives a signal from the hypothalamus that causes muscles in the stomach wall to contract, but the hypothalamus isn't working normally. With FMS, the adrenal glands appear to secrete a lot more adrenaline in response to blood sugar changes.

23. Do you bruise easily, and do your bruises take a long while to come out and a very long time to go away?

These symptoms may be due to constrictions in the myofascia, or to capillary fragility from medications, or to something else, as yet unknown.

I have found a subset of people who have FMS/MPS Complex exhibit these jumpy muscle symptoms, and are also very tall and thin. Perhaps for them the growth hormone isn't implicated in the same way as it is with other fibromites. These people seem to respond well to Klonopin.

Klonopin is an anticonvulsant which often has good results with teeth clenching, muscle twitching, restless legs and night-time muscle jerks (myoclonus) in cases of FMS and/or MPS. Note that this is true not just for the subset of tall thin people, but for any patient with FMS and/or MPS with these symptoms.

D.J.S.

24. Do you have jumpy muscles?

Your muscles may cause you to "jump" when you're nearly asleep. This is often found in combination with teeth grinding (bruxism) and restless legs (see Chapter 10, Sleep). These symptoms are common in both FMS and MPS.

25. Do your hands feel painful in cold water?

This may be due to peripheral vascular spasm, as it is in cases of Raynaud's phenomenon, but we don't really know why it occurs.

26. Have you experienced a recent weight gain or loss?

If you have experienced a recent weight gain, it may, in part, be due to the medications you have been taking. Elavil (amitriptyline), for example, has a tendency to give folks the munchies. Sometimes, your eating may be activated by a need to chew. Jaw grinding is a common symptom in FMS/MPS Complex. Carbohydrate craving is another common symptom. So it goes. There is also a subset of fibromites who lose weight and have to struggle to regain it. Many of these people are quite tall.

27. Are you very sensitive to light?

Light sensitivity can be a real problem. Some fibromites can't go anywhere unless they wear dark glasses. Others have Seasonal Affective Disorder (SAD) and need to experience certain amounts of daylight to prevent depression. In the winter they become very depressed when the amount of light dwindles. In FMS, part of this problem may be due to a connection between the hypothalamus and light sensitivity. (For more information, see Chapter 16, Coping Day to Day.)

Often, people with FMS have too little of the neurotransmitter, melatonin, which helps to regulate sleep. This lack may also be connected to light sensitivity. People with SAD have too much melatonin, and they don't always have the necessary night/day fluctuation of melatonin production. (See Chapter 19, Postive Change and Chapter 22, Enhancing Your Medications for more information about melatonin.)

28. Does the *noise* of fluorescent lights bother you?

The sound a fluorescent light makes can be more than irritating to fibromites. It can be positively disruptive in the workplace. We can get massive headaches or become terribly irritable because of this noise that others rarely notice. Also, the flickering of these lights as they wear out can be hazardous to our peace of mind. People on the Internet have reported varying responses ranging from very mild irritation and disquiet to near seizure and petit-mal-type fugue states.

29. Do some patterns (stripes, checks) make you dizzy?

Some people have reported becoming dizzy and vomiting from looking at patterns. It can cause dizziness to the point of falling over. These people have had to leave fabric stores and avoid using escalators because of it.

30. Do you have electromagnetic sensitivity?

Perhaps you become "wired" by electrical storms, are up all night when the moon is full, and seem to sense the feelings of others. This is part of your empathic connection that is called "electromagnetic sensitivity." Some people with FMS or FMS/MPS Complex appear to be very sensitive to electomagnetic transmissions, especially when they are experiencing a flare. They have reported stopped watches, computers, phones that come on, and VCRs that are affected, but they have been *afraid* to mention this to their doctors, which is unfortunate because this can be very important in terms of treatment (see Chapter 26, Bodyworkers). A Russian study on the skin's electromagnetic potential indicated that one-fourth of the people tested were electromagnetically sensitive, one-fourth were electromagnetically null, and the remaining half were considered "average."

It seems likely that most people with FMS and FMS/MPS Complex, at least those with extreme dysregulated neurotransmitter activity, are electromagnetically sensitive due to their enhanced autonomic nervous system activity, souped-up receptors, and so forth. (For more information, see Chapter 28, Alternatives: Other Cultures Other Ways.)

31. Do you experience numbness or tingling?

If electrolytic dysregulation occurs, that may contribute to the symptoms of numbness and tingling. For nerves to conduct sensations, ions such as potassium, chloride, and sodium (called electrolytes) must pass back and forth across the nerves' outer sheath. When a nerve is compressed, this transfer stops. When the pressure is released, the sudden movement causes pain and tingling. Numbness and tingling in referred pain zones are common symptoms with some TrPs.

32. Have you had any serious illnesses, surgeries, or physical traumas?

Illnesses such as diabetes, arthritis, and others, as well as surgeries and physical trauma, can be the original sources for perpetuating factors in FMS/MPS Complex. (See Chapter 7, Perpetuating Factors.)

> I believe that the dizziness caused by looking at patterns has to do with the TrPs in the internal eye muscles, and the fight that the eye has to make to attempt to accommodate the inaccurate and changing visual field.
>
> I have to be very careful when I'm around some kinds of fabric. I can't look at people who are wearing certain small check patterns or some stripes. This seems to go along with astigmatism. I must also make sure that I don't look at escalator steps. They are ridged, and the lines and movement are enough to drop me in my tracks. I imagine none of us would do well in a job with moving conveyor belts. (It could be dangerous.)
>
> D.J.S.

Section II: The Head Bone's Connected to the Neck Bone

1. Do you have motor coordination problems?

If you have motor coordination problems, that joker, the sternocleidomastoid (SCM) group of muscles, could be a part of your problem (see Figure 3-2). SCM trigger points occur in the neck and can cause any (or all) of the following problems: dizziness, imbalance, neck soreness, a swollen glands feeling, runny nose, maxillary sinus congestion, "tension" headaches, eye problems (tearing, "bug-eyes," blurred or double vision, inability to raise the upper eyelid, and a dimming of perceived light intensity), spatial disorientation, postural dizziness, vertigo, sudden falls while bending, staggering walk, impaired sleep, nerve impingement, and disturbed weight perception. This last symptom can result in spilling food and drink, and throwing an object across the room when you are just trying to pick it up. People with MPS may seem to have poltergeists. What we really have is disturbed weight perception.

If you have SCM TrPs, be careful how you move in bed. When you turn, roll your body with your head remaining flat on the bed, and use your arms to help. Don't lift your head and "lead with it" as you roll. That puts a great strain on your neck area and electrically "loads" the SCM TrPs, just as climbing steps or walking uphill "loads" the muscles of your thighs. This means that the electrical potential of your muscles is changed, and the change is not to your benefit. This also adds to the static and electromagnetic sensitivity that you experience.

2. Do you experience an unusual degree of clumsiness?

Many fibromites bump into doorjambs, walls, and other stationary objects, and knock things over often. If "klutziness" were an Olympic event, your closet might be filled with gold medals. (People with SCM TrPs would have to be barred from entering—they'd have an unfair advantage.) All of us with FMS and/or MPS go tripping through life, cleaning up one mess after another. We learn to keep our sense of humor activated and a good supply of absorbent paper towels handy. This clumsiness can be caused by a combination of internal eye muscle TrPs, gluteus minimus TrPs, FMS lack of optical accommodation, and SCM TrPs.

> My theory is that with muscle tightening, normal fluid passages become constricted, and fluid backs up in the sinuses, so we get a constant post-nasal drip all night long, although the membranes of the nose may feel very dry and even may bleed on occasion.
>
> D.J.S.

3. Do you have sinus stuffiness?

Sinus stuffiness might well be termed FMS/MPS Nocturnal Sinus Syndrome, although this is certainly not an official name; it has never been described elsewhere. The symptoms include a nighttime sinus stuffiness on one side, that *moves* to whichever side of your head is lowest. Gravity drains the congestion to the lower side. This condition goes along with post-nasal drip and, often, a constantly runny nose.

4. Do you frequently have a runny nose?

Almost all FM/MPS patients have this form of "vasomotor rhinitis." That's a runny nose without a bacteria or virus.

The side with the worst head and neck rigidity is often the side the person with FMS sleeps on most, and it is subjected to more of the drip . . . drip . . . drip . . . on the back of the throat, all night. (It's like water torture.) The SCM TrPs and the scaleni become tight in order to "splint" the sore throat and digastric TrPs. See Chapter 4 for an explanation as to how the myofascia hardens to splint a painful area, thus restricting movement and preventing more pain. (See also Figures 3-1, 3-2, and 8-1.)

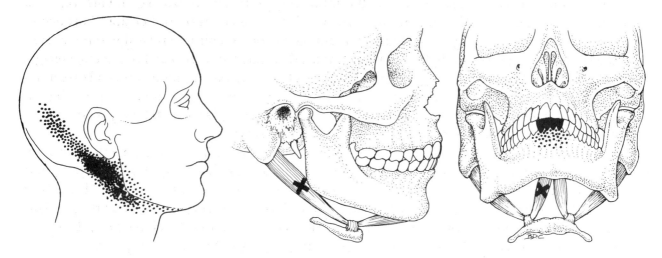

Figure 8-1: Trigger points in the right digastric; stippled and dark parts show areas of referred pain.

Using very warm saltwater for nose drops to clean off the throat and nasopharyngeal area before going to bed will prevent or at least minimize this difficulty without the need for any further medication. Just be careful. If you suspect the area is raw, don't use much salt or too high a temperature.

5. Do you have trouble swallowing?

If the post-nasal drip described in Question 4 above isn't treated, trouble with swallowing develops due to the presence of digastric TrPs. (See Figure 8-1.) This leads to head and neck pain, and a "swollen glands" feeling.

Warning—it hurts to work the digastric TrPs. Sometimes it's best to "milk" the area of its excess fluid, using a gentle downward motion from the base of the chin to the base of the throat. Start lightly and listen to your body. It will tell you how much pressure to use.

6. Do you have ear pain?

Medial pterygoid TrPs can cause deep ear pain and also stuffiness in the ear (see Figure 8-2). The sternal portion TrPs of the sternocleidomastoid muscle group can also cause deep ear pain (see Figure 3-2).

> When I go clothes shopping, I don't even look at anything unless it has pockets for handkerchiefs. I use cotton ones—the old-fashioned kind. They are easier on the nose and the pocketbook—if you can find them.
>
> D.J.S.

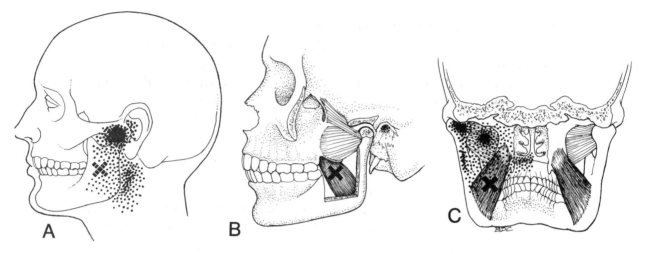

Figure 8-2: Trigger point in the left medial pterygoid (A) stippled parts show external areas of referred pain (B) location of the TrP is on the inner side of the mandible (C) looking forward, showing internal areas of pain.

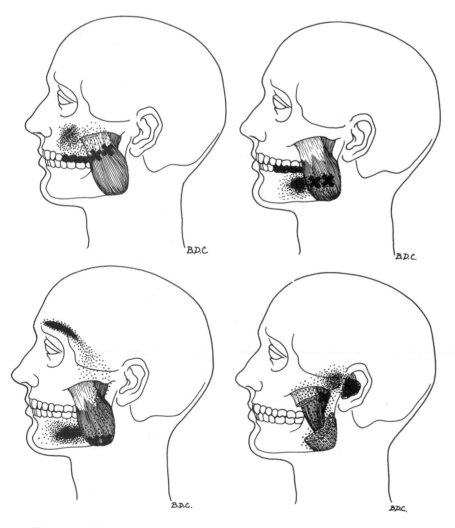

Figure 8-3: Trigger points located in various parts of the masseter

7. Do you experience ringing in the ears?

Deep masseter TrPs may cause a ringing or low roaring sound in the ears (see Figure 8-3). The sound may vary, you may experience a crackling noise, or the sound the phone makes when it's off the hook.

8. Do you have a chronic dry cough?

A chronic dry cough is often due to a TrP at the lower end of the sternal (breastbone) division of the SCM (see Figure 3-2). The sternocleidomastoid is not a muscle, but a muscle group. Trigger points in different areas of this muscle group cause different symptoms. To further complicate matters, a chronic dry cough can also be caused by esophageal reflux. (See Question 4 in Section III for an explanation of esophageal reflux.)

9. Do you have fluctuating blood pressure?

This is a symptom currently under study. There are several possible mechanisms involved. One possibility is mechanical. There are blood vessel swellings in your neck called the carotid sinuses. These sinuses, or cavities, in the blood vessels occur where the common carotid artery splits into two parts; one on each side of the neck. These sinuses are lined with pressure receptors that help to control the blood pressure by constricting and dilating the blood vessels. TrPs could affect them. Other physicians are looking at this from the biochemical angle, and we expect to see more research on this published within the next year.

10. Do you have dry eyes, nose, and mouth?

The symptoms of dry eyes, nose, and mouth are called *sicca syndrome,* which simply means that you have dry eyes, nose, and mouth. With FMS/MPS, all of the mucous membranes can become excessively dry, including the lining of the vagina and the gastrointestinal tract.

11. Do you have problems with swallowing and chewing?

Many people with FMS/MPS Complex have problems swallowing and experience the following symptoms: pain when chewing, jaw clicking, temporomandibular joint dysfunction (see Question 14 in this section), soreness inside the throat, excessive saliva secretion, and sinusitis-like pain. They may drool in their sleep and choke on saliva. All these symptoms can be caused by the internal medial pterygoid TrP, which is often overlooked in therapy (see Figure 8-2).

12. Do you have a prickling "electric" face?

The pain of a prickling, "electric" face is most often due to the platysma TrP. This TrP refers the prickling pain to the skin that covers the jaw. The platysma is a flat, sort of thin muscle over the throat area (see Figure 8-4).

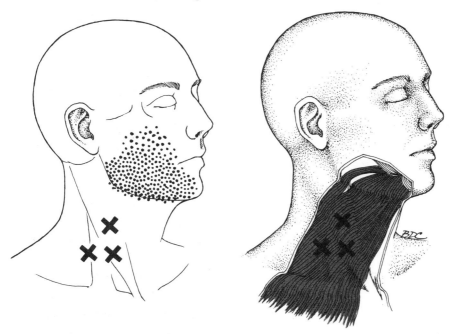

Figure 8-4: Trigger points in the platysma. The stippled area shows the prickling pain in the skin over the jaw.

13. Do you have red and/or tearing eyes?

Red and/or tearing eyes can be caused by TrPs in the SCM. (Hearing impairment and a disturbed sense of weight perception can also be caused by these TrPs.)

14. Do you experience popping or clicking of the jaw?

The symptoms of popping or clicking of the jaw are called temporomandibular joint dysfunction (TMJ). Jaw pain and dysfunction are usually

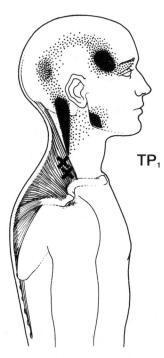

caused by the *masseter* TrP (see Figure 8-3), although the trapezius and temporalis TrPs are often involved, too. (See Figures 8-5 and 8-6.)

15. Do you have itchy ears?

The masseter TrP can also cause itchy ears (see Figure 8- 3). The itch, which can drive you to distraction, can be relieved by acupressure on the TrP.

16. Do you grind and clench your teeth?

You may find that you grind your teeth at night and clench them during the day. Teeth clenching is the brain's default mechanism. When the brain doesn't know what to do in response to the mixed or erratic signals that it often receives from the poorly regulated neurotransmitters and hypersensitive, and occasionally, dysfunctional receptors of those with FMS/MPS, it clenches the jaw. It's sort of a cerebral twiddling of the thumbs. The masseter TrP may be responsible for this symptom (see Figure 8-3).

Figure 8-5: Trigger points in the upper trapezius

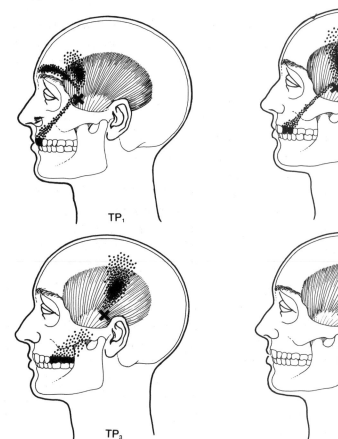

Figure 8-6: Trigger points in the temporalis; stippled and dark parts show referred pain patterns.

17. Do have unexplained toothaches?

If you have toothaches that cannot be explained, they may be caused by several TrPs, chiefly the digastric, masseter, and temporalis (see Figures 8-1, 8-3, and 8-6, respectively). Each TrP has its own particular toothache pattern. A TrP-induced toothache is usually intermittent. During a long dental procedure, which often activates these TrPs, you should take periodic rests to exercise and relieve your jaw muscles. Anterior digastric TrPs refer pain to the two front lower teeth, and can have you running to the dentist with no apparent cause.

18. Do you have eye pain?

Cutaneous (on the skin) facial TrPs can cause pain in the ears, eyes, nose, and teeth. These TrPs are shallow and can occur in many places on the face. Try some pressure-point work on your face. If the TrPs are there, they will let you know.

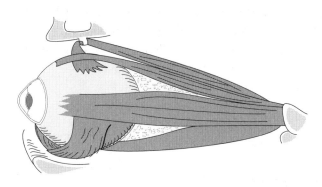

Figure 8-7: Trigger points can occur in any of these extrinsic eye muscles.

19. Do you have double vision, blurry vision, or changing vision?

For vision to be clear, both eyes must take the same picture at the same time. When this doesn't happen, vision problems result. One theory holds that a misalignment of the eyes may be caused by TrPs contracting the muscles that hold the eyeballs in place. If these muscles are being contracted at different amounts of tension, that could cause all the vision irregularities addressed in this question. Muscle fatigue makes things worse. The culprits may be TrPs in the extrinsic eye muscles (see Figure 8-7), or the SCM, trapezius, temporalis, or cutaneous (not shown) facial muscles (see Figures 3-2, 8-5, and 8-6, respectively; note that the cutaneous facial muscles are not shown).

To check your inner eye muscles, stretch them. Put one hand on your head, above your forehead. Then try to look at your hand. This shouldn't hurt. If it does, it's the TrPs in your muscles telling you that they are there. With your eyes still looking upward at your hand, look from one upper corner of your eye to the other. This will probably hurt too, which is a good sign because it signifies the presence of contraction and of possible TrPs. That means you need to stretch these muscles, and they could be causing all or some of your symptoms.

Splenius cervices TrPs can also cause blurring of near vision, as well as pain in the side of the head to the eye on same side, and in the eye orbit (see Figure 8-8).

20. Do you have dark specks that float in your vision?

This is a very common symptom for people with FMS/MPS Complex. We don't know why, but it may be

I have had Internet "patients" who have reported a 50-percent improvement of their vision from doing the eye exercises I suggested. I never knew this would happen, I just wanted the pain to ease, which it did. The vision improvement was a huge bonus.

D.J.S.

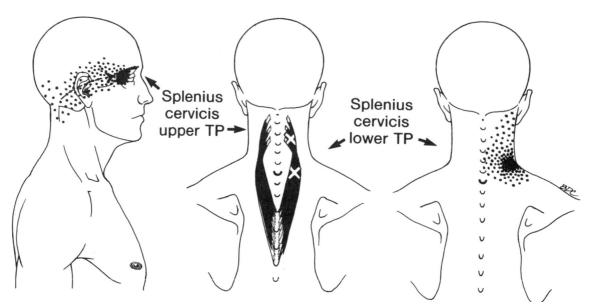

Figure 8-8: Trigger points in the upper and lower splenius cervici

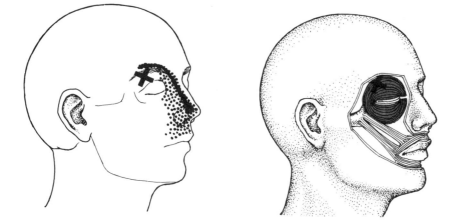

Figure 8-9: Trigger points in the orbicularis oculi

associated with the overgrowth or dysregulation of connective tissue growth, due to myofascial problems.

21. Do words jump off the page or disappear when you stare at them?

The orbicularis oculi TrPs (see Figure 8-9) will refer pain to your nose, cheek, and above your eye, and cause "jumpy pages" when you try to read. (Putting clear plastic over the page to decrease print contrast may help with this problem.)

22. Do you have frequent headaches?

TrPs in the sternocleidomastoid (SCM) are common causes of headaches. So, indirectly, are any of the causes of sore throat, for often a sore throat refers pain to the head. The posterior cervical TrP is also suspected of causing headaches if it entraps the occipital nerve (see Figure 8-10). This will cause a numbness, or a tingling, burning pain—like a band around head. Other posterior cervical TrPs can refer pain to the back of the neck down to the shoulder blade, and in

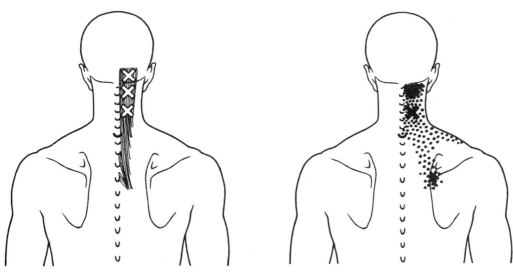

Figure 8-10: Trigger points in the posterior cervicals

the back of the skull on the involved side. These TrPs are often aggravated by reading or working at a desk with your neck bent over for a long time. Many upper body TrPs are implicated in headaches. (See Chapter 33, The Workplace.)

23. Do you experience migraines?

Migraines often occur due to constricted blood vessels inside the skull that suddenly expand. There is a strong correlation with food sensitivity, and with neurotransmitter imbalances. Serotonin regulates the constriction and dilation of blood vessels, and serotonin is regulated in delta-level sleep, which is frequently disturbed in people with FMS. The heralding or warning aura of visual disturbances that often precedes a migraine, which can include zigzag lines and flashes of light, occurs because the trigeminal nerve pathway involved runs very close to the reticular formation in the eyes (Xenakis 1993). The constant stimulation of both decreased blood flow and increased nerve involvement common in migraines causes the light show.

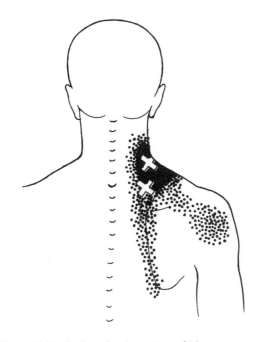

Figure 8-11: Referred pain pattern of trigger points in the right levator scapulae

The sternocleidmastoid (SCM) and the digastric, cutaneous facial, temporalis, trapezius, splenii, and posterior cervical, are all possible migraine-inducing TrPs. (See Figures 3-2, 8-1, 8-5, 8-6, 8-8, and 8-10, respectively.) Note that there is no illustration of the cutaneous facial trigger points.

24. Do you ever get a stiff neck?

Levator scapulae TrPs (see Figure 8-11) are the most common cause for a stiff neck, although

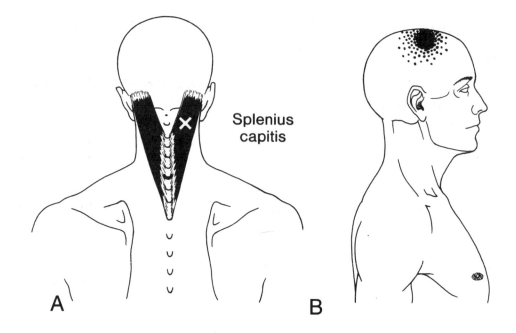

Figure 8-12: (A) Trigger point in the splenius capitus (B) referred pain on the crown of the head

this can also be caused by trapezius and posterior cervical TrPs (see Figures 8-5 and 8-10).

25. Do you experience dizziness when you turn your head or move?

Here's that busy sternocleidomastoid (SCM) muscle group again (see Figure 3-2). Active TrPs in this group can make heading into traffic miserable; you try to look both ways while holding your head in your hands to avoid dizziness. Or you can be stooping over to change the cat litter, and when you stand up, you can tumble right over—backwards.

It is important to keep your neck warm and away from drafts if you have an SCM TrP problem. If the TrPs are active (see Chapter 3, Trigger Points), it is a wise precaution to use a soft, triple-folded handtowel pinned as a splint or "chin rest" before riding over bumpy roads.

26. Do you have a sore spot on the top of your head?

This is often caused by the splenius capitis TrP (see Figure 8-12). With FMS/MPS Complex, just the motion of the wind on your hair can produce a tremendous soreness on the crown of your head.

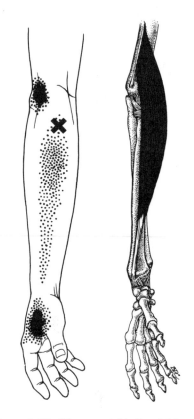

Figure 8-13: Trigger point in the right brachioradialis

Section III: The Shoulder Bone's Connected to the Back Bone

1. Do you experience extreme discomfort when you wear heavy clothing and/or discomfort or pain mid-shoulder when you carry a purse?

This is caused by the upper trapezius TrP (see Figure 8-5). The trapezius muscle is the most common muscle to get TrPs. It can get many TrPs, and each one has its own pain pattern or symptoms. One trapezius TrP, for example, can cause a queer shivery feeling with gooseflesh appearing on your arm or leg.

2. Do you have pain when you write, a changing signature, and/or illegible handwriting?

These problems can be most frustrating if you work with your hands and depend on them. Pain is caused by the lack of blood flow to the muscles, which causes severe disruption of handwriting skills. This can be due to many shoulder and arm TrPs. Thumb pain and tingling numbness are often due to brachialis entrapment of the radial nerve (see Figure 8-13) and adductor and opponens pollicis TrPs (see Figure 8-14).

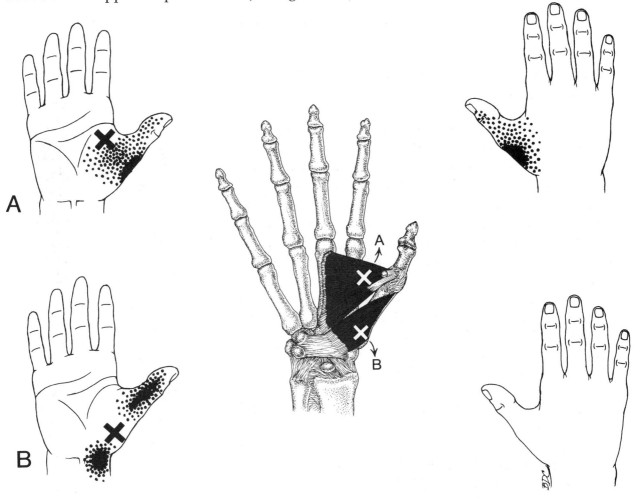

Figure 8-14: (A) Trigger point in the adductor pollicis (B) trigger point in the opponens pollicis

Adductor and opponens pollicis TrPs also can cause "trigger thumb," "weeder's thumb," clumsiness, and handwriting that is both painful and illegible. The brachioradialis is most often responsible for writer's cramp and for the weak grip that allows objects to slip out of your hand or causes spills from a cup when you're trying to drink something, and you end up wearing it instead.

> Writing a book can be frustrating when you are limited to 20-minute segments, broken up by physical therapy so that you can do another 20-minute segment. The use of "Hand-eze" supports makes it possible for me to write at all.
>
> D.J.S.

3. Do your fingers turn color with the cold?

If your fingers and/or toes turn red, then white, and then a bluish color when the weather outside is icy, ask your physician to investigate Raynaud's phenomenon, a peripheral vascular condition, common in FMS. This condition is caused by spasms of the blood vessels in response to cold—or stress.

4. Do you have esophageal reflux?

Reflux means a backwards flow, which is exactly what happens to the contents of the stomach in this condition. It starts with just the stomach gases—hydrochloric acid fumes—which can cause severe heartburn, sore throat, and TrPs. The next phase of this process involves the stomach juices. If you lean over, or strain at a bowel movement, or put pressure on the stomach, in any way, some of the fluid—also highly acidic—comes up to burn your esophagus and throat. The next stage, vomiting, occurs with the same actions. Sometimes, even lying down after a big meal can cause vomiting. There are many over-the-counter medications now available for reflux. Reflux perpetuates TrPs.

This is a thoroughly irritating condition. It often starts as simple heartburn after you eat. Back pressure from the stomach opens the muscular valve between the top of the stomach and the bottom of the esophagus, which is called the cardiac sphincter. The acidic gas from the stomach begins to irritate the end of the esophagus, causing heartburn. If this continues, stomach gases are burped up, which are damaging to delicate throat tissues. You then might get a sore throat which might give you a headache. Bending over or lying down often adds just enough gravitational pressure to cause reflux. In severe form, the actual stomach contents are regurgitated.

> Before I started on guaifenesin (see Chapter 23), I would vomit or come close to vomiting every time I bent over. It made gardening, one of my favorite activities, very difficult. Eventually, it was happening even when I was taking medicine for reflux.
>
> D.J.S.

A hiatal hernia adds to the pressure, as does obesity. More than 30 percent of people with FMS have a hiatal hernia.

Overeating, some medications, certain foods, and heavy drinking will aggravate reflux. Raising the head of your bed about six inches may help. Limiting coffee (regular or decaf), and other caffeine-containing liquids, stopping bedtime snacks, quitting smoking, avoiding certain foods such as chocolate and fried foods also helps, as does avoiding peppermint, spearmint, and onions (one exception to this rule is enteric-coated peppermint). If a food makes you belch, it probably can give you

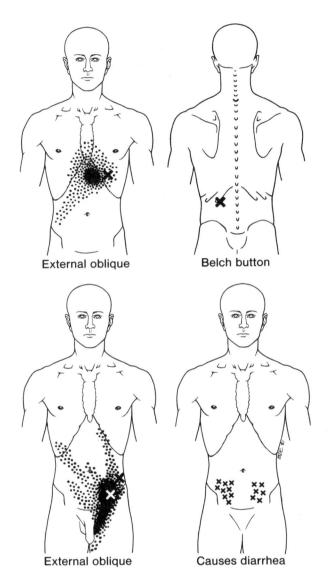

External oblique   Belch button

External oblique   Causes diarrhea

Figure 8-15: Trigger points for the external oblique (heartburn), lower quadrant oblique, "belch button," and abdominal muscles; stippled and dark areas show referred pain pattern.

heartburn. Avoid eating too fast, chew carefully, and eat small portions. The external oblique muscle TrP often aggravates reflux (see Figure 8-15).

5. Do you experience shortness of breath?

This symptom, often due to TrPs in the serratus anterior muscle, is commonly identified as a "stitch" in the side (see Figure 8-16). This TrP can contribute substantially to the pain of a heart attack. It can also cause a "catch" in the lower inner side of the shoulder blade. The pectorals are often involved as well. There is a reduced tidal volume in the lung due to restricted chest expansion, which means that less air is taken into the lung because the breath is shallower.

6. Do you have hypersensitive nipples and/or breast pain?

This is commonly due to TrPs in the pectoralis muscles (see Figure 8-17). Many of us have latent pectorals and sternalis (see Figure 8-18) TrPs. You can do "doorway stretches" to help these points (see Chapter 27, Bodywork You Can Do Yourself).

7. Do you have a "frozen shoulder"?

Subscapularis TrPs (see Figure 6-1) can cause what is termed "frozen shoulder." This TrP severely restricts rotation movement of the arm at shoulder level. Hanging curtains, folding sheets, throwing a ball overhand, raising an arm at school to answer a question—these things are out of the question. Driving long distances aggravates this TrP, as does anything that causes your arms to remain in a shortened position. The in-doorway stretch (see Chapter 27, Bodywork You Can Do Yourself) is good for this TrP, and for the pectorals TrPs.

8. Do you have a painful, weak grasp that sometimes just lets go?

This is the result of infraspinatus (see Figure 8-19), scaleni (see Figure 3-1), hand extensors (not shown), and brachioradialis TrPs (see Figure 8-13). The pain felt when turning a door knob

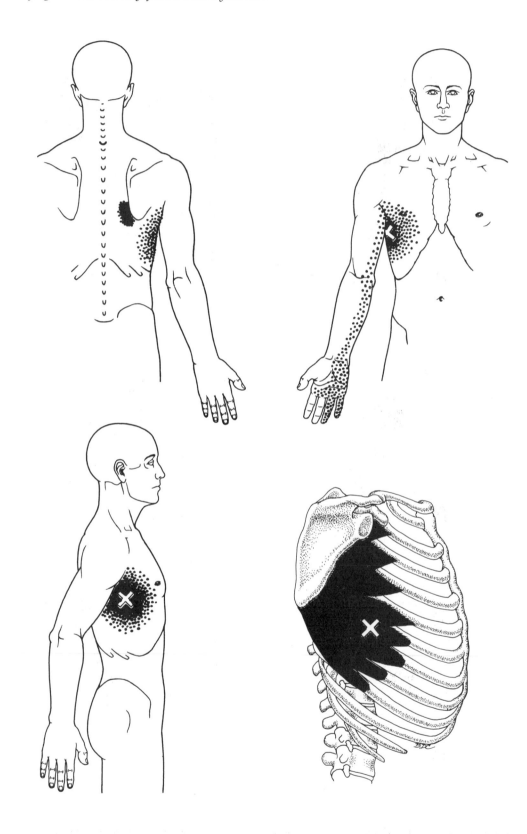

Figure 8-16: Trigger points in the serratus anterior; stippled areas show the referred pain patterns.

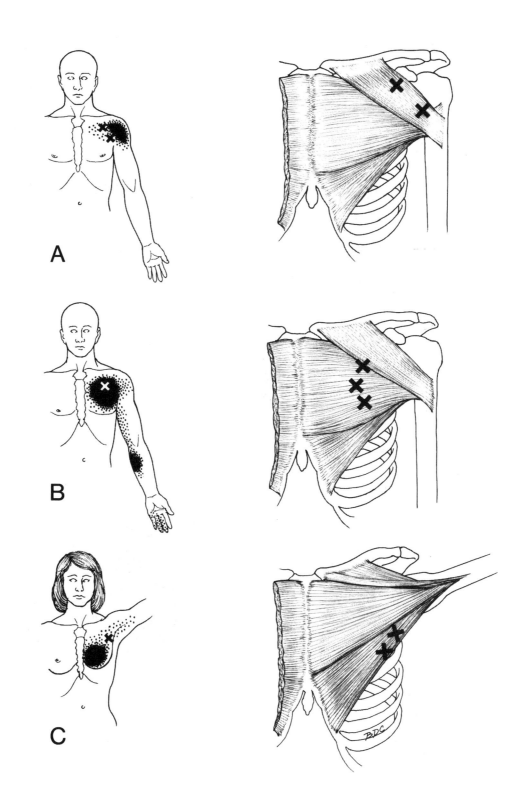

Figure 8-17: Trigger points in the left pectoralis major (A) the clavicular section, (B) the intermediate sternal section, (C) the lateral free margin of the muscle

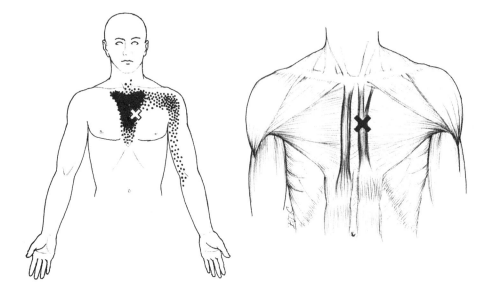

Figure 8-18: Trigger point in the left sternalis; stippled and dark areas show referred pain patterns.

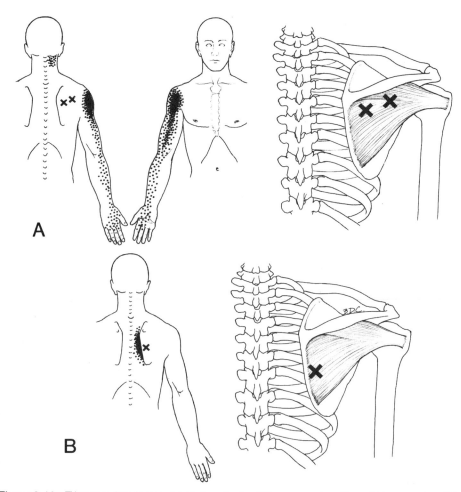

Figure 8-19: Trigger points in the right infraspinatus (A) common location of trigger points (B) a more unusual location for a trigger point

or using a screwdriver can be intense if you have these TrPs. You may also experience extreme weakness in your hands. Loss of control when drinking, pouring liquids, and so forth is common. People with FMS and/or FMS/MPS Complex really have a "drinking problem"—there are days when you'll just have to rely on straws to get liquids to your mouth.

Trigger points in the scalene muscles (see Figure 3-1) also can cause hands to drop objects, numbness, or tingling (usually in the little finger and the finger next to it), and hand swelling (noticeable when wearing rings). This muscle group causes compression of arteries and sensory nerves, shoulder pain, and pain in the upper half of the arms. It is also responsible for sleep disturbance and ulnar and median nerve numbness, and, in addition, can entrap some of the spinal nerves in the neck.

9. Do you have chest tightness?

This is usually due to the pectoral TrPs (see Figure 8-17). Often these will pull down the sternocleidomastoid (SCM) muscle group and work to perpetuate TrPs there. If involved, the pectorals' TrPs must be treated before the SCM TrPs can be successfully treated.

10. Do you have a hiatal hernia?

This is a protrusion of the stomach upward through the diaphragm in the space where the esophagus goes through. Symptoms of a hiatal hernia are reflux (see Question 4 in Section III for a discussion of reflux) and heartburn. The abdominal oblique TrP (see Figure 8-15) can produce a "stitch" in the side and hiatal hernia symptoms.

11. Do you experience heart attack-like pains, rapid heartbeat, and/or a fluttery heartbeat?

This alarming set of symptoms can be caused by pectoral and sternalis TrPs (see Figures 8-17 and 8-18). Trigger point pain following recovery from a heart attack can often be eased by using a vapocoolant spray, such as Fluori-Methane (Travell and Simons 1983; Travell 1968). (See Chapter 21, Fibromyalgia/Myofascial Pain Syndrome Medications.)

12. Do you have mitral valve prolapse?

As mentioned in Chapter 6, Coexisting Conditions, this valve in the heart consists of connective tissue. When connective tissue loses its elasticity, the valve doesn't flex as it should, and thus doesn't fit as it should. This allows some of the blood to flow backward in the heart. This is not a desirable condition.

13. Do you have intestinal cramps, bloating, etc.?

Active TrPs in the abdominal muscles may cause a lax, pendulous abdomen filled with gas. The gut can't be

When I was a child, we had a piece of playground equipment at school that was potentially very dangerous. (It's probably not used anymore.) It was a metal pole with a movable circle of rings at the top. Chains were suspended from each ring, and each chain had a handle. The object was for each child to grab a handle and run in one direction, around and around the pole.

When we built up sufficient speed, we'd lift our feet off the ground and "fly" around the ring, holding on to the moving chains. It was like the centrifugal motion rides at amusement parks, only scaled down. But we wanted more. So one of us would walk around the others, wrapping one chain around all the others' chains, so that when everyone began to run, this child would "fly" higher, over the other kids' heads, still gripping the handle. At that point in time, I already had trigger points. When it was my turn to whip around, my hands couldn't hold on, and I quite literally flew. I landed on my back some distance from the pole, and scared several teachers quite badly. I was flat on my back for more than half an hour.

Kids with TrPs that affect their grasp are at real risk of "losing their grip," and maybe their lives, in gymnastics and other sports.

When I was older, I attempted a flying dislocate from the high bar. Again, I really flew, and I landed on my back on the mat. (Perhaps I was a bird in a former life.)

As an adult, I found it impossible to maintain a grip to water ski. At least now I know why. Nowadays, the big crises in my house occur when my hands don't work well enough to open the cat-food cans; I no longer risk life and limb on questionable gymnastic feats.

D.J.S.

pulled in because the TrPs inhibit contraction. A fat pad forms right over the abdomen. This fat pad is hard to get rid of, due to the TrPs. The first thing to do is to find and eliminate the back muscle TrPs that refer pain to the abdomen. These can cause burning, fullness, bloating, and swelling. Only then can you hope to eliminate the abdominal muscle TrPs in the gut.

14. Do you experience nausea?

The abdominal TrPs and multifidi TrPs (see Figure 8-20) can cause severe nausea. Vomiting can be caused by the upper rectus abdominis TrPs (not shown).

15. Do you experience appendicitis-like pains?

This is another symptom that can have you running to a hospital's emergency department. It can be caused by TrPs in the iliopsoas (see Figure 7-1), rectus abdominis (not shown), piriformis (see Figure 7-2), or iliocostalis (see Figure 8-21) muscle groups. There is one TrP that forms right at McBurney's point (see Figure 8-22), which can cause pseudo-appendicitis or can refer pain to the pelvis or to the penis.

Note that pain caused by TrPs in the iliopsoas (see Figure 7-1) muscle may seem like appendicitis, but it often radiates down the leg.

16. Do you have an irritable bladder and/or bowel?

This can be due to the pyramidalis (not shown), multifidi (see Figure 8-20), and abdominal TrPs (see Figure 8-15), as well as to yeast overgrowth in the gastrointestinal tract. Trigger points in the upper rim of the pubis appear to add to the irritability and spasming of the genital-urinary tract. This is as least part of the reason why so many of us have to urinate so often. With FMS/MPS Complex, not only is the bladder hypersensitive, it won't hold as much. In addition, we can't empty our bladders totally. Below normal electrical activity in the muscles of the gut, common in FMS, can lead to constipation and intestinal cramps, as well.

There are specific TrPs that may cause or intensify diarrhea, nausea, vomiting, food intolerance, colic, burping and/or painful menstrual periods. (See Figure 8-15 for the external oblique, lower quadrant oblique, "belch button," and abdominal TrPs.) (For more information see Chapter 11, Irritable Bowel Syndrome.)

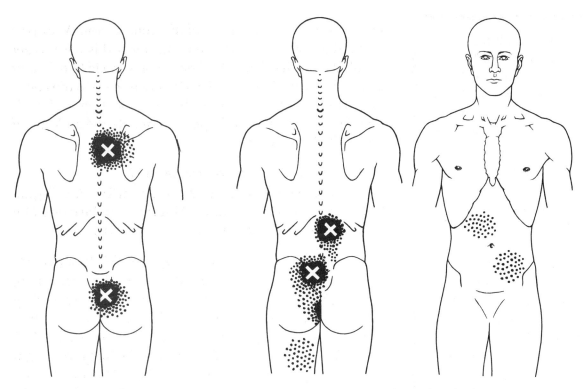

Figure 8-20: Trigger points in some of the multifidi; stippled and dark areas show referred pain patterns.

17. Do you have burning or foul-smelling urine?

This is a fairly common symptom for people with FMS and can intensify with MPS. It also occurs with guaifenesin treatment (see Chapter 23, Guaifenensin). This symptom can mimic a true urinary infection.

18. Do you experience pain with intercourse?

This symptom may be caused by vaginal TrPs (not shown) and pelvic floor TrPs (not shown). In addition, abdominal and low-back TrPs may be the cause of aching discomfort and cramps during sex. Where there is sharp pain, the culprit may be the piriformis TrP (see Figure 7-2) with pudendal nerve entrapment. (For more about this, see Chapter 30, The Home Front.)

19. Do you have menstrual problems such as severe cramping, delayed periods, irregular periods, long periods with a great deal of bleeding, late periods, missed periods, membranous flow, and/or blood clots?

Some of these problems can be caused by coccygeus (not shown), iliocostalis (see Figure 8-21), rectus abdominis (not shown), pyramidalis (not shown), and other pelvic and vaginal TrPs, as well as the adductor magnus (not shown). There may also be thick secretions to deal with, and a lot of hormone problems. (These hormone problems are due to faulty neurotransmitter functioning, which is common among people with FMS.)

20. Do you experience impotence?

This problem can be created by piriformis entrapment of the pudendal nerve. Piriformis TrPs can also create sciatic radiating pain, lumbago, and low-back pain. Pain from the entrapped

There is a theory that people with FMS/MPS Complex can lose bladder elasticity as the myofascia in the bladder area tightens. This loss of elasticity is also a common occurrence even in healthy people as they age. Often, in cases of irritable bladder and bowel, the lower internal oblique muscle TrPs (not shown) and possibly the lower rectus abdominus TrPs (not shown) are involved.

D.J.S.

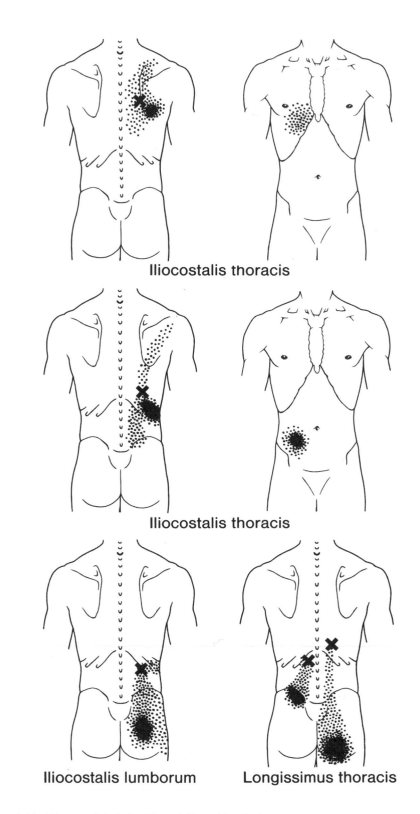

Iliocostalis thoracis

Iliocostalis thoracis

Iliocostalis lumborum   Longissimus thoracis

Figure 8-21: Trigger points in the iliocostalis and longissimus

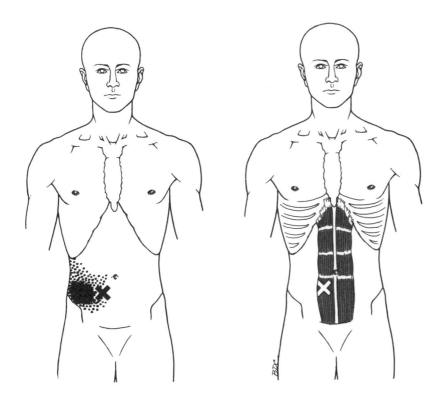

Figure 8-22: McBurney's point

nerve may extend down to the sole of foot. Blood vessels may also be entrapped by this small but very busy muscle.

21. Do you have low-back pain?

This is a tiger with many claws. The quadratus lumborum TrP (not shown) is usually the main claw. It causes pain when walking, when turning in bed, when getting up from a chair, and when coughing or sneezing. It (along with the iliopsoas; see Figure 7-1) is often the cause of "failed low-back postsurgical syndrome"(Travell and Simons 1992). You can get a deep "lightning bolt" pain from the quadratus lumborum to the front of the thigh. Pain may extend to the groin, testes, scrotum, or down the leg like sciatica pain.

If this tiger gets its main claw in your back, you may feel a heaviness in your hips, a cramping of your calves, and burning sensations in your legs and feet. This can cause TrPs in those areas, which then become additional claws for the tiger. Sleeping conditions can affect the quadratus lumborum very strongly. (For more information see Chapter 7, Perpetuating Factors, and Chapter 10, Sleep.)

Section IV: The Hip Bone's Connected to the Leg Bone

1. Do you have sciatica?

This throbbing ache can feel like a "toothache" festering in the hip. There are a lot of muscles in the hip, and it's hard to be sure you have found the precise culprit. Often the TrPs work as a team, egging each other on. The thoracolumbar paraspinals, (not shown) gluteus minimus (see Figure 8-23), hamstrings (see Figure 8-24), piriformis (see Figure 7-2), and iliopsoas (see Figure 7-1) TrPs are often the villains of sciatic pain. The other gluteals are also often involved.

Using pillows under your knees during the night, if you sleep on your back, or between your knees, if you sleep on your side, will prevent overextension of the hip muscles.

2. Do you have weak ankles?

The peroneus (see Figure 8-25) and tibialis (see Figure 8-26) TrPs are the most common TrPs that can cause the ankle to buckle outward, often causing soft-tissue damage and even falls. The problem can begin with some kind of trauma, such as immobilization of the leg in a cast, or with variations of foot structure, such as in Morton's foot (see Figure 7-6). The inner ankle pain is usually due to the tibialis TrP.

3. Do you get shin splints?

The same TrPs that cause weak ankles are responsible for the sharp pain you get when you kneel or get up from kneeling. The pain travels like electricity up your lower leg. Sometimes this pain can be avoided if you make sure your feet stay at right angles to your legs, that is, your

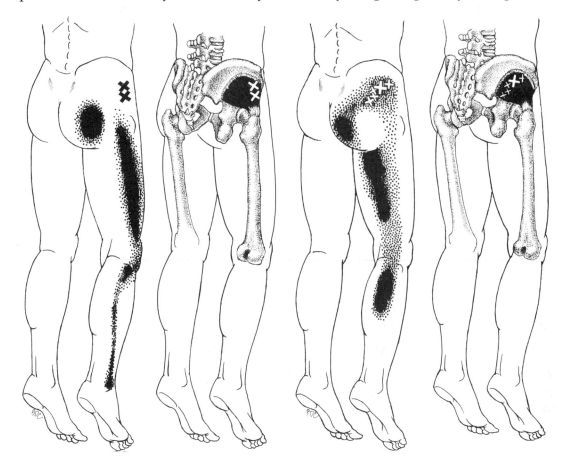

Figure 8-23: Trigger points in the gluteus minimus; stippled and dark areas show referred pain patterns.

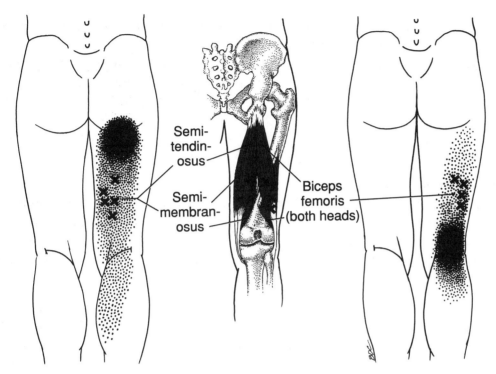

Figure 8-24: Trigger points in the hamstrings; stippled and dark areas show referred pain patterns.

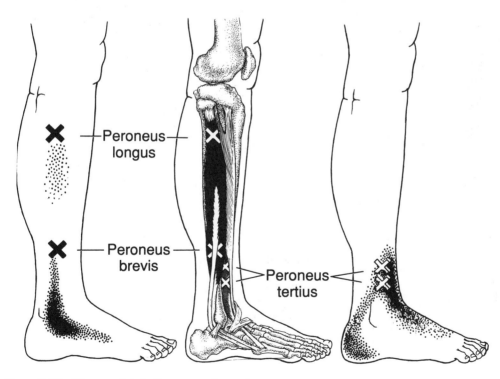

Figure 8-25: Trigger points in the peroneal muscles

toes stay bent while kneeling and the top of your foot is not touching the floor. If your muscles are rigid, it can be difficult to feel the peroneal and tibialis TrPs. (See Figures 8-25 and 8-26.)

4. Do you "stumble over your own feet"?

The tibialis TrP (see Figure 8-26) is often responsible for what is called "foot slap" and "foot drop." This is the loss of foot clearance when one takes a step. The brain doesn't receive the proper feedback signals from the body that tell it how high to raise the foot in order to clear the ground. The tibialis TrP can also cause big toe pain.

5. Do you have upper/lower leg cramps?

Trigger points in the sartorius muscle (see Figure 8-27) are mostly responsible for upper leg cramps, and TrPs in the gastrocnemius muscle (see Figure 8-28) are usually the culprits in calf cramps. Note, however, that these cramps can be caused by other problems, as well. For example, dehydration, electrolytic imbalance, and heat stress can all cause calf cramps. Also some drugs, such as lithium or cimetidine, can cause leg cramping.

There is a muscle "pump" in the legs, the soleus muscle (see Figure 8-29); it helps the heart by returning blood from the lower legs. This soleus pump "sleeps" when you do, which contributes to pooling of blood in the lower legs and to circulatory insufficiency in the calf muscles.

Myofascia from the gastrocnemius and soleus (see Figures 8-28 and 8-29) muscles join to form the Achilles tendon. Large cavities in the deep veins beneath the soleus, the tough fascia, and the veins above the soleus form an "effective musculovenous pump that serves as a 'second heart'" (Travell and Simons 1992). The soleus muscle acts as a pump and helps the heart by returning blood from the lower legs. This "pump" "sleeps" when we are sleeping, which contributes to blood pooling in the lower legs and to circulatory insufficiency in the calf muscles. This is one reason that calf cramps often occur when we lie down, or when we first arise from sleep. When there are TrPs in the soleus muscle, this problem becomes more common (Travell and Simons 1992).

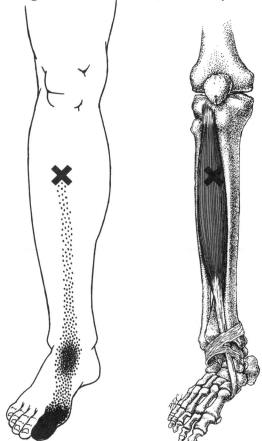

Note: Soleus TrPs usually cause referred heel pain and tenderness, but there is one most unusual pain pattern that refers pain from the soleus to the jaw. Travell and Simons (1992) mention that they have seen this twice. In one occurrence of this pattern, the patient had jaw pain but no typical jaw TrPs, and had been tooth grinding at night. There was no leg pain, but when the soleus TrP was touched, the jaw pain was activated. It isn't clear why this connection exists, but, in this case, at least, "the leg bone's connected to the jaw bone" to paraphrase the old song.

Figure 8-26: Trigger points in the tibialis

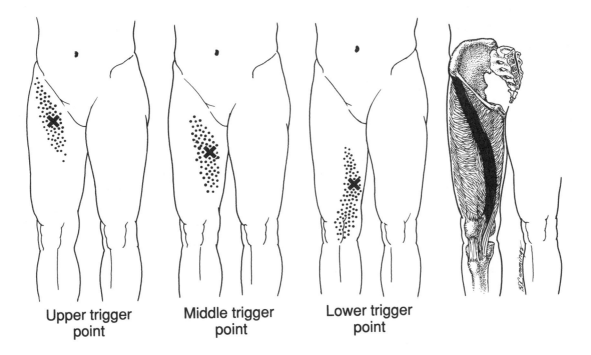

Figure 8-27: Trigger points in the sartorius; stippled areas show referred pain patterns.

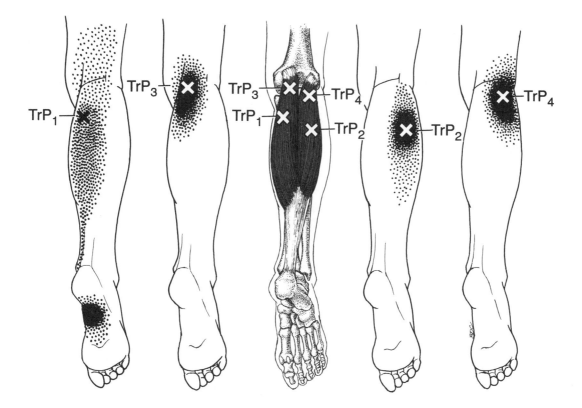

Figure 8-28: Trigger points in the gastrocnemius muscle; stippled and dark areas show referred pain patterns.

Most people are unaware that the soleus is so important to good circulation. Military professionals, however, learn that if they alternately tense and relax their lower legs while standing at attention for any length of time, they will avoid fainting. (Cadets often learn this the hard way.)

The central nervous system also plays a role in nocturnal cramps by dictating the dilation of the blood vessels. Even TrP-induced cramps are worsened by impaired circulation. With these TrPs, there is difficulty in walking fast or on uneven ground. Vitamin C may help (Travell and Simons 1992).

At night, placing a firm pillow or blanket roll under your feet to keep them in a neutral position may help. (Do not point your toes, as in ballet; keep your feet at right angles to your legs.) When you make the bed, try tucking in the bottom end of the cover sheet very loosely, to allow room for your feet. Don't ever sacrifice function for packaging. Your feet will become riddled with TrPs.

6. Do you experience muscle cramps and twitches elsewhere?

Check the trigger point charts for a pain referral pattern that is in the area of the cramp or twitch. Then, find the location of a TrP affecting that area. Check your body to see if a TrP is causing the cramp or twitch. Muscles function in groups, but the TrPs must be treated one at a time. Ordinary muscle cramps are caused by overstimulation of a muscle by nerves, unlike spasms, which are caused by a chemical imbalance in the muscle.

7. Do you have a buckling knee?

This "falling failing" is often due to a combination of vastus medialis and quadriceps TrPs (see Figure 8-30), and adductor longus TrPs (see Figure 8-31). This can arrive as a secondary symptom to abdominal congestion and pelvic pain, often during the menstrual period. The knee will ache, frequently on the inner side, and then it will "give out," especially when walking over rough ground.

Phantom limb pain can be induced by residual (meaning "left over" from before amputation) muscles in the thigh (Travell and Simons 1992). When treating these TrPs, it is important to treat the hamstrings also, as they are usually tight because of deep TrPs (see Figure 8-24). Avoid prolonged immobility, which will worsen the buckling knee. A buckling knee from a vastus medialis TrP seems to result when the quadriceps is con-

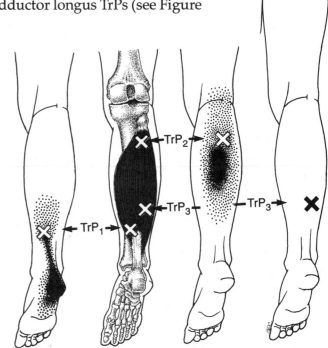

Figure 8-29: Trigger points in the soleus

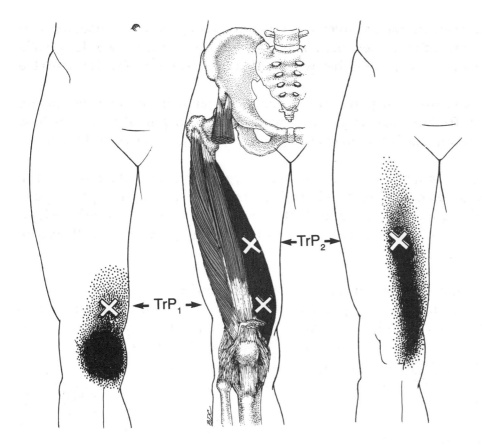

Figure 8-30: Trigger points in the vastus medialis and quadriceps

stricted by TrPs and can't do its job. The vastus medialis muscle tries to take up the slack, until it can no longer cope (see Figure 8-30).

8. Do you have difficulty climbing stairs?

This can be due to sartorius (see Figure 8-27), quadriceps femoris (see Figure 8-32), and/or vastus medialis (see Figure 8-30) TrPs. The first two muscles ache in the thigh. The vastus medialis usually causes pain in the knee. One way to avoid aggravating these TrPs is to climb steps with your feet and body held at a 45-degree angle to the steps. Don't face them head on.

Trigger points in the thoracolumbar paraspinals (not shown) can also cause difficulty walking up stairs. They produce a form of sciatica that is aggravated by prolonged immobi-

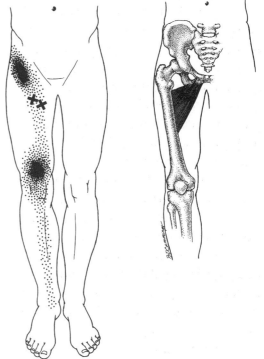

Figure 8-31: Trigger points in the adductor longus; stippled and dark areas show referred pain patterns.

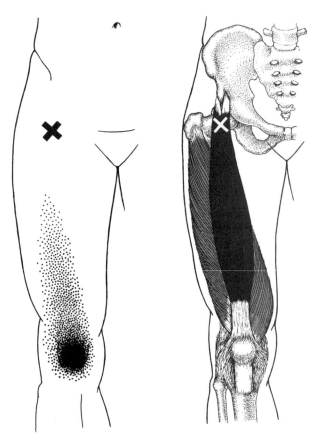

Figure 8-32: Trigger point in the quadriceps femoris

lity—for example, during and after airplane or auto trips, sitting at a computer, or sitting during long meetings without moving around.

9. Do you have foot pain?

This can come from a variety of causes. Heel pain is often caused by TrPs in the soleus (see Figure 8-29). The soleus muscle is an important one.

Frequently, people are treated surgically for a heel spur. There may be a heel spur on the other heel, too, but it gives the patient no problem, and is usually ignored. After the painful heel spur is removed, however, the pain often remains, because the TrP, which is the actual cause of the heel pain, has not been treated. The pain remains until the TrP is defused and the perpetuating factors are remedied.

Pain in the sole of your foot when running or walking can also be caused by TrPs in the tibialis posterior (not shown), although the intrinsic foot muscles are also implicated in sole pain. Pain from the tibialis posterior is usually most severe in the arch of the foot, but it can also occur in the heel, toes, and calf.

Tibialis posterior weakness causes severe pronation. *Pronation* means that when you stand, your feet point out at an angle rather than straight ahead. The pronation is a symptom, not the cause, of the TrP. Too often, expensive orthotics (inserts) are placed inside the shoes to correct pronation, and the cause of the pronation is overlooked.

10. Do you have feet that are wide in front and narrow in the back, with a high arch?

We call this the "FMS/MPS foot," for want of a better term. The great toe is often slanted in toward the little toe, and the space between the big toe and the second toe is wide. This is a perpetuating factor of foot and leg TrPs, as is Morton's foot, another foot shape variant. Morton's foot has a second toe longer than the big toe, with a wide web between the second and third toes (see Figure 7-6). These conditions, along with Morton's neuroma, are discussed in Chapter 7, Perpetuating Factors.

11. Do you have tight hamstrings?

If back pain is a tiger, then the hamstrings are an enraged pit bull. The hamstring complex (see Figure 8-24), adductor magnus (not shown), quadriceps femoris (see Figure 8-32), iliopsoas (see Figure 7-1), and gastrocnemius (see Figure 8-28) are often involved with TrPs. Defusing the

TrPs in this area is a very complex procedure. As with many areas of thick musculature, there is one layer of muscle after another, crossing over each other, and layers of TrPs.

12. Do you experience strange sensations—numbness, hypersensitivity, "running water," "ants crawling under your skin," and so forth, on the outer thigh area?

This condition is called *meralgia paresthetica*. It occurs because of a very large, superficial nerve on the outer thigh, called the lateral femoral cutaneous nerve. This nerve can be entrapped by several muscles as it leaves the pelvic area—the quadriceps femoris (see Figure 8-32), vastus lateralis (not shown), sartorius (see Figure 8-27), and tensor fascia latae (not shown).

Meralgia paresthetica is often associated with a lax, pendulous abdominal wall. As noted in Section III, Question 13, above, the lax, pendulous abdomen is often caused by TrPs.

13. Do you experience burning or redness on the inner thigh?

This is another TrP in a muscle that very few people are familiar with. (It is mind-boggling how little we know about our own bodies, until they start malfunctioning.)

The gracilis muscle TrP (not shown) causes a superficial hot, stinging pain in the middle thigh, and no change of position reduces the pain. Walking tends to relieve it, but one of our local support group members found that taking long walks actually caused the pain.

14. Do you have restless leg syndrome?

This is the name used to describe a constantly moving leg. The movement can happen just at night, when the jiggling will drive your spouse or "significant other" up the wall, and/or it can occur during the day, when it will drive just about everyone else up the wall. It can be caused by TrPs in the gastrocnemius or soleus muscles. (See Figures 8-28 and 8-29).

15. Do you have a staggering walk and balance problems?

If caused by MPS, these symptoms are usually due to sternocleidomastoid (SCM) (see Figure 3-2) and/or gluteus minimus (see Figure 8-23) TrPs. The use of flexible shoes with good support will aid in controlling some of the balancing problem.

16. Do your first steps in the morning feel as if you are walking on nails?

This can also happen after a meal or at other times when you stand up after sitting for a while. In Travell and Simons' Trigger Point Manual, Volume II, this condition is listed (in Chapter 22) as commonly occurring with flat feet, but it also occurs with cases of the wedge-shaped FMS/MPS foot, which is characterized by high arches as well. The condition occurs as the foot first flattens during the stride, due to the weight of body.

When the plantar fascia (fascial tissue on the bottom of the feet) stretches more than it should, it starts to contract whenever you are off your feet for any length of time. It sometimes shortens to the point that walking can become very painful. This condition is usually caused by TrPs in the long flexor muscles of the toes. These TrPs are to be found in the calf area, not the foot itself. Morton's foot or any other foot deformity that causes *hyperpronation* (walking with toes pointing further out than normal) can become perpetuating factors for these TrPs.

Check your calf, toward the inner side of the knee and about a handsbreadth down from the knee. The TrP pain will radiate down the calf over the ankle and to the underside of the foot. Toe cramps can be caused by intrinsic flexors in the foot itself.

17. Do others in your family have these symptoms?

FMS runs in families. It isn't uncommon to have several generations in a family represented at a support meeting, or many members of one family with FMS. People with FMS seem to be born with the tendency to develop it (Pelligrino 1989).

In Conclusion

The signs and symptoms described in this chapter are by no means all of the possible symptoms associated with FMS and / or the FMS / MPS Complex. There are many more trigger points than have been shown. You have your own story to tell and your own pieces of the puzzle to add to the growing body of information. You just need to find doctors who will listen. (See Chapter 37, Finding Your Primary Care Physician.)

PART III

INTERNAL AFFAIRS

CHAPTER 9

Chronic Pain States:
A Different Animal

Pain is a personal and an emotional issue. No one else can know how much you hurt and how overwhelming it can be as pain seeps through the tiniest cracks in your support structure, threatening your stability, your health, and sometimes your life itself.

It has been established that pain itself can suppress the immune system and can encourage the growth of some forms of cancer. Pain alone can also affect blood pressure.

This book offers many ways to help you cope with the chronic pain of FMS and FMS/MPS Complex. In this chapter, the focus is on the doctor/patient relationship when pain is treated with medications. (See also Chapter 22, Enhancing Your Medications.)

Chronic Pain States

Chronic pain states are quite different from acute pain states. When you know the pain is eventually going to end and that you will recover and the pain will be gone, it is easier to tolerate the misery. Hope helps you to carry the burdens.

Endorphins and Pain

Normally, physical and emotional trauma releases the body's own painkillers—the endorphins. These are produced in response to orders from the hypothalamus and the pituitary, as well to as one type of "gray matter" in the nervous system. These glands, with the adrenals, form the HPA axis (see Chapter 14 for a description of the HPA axis), the functioning of which is disrupted in FMS. When the "fight or flight" stress response is triggered by acute pain, endorphins flood the body, dampening the pain to allow the body to respond to the threat.

You may have read about injured people at an accident site who performed physical actions that should have been impossible, because of their severe pain. This is due, in part, to endorphins. *Chronic pain does not provoke this kind of response.* After a time, less endorphins are produced to counter the same amount of pain. The body cannot remain in a "fight or flight" mode for long without exhaustion.

Endorphins, along with ACTH—a hormone secreted by the adrenal glands—bind themselves to nerve cell receptors, just as narcotics do. This not only changes the way you feel pain, it changes the way you *feel about* the pain you feel. The pain is much less intense. And you feel more detached from it. The pain is still talking to you, but it is no longer screaming for all of your attention. You do not "get used" to the pain if you have a chronic pain condition. It becomes harder to endure (McCaffrey 1989).

The scientific / medical community is just now slowly unraveling what the nature of pain is. Some researchers are looking at the body's mechanism for dealing with physical pain as an "organ system" that is subject to malfunction just as any other organ system. These researchers feel that some chronic pain states are caused by a malfunction in this mechanism, rather than by another type of illness (Sedgewick 1991).

Neurotransmitters and Pain

Many of the medications used in FMS work by affecting the biochemicals known as neurotransmitters. As mentioned in several previous chapters, neurotransmitters play a large part in running the body. They do so in the following manner: There are no direct connections between two nerve fibers, or between a nerve fiber and a muscle or gland. But at the end of the nerve, the electrical signal causes the release of a neurotransmitter, which bridges the gap between two cells. Each neurotransmitter has a specific receptor site, like jigsaw puzzle pieces made for each other. But in a puzzle, each puzzle piece fits with other specific pieces. That is not true in the body.

This is how many medications work: They fit into these specific receptor slots. Some medications trigger a response, and others just plug the receptor site so that no neurotransmitter can "communicate" with it (Mann 1994).

Serotonin

Serotonin is a neurotransmitter with many different receptor sites. It controls sleep states, vomiting, moods, migraines, and depression. Some of the "anti-anxiety" medications used for FMS are "specific serotonin re-uptake inhibitors" (SSRIs). These medications block the receptor sites, leaving more serotonin actively moving in the body.

Medications and Pain

Medications that affect neurotransmitters can work in other ways. They can prevent or increase the release of neurotransmitters, change the permeability of the various cell membranes involved, or mimic the action of the neurotransmitter.

Many pain medications function as filters, covering the pain receptors so that the pain impulses cannot get through. Some researchers believe that people with FMS/MPS Complex have a reduced ability to filter out pain both at the spinal cord level and in the brain (*Fibromyalgia Network Newsletter* January 1995).

Chronic Pain and Depression

Chronic pain can also cause depression. Depression is a normal response to chronic pain. If a depressive state already exists, chronic pain will intensify the normal depressed reactions and must be dealt with, and not just in the obvious, psychological way. It makes sense that someone who hurts all the time can become depressed. But it now appears that the same biochemicals that intensify pain can also cause or intensify depression.

People who take tricyclic antidepressants for primary depression may need to be on the medication for weeks before the effects of the drug become noticeable. However, when these medications are prescribed (at a much lower dose) for chronic pain, they often take effect in a day or two. This leads us to believe that the pain receptors may double as depression modulators. (Carol Warfield, M.D., Director of Beth Israel Hospital's Pain Center in Boston, quoted in Sedgewick 1991.)

Chronic pain by itself can also cause fatigue, problems in concentrating, changes in appetite, and, ultimately, withdrawal from life. Chronic pain is one of the chief sources of stress in life. It is an aggressive condition that must be vigorously treated as soon as possible, before it leads to further muscle tightness and thus to more pain.

Like most people, you are probably unprepared for the totality of a chronic pain condition. Your old life dies. The new life that is born is not the comfortable life you used to live. It is prickly, with sharp edges that can wear away the spirit and endurance of the unprepared. But you can prepare yourself!

Doctors and Chronic Pain in FMS and FMS/MPS Complex

Because of all the cognitive symptoms that accompany FMS/MPS Complex, too many doctors dismiss the debilitating pain that often accompanies the physical symptoms. They blame the pain on depression. "You look okay to me," they say, and tell the suffering patient to put on a happy face, lose some weight, and get on with life. It's no wonder that pain can lead to murder. Patients suffering from chronic pain have, indeed, killed or tried to kill doctors who refused them adequate medication. "Pain can drive people to murder. Distraught patients have killed or tried to kill the doctors who refused to give them medicine for it." (Batten 1995).

One person on the Internet described her experiences with chronic pain like this: She wrote that at first she thought FMS/MPS was like a bad bruise and that it would go away in a few days. Then, she felt it was like a broken arm, and her body would mend in a few months. Now, she knows that it is more like having both arms amputated.

D.J.S.

One woman with FMS I spoke with could not get any pain relief from Darvocet or other more standard FMS/MPS medications. Her doctors didn't want to prescribe anything stronger, but she couldn't sleep because of the pain she was experiencing. When her doctors found cancer, suddenly she was prescribed all the pain medications she needed. The pain hadn't changed at all—only her *doctors'* perception of it.

D.J.S.

Bodywide chronic myofascial pain syndrome (MPS) can be extremely disabling, and fibromyalgia is a pain amplification syndrome. These facts translate into agony when they occur together, as they frequently do. Sometimes, it seems as though the doctors who don't believe in the reality of fibromyalgia choose not to do so, because if they did admit its reality, they would have to also admit to complicity in torturing so many chronic pain patients.

Margo McCaffrey and Alexandra Beebe, two remarkable nurses, have written a text, *PAIN, A Clinical Manual for Nurses* (1989) that should be required reading for doctors as well, especially the chapter on chronic nonmalignant pain. McCaffrey and Beebe share a philosophy with Janet Travell: They start out by believing their patients. The following quoted material is from McCaffrey and Beebe's book:

"Only the patient knows when and how much he hurts. Therefore the patient is in control, i.e., [he is] the final authority about his pain . . . .

Although the patient may report severe pain, the patient is not always acting like he is in pain since he has been in pain for so long. However, the patient is often depressed and there may be signs of anxiety . . . .

In programs for chronic pain management, an attitude of self-control and control over pain is fostered. If a patient with diabetes or chronic hypertension knows all about his medications and when he should take them, this is viewed as desirable. When the patient with chronic pain has the same information and has learned to use it to manage his pain, ironically this tends to upset the health team . . . .

They [doctors] tend to believe that pain is less intense in patients with chronic vs. acute pain, especially if there are no signs of pathology . . . .

There is also a tendency for nurses to believe that pain relief measures are less effective when the patient is depressed, failing to appreciate that the pain may cause the depression . . . .

Patients seem to be aware that expressions of depression may be viewed negatively. They may defend themselves against the possibility of their pain being psychologically interpreted by making a great effort to represent themselves as cheerful and nondepressed. Thus the patient is in a no-win situation. If he acts like his pain is emotionally disturbing, he may be diagnosed as having a 'mental problem,' and his pain may be labeled as largely psychogenic [originating in the mind]. If he does not appear depressed, the intensity of his pain may not be believed."

The fact that there is no way to measure chronic pain does not justify the "it's all in your head" response. Patients who exaggerate their pain and other symptoms may just be trying to get their health care team to believe them. When patients sense their doctors' disbelief, they may increase their overt reactions to their pain in their efforts to convince the medical staff that they really hurt.

A patient who is a "frequent flyer" to the emergency room and who is regularly in a pain crisis state may have poor coping behavior and/or an ineffective support strategy, but the pain is still there. There is no excuse for blaming the patient. Patients may need extensive counseling and/or other intervention but presently they are doing the best they can. That's all that can be asked of anyone.

The Dependence Factor

Of course, you must do what you can to minimize your pain, by being good to your body, avoiding overwork, and refusing to perform activities when you are exhausted or in pain. Often, however, these preventive measures aren't enough.

With FMS and FMS/MPS Complex, *you need a primary care doctor who understands pain, and a pharmacist to match.* They must understand and agree that a physical dependency is the body's natural adaptation to some types of medication. If someone stops taking a medication that has been taken regularly, for some length of time, a withdrawal effect will occur; but this is not an addiction, as addiction is commonly understood.

"In recent years the term addiction has been redefined. Not too long ago it was thought that addiction was both psychological and physiological dependence. Now physiological changes from repeated use of narcotics are recognized and treated as separate entities."(McCaffrey 1989)

If you have a chronic pain condition and no history of drug abuse, you should not be denied adequate pain control because of a fear that you will become addicted. You have a great deal of pain. It doesn't ease your pain to compound it by adding guilt.

It is the rule rather than the exception that FMS/MPS Complex patients will save strong pain medications after a surgery or an injury for the times when they will *really* need them—those times when they have an FMS/MPS flare (see Chapter 12, Flare). Rather than having to resort to this tactic, you should ask your doctor for a small amount of stronger medication to have available for short-term use when you really need it.

". . . Several studies have shown that prolonged narcotic therapy for selected patients with chronic nonmalignant pain can be a safe and humane alternative to surgery or no treatment." (McCaffrey 1989) If other alternatives have been tried with no effect, and if the patient is doing everything possible otherwise, mild narcotics may be the answer for proper pain management.

> I would not have been able to write this book without the help of adequate pain medications, other medications, and tons of physical therapy. I am looking forward to the time when I can cut back on the medications and still improve my quality of life.
>
> D.J.S.

Describing Chronic Pain to Your Doctor

To help yourself, you need to learn how to communicate to others, especially to your doctors, how you feel. You need to understand the language of pain.

The words you choose are important because they can give your doctor clues as to what the pain is like. Your motions are also important. A man describing a crushing pain may clench his arms tight to his body. A woman talking about a radiating pain may spread her fingers in the direction of the radiation.

The Language of Pain

There are many words to describe pain. Words such as pulsing, throbbing, pounding, shooting, prickling, stabbing, lancing, electrical, sharp, pinching, pressing, gnawing, cramping, crushing, tugging, wrenching, hot, cruel, vicious, killing, blinding, intense, unbearable, spreading, radiating, piercing, tearing, agonizing, and torturing all describe different types of intense pain.

Tingling, itchy, smarting, stinging, dull, sore, aching, heavy, tender, taut, tiring, exhausting, sickening, suffocating, frightful, annoying, troublesome, miserable, tight, rigid, numb, drawing, squeezing, cool, cold, icy, nagging: These are other words to describe different kinds of pain more precisely.

Then, there is the kind of pain that brings on other symptoms such as vomiting, shaking, distractibility, and / or an inability to concentrate. Important questions to ask you doctor may be: "Do you believe that I have this pain? Do you understand its severity and the disrupting influence it has on my life?"

In Conclusion

Chronic pain is different from acute pain, and it must be treated differently. It may be accompanied by a number of other symptoms, including depression. The key to treating the chronic pain of FMS and FMS / MPS Complex lies in the ability of people with these conditions to describe their pain symptoms *and* the ability of their *doctors* to understand and respond appropriately.

CHAPTER 10

Sleep

We don't know enough about the nature of sleep. Some researchers even believe that sleep is a state when the mind is awake but the body is not (Alvarez 1995). We do know that sleep plays a vital role in memory and that new skills can be consolidated during sleep. Many people seem to be able to solve some of their problems in their dreams, during sleep.

We also know that sleep dysfunction is an integral part of many illnesses. FMS and MPS are two of these.

Most of us think of sleep as a time when we are "just resting." This is not true. Even in sleep, the body and mind are continually communicating at a rate that can be difficult to grasp.

Think of a picture of the surface of the brain—the thin, convoluted outer part that looks somewhat like the meat of a walnut. This outer surface is called the cerebral cortex. In this part of the brain alone, there are about 10 billion nerve cells. Each of these nerve cells is communicating by neurotransmitter with at least 10,000 other nerve cells next to it, and sending between 100 and 300 communications a second. Each of them, no matter whether we are awake or asleep, is active to that degree (Alvarez 1995).

When you realize that FMS or FMS/MPS Complex creates a great deal of extraneous "noise" along these "transmission lines," you begin to see the picture. The picture is one of chronic sleep deprivation.

Sleep and Trigger Points

People who have suffered from trigger points (TrPs) for months or years are likely to have developed some sleep problems and to have restricted their activity and exercise because of pain and other symptoms. These restrictions aggravate the TrPs, causing a vicious cycle.

Your physical therapist should give top priority to inactivating those TrPs that are chiefly responsible for your sleep problems. Chronic sleep deprivation is a prime TrP perpetuating factor and, sadly, disturbed sleep is a way of life for many chronic pain patients—especially those with FMS/MPS Complex.

According to a Cornell University. Medical Center study, by Daniel Wagner, M.D., it takes four to six weeks of getting enough sleep to fully recover from prolonged sleep deprivation. If, like many people with FMS or FMS/MPS Complex, you have had years of sleep deprivation, you have a lot of catching up to do.

The Stages of Sleep

Sleep is different for each individual, but most people, to a greater or lesser extent, experience certain specific stages while they are sleeping.

> Someone once told me that successful people are those who can eat when they are hungry and sleep when they are tired. I try to go to bed when I'm sleepy and stay up (and busy) when I'm not. This philosophy may also help you.
>
> D.J.S.

Just before you fall sleep, you pass through a period known as the *hypnogogic stage*. It is matched by an after-sleep awakening period known as the *hypnopompic stage*. Unusual things can happen to you at these times. You are more suggestible, for instance, and, if you can focus on them, affirmations work particularly well at this time. Some people even hallucinate during this stage.

The onset of sleep is often heralded by a feeling of floating or falling, and sometimes this stage ends abruptly with a startled wakefulness. At times, the whole body can twitch or jump; this is called a *sleep start*.

REM Sleep

Dreaming takes place during Rapid Eye Movement, or REM, sleep. Stage One sleep is a drowsy non-REM (NREM) sleep. Stage Two is a light NREM sleep. There are also deeper stages of NREM sleep, times of delta-brain wave rhythm, when much of the body's regulatory work and biochemical balancing take place, and antibodies are produced in greater numbers. These stages are punctuated by periods of REM sleep.

During REM sleep, there is a complete loss of muscle tone, called *flaccid paralysis*. While dreaming, the body cannot move. Body movements take place in the lighter stages of sleep but not in deep NREM sleep or in REM sleep's "flaccid paralysis stage."

NREM sleep is always the first stage in each sleep cycle. At the onset of REM, small convulsive twitches of the face and fingertips can be observed much as what can be seen in a sleeping cat or dog, but it is during NREM that snoring occurs.

Chronic Pain, Stress, and Insomnia

Chronic pain worsens sleep difficulties. In chronic pain conditions, alpha rhythms often intrude, especially into delta sleep, disrupting slumber. (Alpha waves are normally generated during waking hours. Delta brain waves are associated with deeper levels of sleep.) A high proportion of alpha waves during sleep means that there will be a more sensitive perception of pain. More delta waves during sleep lessen pain sensation and improve energy levels. When a pattern of chronic alpha-wave intrusion into delta-level sleep is established, it is called the *alpha-delta sleep anomaly*.

The Alpha-Delta Sleep Anomaly

Brain cells generate alpha-wave activity during average waking hours. During light sleep, the brain waves are mixed. As sleep becomes deeper, more delta-level waves appear. Stage Four sleep, the deepest, is basically uninterrupted delta waves, *unless* the sleeping person has FMS or FMS/MPS Complex. The alpha-delta sleep anomaly is one of the most commonly occurring symptoms in FMS.

Whenever people with FMS reach delta-level sleep, alpha (waking) brain waves intrude. These alpha waves can jolt them awake, or rouse them to a lighter level of sleep. If this sounds similar to a torture used on prisoners of war, you've gotten the idea. It is exactly the same. And chronic sleep deprivation can cause chronic pain.

Stress and Sleep

Stress is a leading cause of insomnia. Stress can lead into a repeating cycle, i.e., stress causes sleep loss which causes further stress, which causes further sleep loss, and so on. Stress itself is a symptom with many causes. Some of these are as follows: illness, psychological problems (Post-Traumatic Stress Disorder, Panic Disorder, and so on), medications, the environment (noise, interruptions, and so on), sleep disorders, faulty sleep associations from temporary insomnia, disturbances of circadian rhythms (jet lag, shift work), and more. These are all currently being studied in the fairly new field of chronobiology.

Forms of Insomnia

There are three main *forms* of insomnia, although there are several types of insomnia within each form. Difficulty in falling asleep is called *sleep onset insomnia*. If your problem is waking up many times during the night, it is called *maintenance insomnia*. Waking very early and being unable to go back to sleep is called *early a.m. insomnia*. (Note that early a.m. insomnia is often a symptom of underlying depression.)

There is also *mixed insomnia*, which is most commonly a combination of sleep onset and maintenance insomnia or sleep onset and early a.m. insomnia. *Conditioned insomnia* occurs in people who are predisposed to sleep disorders after a period of poor sleep, such as might happen with a new baby in the household.

A type of insomnia called *compulsive urination insomnia* appears to be very common in people with FMS/MPS Complex. Most people urinate before they go to bed, and a small amount of urine is usually left in the bladder. But because people with FMS/MPS Complex have hypersensitive nerve endings, they feel the bladder pressure, so they get up to urinate again. Because they are conscious of how hard it is for them to get to sleep, they don't want to take a chance on being awakened in the night by having to urinate again. For this reason, whenever they wake (sometimes with every alpha intrusion), they go to the bathroom. This can happen more than 30 times a night! Lidocain ointment on the urinary opening will stop some of the sensitivity. If you experience urination imsomnia, however, first get checked out for a possible yeast or low-grade bacterial infection before trying Lidocain.

Another type of insomnia called *dream-interruption insomnia* is caused by deep anxiety. People with this type of insomnia wake up during REM sleep, with residual paralysis. In some cases, a person may wake up with voice box muscle spasms and be unable to speak. This can be terrifying.

Factors Affecting Sleep

Nicotine can play a role in insomnia. Nicotine is a stimulant that causes the release of epinephrine, a neurotransmitter, which interferes with sleep. Withdrawal from nicotine begins two or three hours after smoking and can also promote insomnia.

Some people have sleep problems that aren't true insomnia but can easily turn into it. They don't want to go to bed. Some of these people are either high-energy achievers or high-anxiety worriers who don't want to let go of the day to "waste time" sleeping. Some are having marriage problems. Some were abused in bed. Any kind of extreme long-lasting stress or abuse may trigger fibromyalgia. Such people often develop FMS (van Why 1994). If you suspect you are one of these, it is important that you get to the root of your problem. Find out what it is about going to bed that you don't like. This kind of sleep problem is a wake-up signal for the practice of meditation and mindfulness, relaxation techniques, breathing exercises, and affirmations.

Nerve Entrapment

During the night, parts of your body may become numb if they have had the slightest weight on them. This becomes very noticeable when you wake up. You may discover you cannot lie with one part of your body under another, e.g., one arm lying on top of the other, because you will experience nerve entrapment.

Nerve entrapments may occur because of pressure on the nerves by the palpable bands of taut muscle fibers that are associated with trigger points. When a nerve passes through the muscle between taut bands of myofascia, or when it is compressed between such a band and bone, *neurapraxia*, which is the loss of nerve conduction, may result.

FMS/MPS Complex and Sleep Patterns

People with FMS and FMS/MPS Complex need to sleep well for more reasons than just to banish fatigue. Even relatively moderate sleep loss during one night can cause a drastic reduction in the activity of the natural killer cells of the immune system.

Fibromites often get sleepy at inappropriate times, such as in the afternoon and again around 8 p.m. If they push themselves past the hump, they become "wired," wide awake again, and unable to fall asleep when they become fatigued. Some fibromites get terribly sleepy just before a rainstorm. This may be related to electro-magnetic disturbances. Relief from an extreme form of weariness can come with the rain.

If you start yawning and need to rub your eyes, these are the early warning signs of approaching sleepiness. Go to bed and settle in your preferred going-to-sleep position. If you don't get right to bed, the "reflex arousal" will put you into an alert state again. (The reflex arousal occurs when you are sleepy, but your continued actions signal that you aren't going to sleep. Then, you start manufacturing biochemicals to overcome the sleepy feeling.)

Note: A compound recently discovered in sleepy cats may be the sleep aid of the future. It fosters a natural deep sleep without side effects. It is a neurotransmitter-like biochemical also found in human beings. Some FMS researchers, notably Harvey Moldofsky, believe that FMS is caused by sleep deprivation in susceptible individuals. If so, this substance may help prevent FMS from developing (Moldofsky 1989).

Many fibromites "crash and burn" with the switch to daylight saving time. Our Internet (fibrom-l listserv) resident sleep expert, David Nye, M.D., has kindly given us permission to publicize his plan to minimize sleep disruption. Follow the instructions below to minimize sleep disruption during the time changes in the spring and fall.

A week or so before the time change goes into effect, begin to prepare your body. In the fall, when the clock moves back, start your night medications and bedtime preparations 15 minutes or so earlier than usual, and increase the time by 15-minute increments until you are on "winter time." This will make the change easier.

In the spring, when the clock moves forward, start bedtime preparations and medications 15 minutes later than you do in winter and increase the time by 15-minute increments until summer arrives.

Sleep Phenomena

There is no magic pill to provide normal delta sleep for us all. There are, however, many conditions that can co-exist with fibromyalgia, which can add to our sleep disturbances. Dealing effectively with any of these may improve your sleep considerably.

Apnea means temporary cessation of respiration. *Obstructive sleep apnea,* or *OSA,* was explained to us by our Internet sleep expert, David Nye, M.D. The muscles of the throat relax during sleep, and this narrows the air passages. If the walls of the air passages start to touch, the air passing between them, as the sleeper breathes, causes vibration, which causes the sound we call snoring.

If the walls of the air passages collapse to the point that the air flow is obstructed, OSA results. Your spouse or significant other will hear a loud snoring broken by pauses, which is followed by a gasp. The inability to breathe will either wake you up or send you into shallower sleep. *Note that obstructive sleep apnea is a life-threatening condition.* People with OSA are exhausted because whenever they fall asleep, they can't breathe. Yet it isn't unusual to be unaware that the condition exists.

Other conditions can also cause sleep apnea. If you snore, It is definitely something to have checked. It could be that you have a sinus blockage, a need for cervical pillow to support your neck, or perhaps a defect in the septum of your nose that can be easily corrected.

Obesity worsens snoring. So does sleeping on your back. Putting a tennis ball in a sock and taping it to the back of your pajamas can discourage you from sleeping on your back.

Restless Leg Syndrome (RLS) is a condition that occurs as you are trying to fall asleep. It is not the same syndrome as what is termed Periodic Leg Movements (PLM), although nearly every case of RLS is accompanied by PLM.

With RLS, you can't hold your legs still. It starts as an unpleasant feeling in the lower limbs. Then, your legs start to ache and feel as if they are expanding and heavy. RLS can also begin with *fasciculations*, or rapid firing of the motor neurons. These lead to twitches. RLS becomes worse after sitting for long periods. Cold weather also makes this condition worse. You can relieve RLS by shaking or moving the legs, or by walking. Lying on a surface with many hairlike extensions, such as wool, seems to help, although we don't know why. L-dopa, an energizing neurotransmitter used in Parkinson's disease, has also been of help. If pain is present, Tegretol is often prescribed.

RLS often occurs in family clusters. More women than men have it, and it becomes worse with menses, pregnancy, and menopause. It also worsens with age and with sleep deprivation. Often it is most intense during the first half of the night and episodes occur in clusters.

Myoclonus (the plural is *myoclonia*) is a term that includes sleep starts, Periodic Leg Movements, and hiccups. These can be common in FMS, MPS, and FMS/MPS Complex.

Hypnic jerk is a sudden twitch of the whole body, which sometimes occurs in FMS. It indicates a high arousal state. Hypnic jerks accompany anxiety states and indicate a need for relaxation. Potassium supplements are often helpful.

There is a relationship between REM sleep and muscle twitching. Some studies have found that if serotonin is inhibited (as it is in FMS and FMS/MPS Complex), animals are able to learn to sleep without it, but they develop muscle twitching (Charmes 1976).

Muscle contractions often lead to increased mental activity. As your muscles work during the day, they gain a momentum, an electrical "loading," that doesn't stop even when you're asleep. Even slightly tensed muscles send nerve impulses through the spinal cord to your brain. There, these impulses generate thoughts that can be persistent and annoying when you are trying to sleep.

Grinding your teeth during sleep may not indicate stress. *Bruxism*, or teeth grinding, is the way the brain "twiddles its thumbs" and it may indicate no more than neurotransmitter dysfunction. Try tiring your jaws just before going to bed, with a bagel or a crunchy apple. Be sure to balance your snack at a 30 percent protein, 30 percent fat, and 40 percent carbohydrate ratio if you suspect you have reactive hypoglycemia. (See Chapter 24, on nutrition.)

Nocturnal cramps are often strong contractions of leg and foot muscles. You can sometimes relieve them by flexing your foot upward or by leaning forward against a wall with your feet flat. In FMS/MPS Complex, any muscle can cramp. Galvanic muscle stimulation (GMS) and other physical therapy can relieve the cramps (see Chapter 25, Bodywork—Helping Your Body Work), although a reactive cramp can occur after GMS or other therapy first releases myofascial splinting. (Splinting occurs when the myofascia becomes thickened and hard, and tries to splint the hurt area of the body so that it won't move and cause more pain.)

Perchance to Dream?

Chronic pain states often cause more dreaming than normal. Some medications—and withdrawal from some medications—can also cause more frequent nightmares. Sometimes it may be hard for you to figure out what causes your dreams to be so strange.

Nightmares and bizarre dreams usually take place in the second half of sleep during long REM periods. They are not unusual in FMS/MPS, but they often diminish with age (Charmes 1976). Also, depression can be the cause of short, unpleasant dreams.

If you are afflicted by recurring nightmares, try rewriting your script. Write down the details of the nightmare and then change them to program a positive outcome. Go over the new dream script a few times a day. Your dreams should change.

Then there is lucid dreaming. If you are able to program your dreams to some extent, you are part of the lucky 5 percent of the population (Charmes 1976). Lucid dreaming offers a great potential to correct bad habits and program your subconscious during sleep.

Sleep terrors are different from nightmares. They are actually partial arousals from NREM, similar to sleepwalking and to talking in your sleep.

REM sleep, the dream stage of sleep, is essential to learning. Dr. Avi Karni, a neuroscientist at Israel's Weizmann Institute of Science, has found that REM sleep helps to imprint skills on the brain. Increasing REM sleep increases learning skills. This may be another reason why in those with FMS/MPS Complex, short-term memory suffers. It has been said that dreams are unopened letters to ourselves. With FMS/MPS Complex, you sometimes feel as if you are getting someone else's mail.

Some Sleep-Inducing Techniques to Try

When you can't sleep, that's a good time to make a journal entry. (See Chapter 17, Keeping a Journal.) Write down what you are feeling; you don't have to analyze it. The wee hours are a good time for meditation, breathing exercises, body scans, affirmations, and subliminal tapes. (See Chapter 20, Meditation and Mindfulness.)

Have a routine that prepares your body/mind for sleep. One hour before bedtime, unwind. *Before* this hour, make a list of your tasks for the next day. This will give you a head start. Then put the list where you have breakfast and forget it until tomorrow morning.

Become more assertive, and spend less time wishing you had been. Try meditation in bed. Try affirmations in bed.

Speaking of bed, make sure you have the type of bed you need. Many people with FMS or FMS/MPS Complex need a waterbed. There is no bed too soft for them. Some use a Somma bed, which is a pillow flotation bed. Some use futons. Some people need an especially hard mattress. Find out what works for you.

Electric lights can confuse your internal clock. Artificial light has an effect on your energy level. Try moderating the lights in your house an hour before sleep.

Keep regular times for going to sleep. Go to bed only when you are sleepy, but get up at a regular time. Don't vary your routine by more than an hour. You may need the help of specific serotonin re-uptake inhibitor (SSRI) to sleep. (See Chapter 9 for a discussion of this inhibitor.)

Sometimes melatonin helps (see Chapter 22, Enhancing Your Medications). Find out what combination works for you, and don't give up until you find it. Good sleep is worth any amount of effort to achieve.

In Conclusion

The link between sleep phenomena and FMS and FMS/MPS Complex is clear. The various types of insomnia all take their toll. Understanding the source of your sleep problems can lead you to solutions. Solving your sleep problems can alleviate many of your problems with pain and depression. If you cannot solve all of your sleep problems, you can probably diminish the intensity of some of them.

CHAPTER 11

Irritable Bowel Syndrome

People with FMS and FMS/MPS Complex often have major malfunctions of the gastrointestinal system. Some of these occur in the large intestine, causing a condition commonly referred to as Irritable Bowel Syndrome (IBS).

Symptoms of Irritable Bowel Syndrome

Irritable Bowel Syndrome is a smooth muscle dysfunction. Muscles in the gut contract and relax at the wrong time, leading to a number of symptoms. These symptoms include the following:

- painless diarrhea

- dry constipation (one of our locals calls the waste matter "rabbit pellets").

In addition, you may have a crampy "urge to go" but find that you cannot. You may also experience irregular contractions of the large intestines, bloating from gas, and hypersensitivity. Normally, the nerve endings in the gut transmit feelings only of fullness or stretching. When these endings are sensitized, pain is also transmitted. Note that other conditions besides FMS/MPS Complex transmit pain.

Note: With IBS, there is no bleeding, fever, significant weight loss, or severe, persistent pain. If you do have these symptoms, see your doctor right away.

What Causes Irritable Bowel Syndrome

Irritable Bowel Syndrome is probably a disorder of the motor activity of the large intestine, which is controlled by the central nervous system (and neurotransmitters). IBS does not cause inflammatory changes, and it is important to note that IBS is not the same as another serious condition, ulcerative colitis. Stress worsens but does not cause IBS.

Normally, liquids are absorbed from the large intestine, which is responsible for moving and consolidating waste matter. To accomplish this, the large intestine has two kinds of movements, mixing and expulsion. Ring-like areas made of longitudinal muscle fibers contract together, propelling the material along. Not much in the way of digestion occurs in the large intestine. Most absorption takes place in the small intestine. There are some organisms that survive the trip through the stomach acids and intestinal fluid. These create gas in the large intestine.

The large intestine contracts on its contents, mixing them. In addition to these contractions, there are strong propulsion movements called "peristalsis." These normally take place a few times a day, and propel the contents of the large intestine toward the anus. (Peristalsis is regulated by the Central Nervous System, through the actions of neurotransmitters.) It takes about three or four hours for material to travel from one end of the large intestine to the other. Some of the matter from each meal remains, to be mixed with the material from the next meal. With IBS, the normal movements of the large intestine are altered.

In terms of chemical activity, the major synthesis of serotonin in the body takes place both in the brain and the gastrointestinal tract. People with FMS / MPS Complex are already low in serotonin, and IBS further restricts serotonin production. This can worsen the FMS, which in turn worsens the IBS and people with FMS, find themselves in the middle of another spiral. Studies have shown that a large proportion of FMS patients do have IBS (*Fibromyalgia Network Newsletter* July 1995; Triadfiloupolis 1991).

Possible Aggravating Factors

A number of conditions may influence the development of IBS. They are as follows:

- poor nutrition

- abdominal trigger points

- medication sensitivity

- FMS (neurotransmitter) dysregulation

- yeast overgrowth

- Leaky Gut Syndrome

- food hypersensitivity—usually to cereals (mostly wheat and corn), dairy, coffee, tea, chocolate, potatoes, onions, and / or citrus

- stress

- menstruation

Leaky Gut Syndrome

This condition is tied to a lot of FMS/MPS Complex symptoms. Many fibromites report intolerance to medications and also report responses to medications that are the reverse of average side-effects, in addition to food intolerances, multiple chemical sensitivities, and food cravings (usually for food that we should avoid) (Leitchtberg 1995). Even muscle pains can be worsened due to the "leaky gut syndrome."

As with so many symptoms that make up the FMS/MPS Complex, there seem to be many causes. The FMS/MPS gut seems to have a type of muscular dyslexia. The muscles don't work together. This action is under the direction of the Central Nervous System, and neurotransmitters; it is not surprising that we have dysfunction.

In addition, many researchers theorize that the gut mucosal lining becomes hyperpermeable. As larger than average molecules begin to seep through the mucosal lining, the body recognizes these as "not belonging." They are alien invaders, and the body forms antibodies to attack them. It is at this stage that food and chemical intolerances develop. This could be because of FMS, or it could be due to the often large amounts of NSAIDS and other medications that people with FMS and FMS/MPS Complex often take to reduce the pain. (AHCPR Guidelines Recommend NSAIDS and Acetaminophen—But How Safe Are They? February 13, 1993. MPI's *Dynamic Chiropractic* 94(5).)

What You Can Do

Irritable Bowel Syndrome can really disrupt your life. You may become housebound (afraid to go out) because of the unpredictability of your symptoms. IBS can interfere with your travel plans and curtail your ability to work.

As with other symptoms of FMS/MPS Complex, proper exercise and stress reduction are significant factors for relieving the symptoms of IBS. Additionally, in order to effect real change with this debilitating and frustrating problem, it helps to list all of your gastrointestinal-related triggers points and/or perpetuating factors. Then, *one by one*, do whatever you and your health team can to ease and alleviate as many of these irritants and malfunctions as is possible.

When you have a bout of IBS, review the past days' events. Note possible aggravating factors in your journal. For example, you may find that when you eat a meal high in fat content, you get a lot of gas. In such a case, you should seriously consider avoiding fried and fatty foods. Talk to your pharmacist about an over-the-counter simethicone medication for those times when you "just have to have a piece of pizza." There are many brands of anti-gas medication that you can purchase without a prescription at the drug store. Phazyme, Mylanta, and Maalox are some well-known brands.

Study your journal entries to see if you can find a correlation between bouts of IBS and recurrent events. Usually the symptoms of IBS result from a combination of several factors.

Diet

Be sure that your diet is balanced. If you have carbohydrate cravings or just crave sweets—especially chocolate—you should write down your cravings, as well as recording every thing that you put into your mouth. You may soon start to see a pattern relating to how you feel (see Chapter 24, on nutrition).

Many people with FMS or FMS/MPS Complex have a condition called reactive hypo-glycemia. This can make itself known by weakness or even tremors before meals. If the tremors disappear as soon as you eat—especially if you eat sugar—that is a warning sign. Often fibromites overreact to sugar—our insulin shoots up, and then crashes. By 2 or 3 p.m. in the afternoon we are ready for a nap. The same thing can happen after dinner. About 8 p.m. we are drowsy, but if we stay up (often snacking to stay awake), we are up until the wee hours of the morning. (See Chapter 24 on nutrition.)

Medications

Many medications taken by people with FMS/MPS Complex (Elavil, Pamelor, Flexeril, Prozac, Sinequan, Surmontil, and so forth) have the side effect of drying the mucus membranes. This dryness increases the likelihood of constipation. You can reduce this problem by eating high-fiber foods such as whole grains, fruits, and vegetables. Using a dietary fiber additive that contains psyllium husks or cellulose and drinking extra liquid daily also helps to eliminate this problem. The use of over-the-counter stool-softeners and gas relievers may also be helpful.

A medication called Propulsid increases the action of the valve between the esophagus and the stomach, and is often used for esophageal reflux (see Chapter 8, Common Symptoms and Why They Occur). It is being prescribed for IBS with good results.

Peppermint oil—not plain mint—in enteric-coated capsules also helps to relieve the symptoms of IBS. Plain mint breaks down in the stomach, and can cause heartburn, according to several studies quoted by Michael T. Murray (Murray 1994). Enteric-coated peppermint oil is available as "Peppermint Plus," found at natural foods stores.

Trigger Points

Refer to Chapter 3, Trigger Points, for information about abdominal trigger points (TrPs). Many TrPs, such as the multifidi, are located on the back, but refer symptoms to the abdomen. If you have them, you will probably also find TrPs in the belly area. These TrPs will be very tight and/or painful. This will tell you that they are causing at least part of the problem. Try tennis ball acupressure on them. It will hurt when you compress the TrPs, but it should give you some relief. (See Chapter 27, Bodywork You Can Do Yourself.)

Another area that can set up TrPs is the ileocaecal valve. This is the valve between the small and large intestine. Once material is in the large intestine, this valve prevents it from returning. The functioning of this valve is under neurotransmitter control. Irritation, such as that caused by IBS, can cause a great deal of pain in the right lower quadrant of the belly. This can mimic appendicitis pain. Iliocaecal pain can set up TrPs, starting in the immediate area with pain radiating down the right leg, sometimes to the inner aspect of the knee. Cold gel packs on the area, and tennis-ball acupressure, can provide some measure of relief. Lying on your back, with your right leg bent and held to the side, also helps. Constipation often triggers this pain, and should be dealt with immediately. Dietary modification and regulation is the best defense against iliocaecal pain.

Yeast

Talk with your doctor about a yeast-antibody test. If you suspect you have a yeast problem, decrease your mold and yeast burden. We normally have yeasts, bacteria, and viruses living in us. Many of us with FMS/MPS Complex, especially those of us with reactive hypoglycemia, carry a yeast burden way above average. It is the yeast that demands to be fed—with sugars and heavy carbohydrates. (See Chapter 24 on nutrition.) Restrict your consumption of sugars, other carbohydrates, and fermented products (such as tofu and alcohol).

Several people we have communicated with have found that when they put out bowls of bleach in their damp basements, the bleach decreased the number of mold spores in the air. If you try this, and, subsequently, you experience a lessening of symptoms, you will have found one of your yeast/mold sources.

In Conclusion

Irritable bowel syndrome often accompanies FMS and FMS/MPS Complex. To keep IBS from interfering with your daily routine, it's important to take a look at all of the elements in your life that may be setting it off and to deal with each one individually. Through proper diet, bodywork, medication, and attention to aggravating factors, you can often eliminate the problem of IBS.

CHAPTER 12

Flare

Fibromyalgia Syndrome and FMS/MPS Complex are cyclical in nature. Sometimes the symptoms are almost in remission. Sometimes they are very active. And then there are flares.

When you experience a flare, your whole body screams for attention. You may experience new symptoms, as well as all the old ones, and they may *all* be amplified. A flare is a time of high-intensity pain and grief, an overwhelming episode of pain in your trigger and tender points that can either creep up on you or hit you suddenly with all the subtlety of a barreling express train. Flare, like a flash-fire, is all-consuming.

What Causes Flare?

Flares are usually triggered by one or more activities or stressors. It might be something microscopically small, such as a virus or a severe yeast infection, or something large and dramatic, such as a traffic accident. The stressor could be as complex as a divorce or as simple as playing a game of volleyball. A menstrual period, a dip in a swimming pool that is just a little too cold, a draft or a sudden temperature change, or the onset of allergy season—any one of these events, alone or in concert, could cause a flare.

Anything that interrupts or disrupts sleep can be a flare instigator. Injury, a new baby, visitors, holidays, a time change, jet lag, travel, vacations, shift work—all of these situations can cause a major flare.

It isn't unusual for a person with FMS/MPS Complex to suffer a severe flare after an upper-respiratory infection or an allergy attack. Some fibromites have an unusual amount of the neurotransmitter histamine, which may be a factor in setting off a flare.

Flare and Yeasts

When taking an antiyeast medication, such as Diflucan (see Chapter 22, Enhancing Your Medications) you can expect the yeast "die-off" phenomenon. Although you are actually improving your health by killing the yeast, your symptoms get dramatically worse as the yeasts die and release toxic chemicals. This often precipitates a flare.

You may think the medication isn't working, and want to stop it. This makes the yeast very happy. If you are already in a flare due to a severe yeast infection, the yeast die-off side-effects can be extreme. Fibrofog (see Chapter 18) and the worsening of all symptoms can result. It is hard to endure, but if you understand what is happening and take it very easy on your body, you can ride it out. Just make sure you are as prepared as possible. Have a supply of food and other necessities at home. Arrange to have friends drop in and help, if necessary.

Signs of Approaching Flare

Flare has a way of creeping up on you when you aren't expecting it. But, as you begin to pay attention to the signs and symptoms of FMS, as you develop a dialogue with your body, it will give you clues when you are once again on the edge of a major flare.

When small groups of muscles randomly fire, you may experience what are called *fasciculations*. One person on the Internet calls them "butterfly kisses." These are small twitches that usually start by being fairly imperceptible, and they do not involve joint movement. They start with rapid firing randomly located neurons. When enough muscle fibers are involved, a twitch results. Jerks and spasms of the body often indicate that the muscles are not getting sufficient oxygen, and these symptoms can increase before flare.

In addition, you may experience one or more of the following symptoms:

- Your muscle strength may become unreliable, and you may drop things more often than usual. You may also be aware of weakness during certain movements, such as when pouring liquids, turning a doorknob, or opening a can of pet food. This occurs because the muscle involved has learned to limit the force of its contraction to below the pain threshold; as a result, it starts compensating and restricting certain movements.

- An involved extremity may feel cold compared with the other one, due to constriction of the blood vessels.

- You may feel frequent dizziness when you change your posture. This could be restricted to when you get up after lying down, or it could happen every time you move your head. Some people cannot walk without feeling that they are falling forward.

- Another symptom is spatial disorientation. You can no longer tell where you are in relation to the world around you. You bump into walls and fall over curbs. It isn't unusual to come out of this with a sprain, strain, or even a broken bone. You may find it necessary to restrict yourself to one floor level.

Along with or instead of this, you may have disturbed weight-perception. It may be hard for you to judge the weight of objects you pick up. This can result in apparently throwing objects around.

- It may be increasingly difficult to feed yourself without spilling food. You may need to use straws to get liquid to your mouth.

- Fibrofog—the inability to think clearly—may become extreme. The fog may creep up and get so thick that you are unaware even of the fact that you are in flare.

- Depression due to chronic pain may worsen, as may the pain itself.

In FMS/MPS Complex, the Myofascial Pain Syndrome trigger point symptoms may become magnified, even though the flare is a function of the systemic fibromyalgia component.

Note: Note that even when you are aware of the signs of an approaching flare, you may not recognize them if you are experiencing increased cognitive impairment. And, sometimes, you may not want to admit to yourself that you're in a flare.

When you are in flare, judgment can be seriously impaired. One person reported on the Internet that she had put a plate of food on the table and microwaved a bottle of cider instead. It exploded. When things like that start happening more often than normally, a flag should go up. (Of course, if you're going into flare, the flag will probably fall and hit you!)

Preventing Flare

You can use the time between flares to take actions that will improve your chances of avoiding flare in the future. Then, if you find you're on an express train to flare-city, you can grab your journal (see Chapter 17, Keeping a Journal) and read your flare-prevention strategy. Now is the time to draw up a crisis management plan for impending flare. By doing this, you will find it helps to analyze actions or processes that have sent you into flare before.

Use the following suggestions as guides for drawing up your personal plan for preventing or minimizing flares once you've observed the warning signs—or before they appear.

- Avoid immediate unnecessary changes in your life.

- Optimize the quality of your life by practicing healthy behaviors.

- Contact your supporters and mobilize your family. Because flare can often creep in under the cover of growing fibrofog, you may be in deep flare before you know it.

> Because of the changes in cognitive function, it is often difficult for me to decide if I am in flare or if I have some kind of illness on top of FMS/MPS Complex. Nothing seems to work right. I start having problems with all my electronic equipment. Typing is nearly impossible. I get lost on our hill (one road, nine houses). I can't even follow conversations.
>
> D.J.S.

When we have house guests, preparing the house and grounds for a visit invariably launches me into flare. My exercise time is curtailed, as are my meditations and sleep time.

It was logical to think that any of these things could have been causing the flare, but I was going into flare *before* the guests came. By analyzing our pre-guest rituals, I found my flare reaction was not caused by the extra stress of guests. My husband, as he helped me clean the house, would tuck away everything I needed to function. He'd find little nooks and crannies where, using only logic and deductive powers, I would never find them. So we talked about it. The next time we expect guests, we will have someone over to clean. We are also planning to build on a room.

D.J.S.

For this reason it's important to educate your family and friends about flare so they can help you when your own alarm system is not working properly. Organize them into a willing team to help you avoid flare.

- Schedule extra appointments with your chiropractor, physical therapist, massage therapist, counselor, or other health care team members.

- Give yourself extra time for bodywork and mindwork.

- Keep a quantity of food and other necessities in the house for those times when going out will be too much exertion. When you cook, make extra portions and freeze the surplus for times when you won't be able to cook.

- Break your problems into little pieces before you break into little pieces. Handle one piece at a time, and give yourself a healthy reward after you do so.

- Make a list of the negative elements in your life. Divide the list into those things you can change and those you can't. Refuse to worry about what you cannot change. Focus on those elements that you can. Take it one step at a time.

- Work on changing habits or implementing strategies in your life that contribute to overall wellness, but be sure to make each change gradually.

- If your sleep has been further impaired by impending flare, resumption of adequate restorative sleep is essential. If you are overwhelmed by exhaustion, give in to it and take a bath and a nap. "Veg out," if that's what it takes. Read a good book—and make sure that it is a positive one.

- Don't overdo *anything* if you are anticipating a flare. Spend more time having fun. (Sometimes you can avoid flare that way.)

- Avoid toxic exposure. Stay away from people who smoke.

- Prepare for potential problems, such as the twice yearly switch between daylight saving time and standard time (see Chapter 9, Sleep).

- If you live alone, arrange automatic payment of as many bills as possible so you don't have to remember to write and send checks. Write yourself a reminder in your checkbook, and remind yourself that you've done so in your daybook. You may want to sign an agreement that if you miss a payment, a third party—a trusted friend or family member—should be notified.

Preparing for a Flare

Sometimes, no matter how careful you are, events combine into the necessary ingredients to produce flare. If you have had periods of major flare before, be ready for a return.

The study of riding out a flare is a study in crisis management. When you are in flare, you are living in a war zone. Your body and your psyche are battered. It's time for a counter-attack.

The best plan for riding out a flare is the one you have tailored—before the flare—to suit your individual lifestyle and needs. Make a plan listing what you will need if a flare becomes severe, and a plan of actions to be taken on your behalf, if and when you cannot take action or make decisions for yourself.

Make sure your doctors, therapists, and supporters receive copies of your plan. Your list should include the following:

- Health care professionals who can be consulted.

- Treatments to be initiated if flare/fibrofog becomes severe and you cannot make decisions for yourself: physical therapy, added medications, and whatever else you might need.

- Treatments not to be used under any circumstance, and why you choose not to use them.

- Hospital facilities you are and are not willing to use. Explore possible facilities with health care professionals, supporters, health care organizations, and other people who have experienced severe flare—places where you would be safe and could receive appropriate treatment if your FMS/MPS were severe, if you have suicidal thoughts or you feel unsafe, or if your condition needs to be closely monitored. If you have been hospitalized in the past, you may already have first-hand information.

- If your flares have involved severe fibrofog, consider arranging for one or more trusted people to have a durable power of attorney to make decisions for you. You can draw up a legal document that defines the conditions under which such people will have the right to make decisions and carry out your wishes.

Riding It Out

Once you are in flare, here are some suggestions to help you through it:

- The old song, "Accentuate the Positive," could have been written for flare. Baby yourself. Find and repeat affirmations from your journal (filed under "flare," perhaps). Keep telling yourself that you *will* get out of flare soon because you are in control.

- Become aware of your body movements and positions. Avoid strain and immobility. Respect your pain.

- Pick your battles. In other words, simplify your tasks, and save your energy for what must be done. You may have to revise your ideas of what *must* be done. If you feel as if your home has become a "house clutterful," make a note in your journal. When you feel better, perhaps you will want to have a rummage sale.

- Ask for help.

- Write helpful strategies in your journal so that the next time you are feeling low, you won't have to relearn these lessons.

In Conclusion

By identifying the causes of flares, you can keep them from recurring in many cases. The key step is to make a commitment to yourself to do whatever you must do to prevent flare—to take a proactive role on your own behalf. If a flare occurs in spite of your best efforts, be sure you have a plan set up to deal with it—and take very good care of yourself. Remember, it will end.

CHAPTER 13

Pregnancy

Some women who are already stressed by FMS or FMS/MPS Complex must also struggle with the formidable demands of pregnancy. This is a time in their lives when they most need support, yet most of the medications that can help them deal with difficult symptoms are not available for their use. That's because many of the medications helpful to people with FMS or FMS/MPS Complex are not safe to take during pregnancy. If you have either syndrome, consult your doctor if you are thinking of becoming pregnant.

Not a lot is known about the effects of FMS/MPS Complex on pregnancy. In this chapter we will discuss the experiences of some women with FMS during and after their pregnancies. One thing is quite clear, however, for women who have FMS, MPS, or FMS/MPS Complex, a regimen of healthful bodywork and mindwork is crucial during pregnancy.

Remission

One woman said her FMS went into remission for most of her pregnancy but that in last few months, it returned with a vengeance. When it came back the headaches, depression, and pain were particularly severe.

Another woman reported that her FMS went into remission from about the third to the seventh month of her pregnancy. Then, she developed toxemia, her diabetes went out of control, and she was put on a strict bed-rest regime. With careful diet, this did the trick, and after a normal labor she delivered a healthy child.

> It may be that during pregnancy there is actually an increase in MPS symptoms and a decrease in FMS symptoms. I have checked my records, and I can document this in three out of 21 cases. (It is probable in 14 more, but since I followed them through cyberspace I couldn't document them. By taking a careful history, I can usually tell what TrPs are involved. I could not, however, rule out other variables.) This would make an interesting topic for a study.
>
> D.J.S.

Trigger Points

For women with MPS, trigger points (TrPs) get worse during pregnancy, as the body changes to accommodate the added burden. One study (Sola 1985) indicated that the gluteus medius TrPs may cause hip pain in the later stages of pregnancy and also may simulate the pain of sciatica. (See Chapter 8 for references to specific trigger points.)

Great care must be taken to avoid sternocleidomastoid and gluteus minimus TrPs. (See Figures 3-2 and 8-23.) There is a danger of falling due to the dizziness and imbalance that these TrPs cause. Pregnancy and resultant changes in weight distribution can magnify these problems.

Be aware of "foot slap," "foot drop," "buckling knee," and "buckling ankle" TrPs. Resultant falls will do nothing to improve the health of your baby or yourself. (See Chapter 8 for a discussion of these symptoms.)

Joints

Several pregnant fibromites noted that they experienced more joint pains during the night. These pains were mostly in their shoulders, hips, and knees. They had to use extra pillows to prop themselves up and to maintain comfortable positions.

Some women complained of sacroiliac joint dysfunction. Abnormal muscle tension can force the joint into an abnormal, displaced position. The joint can then become locked in place. For proper functioning and for an easier delivery, it must be mobilized again.

Sleep

During pregnancy, sleep changes. So does dreaming. Often there is an increase in dreaming, including the appearance of many dreams dealing with body changes. You may need to take more naps. You may feel sleepier during the first two trimesters. Starting in the fifth month, fetal movements can disturb your sleep even more.

Body changes in late pregnancy, such as bladder pressure and an inability to assume your preferred sleep position, may further impact the depth and quality of your slumber. Insomnia may worsen, especially in the last trimester. You may need to use body pillows to get comfortable. Sleeping in the fetal position, with your legs drawn up, can perpetuate the psoas TrPs. Back pain with psoas involvement is common in pregnancy. You may need to place a small pillow under your knees when sleeping on your back, or put one between your knees when lying on your side.

Nighttime leg cramps can increase during pregnancy. One woman had less of a problem with leg cramps if she consumed a small amount of milk and cheese before going to bed—but not enough to cause reflux. Other women have reported that extra calcium and magnesium decreased or eliminated the leg cramps.

Restless Leg Syndrome often becomes worse with pregnancy, especially at night.

Reflux may get worse. This may start early in pregnancy. Avoid eating two to four hours before going to bed, and see if that helps. Talk to your doctor about antacids.

Morning Sickness

An acupressure study by the Massachusetts Medical Society found that acupressure on a wrist point alleviated nausea and morning sickness in pregnancy (de Aloysio 1992). The acupressure point is located two inches above the wrist fold on the inner aspect of the wrist, a little toward the inside of the center.

A few women have reported that fresh lemon slices before they got out of bed in the morning helped to curb morning sickness. (For the benefit of your teeth, squeeze the slices into water. Straight lemon juice is too hard on the teeth, and will erode them.)

Hormones

Hormone fluctuations may increase for pregnant women with FMS. It appears that FMS may worsen in menopause, and get better during some pregnancies. The October 1995 *Fibromyalgia Network Newsletter* confirms that when you lose estrogen, your HPA-axis is further disrupted, and this could create "problems with the regulation of other systems such as the autonomic nervous system, growth hormone and serotonin production, and others."

Recent studies on cortisol (the corticotropin-releasing hormone (CRH), which fights stress and improves cardiovascular efficiency) indicate that temporary hormone deficiency after birth provokes post-partum depression.

Pregnancy shuts off production of CRH by the hypothalamus gland because the placenta releases large amounts of it during the second trimester. After the delivery, there is a lack of cortisol because the hypothalamus may remain shut off for as long as 12 weeks after birth (*Science News* July 1, 1995).

Other Issues

This section takes a brief look at some additional concerns for pregnant women with FMS or FMS/MPS Complex.

- **Protein levels:** One woman consumed extra protein during pregnancy, yet her protein levels always stayed low. Protein levels may need monitoring, especially if the expectant mother has reactive hypoglycemia.

- **Length of gestation:** Among the women questioned, one's pregnancy lasted 10 months for two different pregnancies—each resulted in the birth of a healthy child.

This may be related to altered hormone levels, other FMS biochemical irregularities, or even myofascial tightening.

- **Immune problems:** One woman had severe immune problems the first four months of her pregnancy. It seemed as though she had one sickness after the other. She became supersensitive to odors, and her skin became very dry.

- **Heat intolerance:** The woman with immune problems also noted that she experienced severe heat intolerance. It makes sense for heat intolerance to be very common in pregnancy. People generate heat, and the tiny being growing inside generates heat, as well. The body is working double-time. Since heat intolerance is not uncommon in FMS, the sensitivity may be magnified during pregnancy.

- **Other symptoms:** Urinary frequency, water retention, shortness of breath, and low-back pain are more common in pregnant women with FMS/MPS Complex than in healthy women.

- **Exercise:** Exercise and gentle stretches are very important during pregnancy. Good posture is vital. Proper exercise during the last trimester can lead to an easier delivery and faster recovery.

After the Birth

A critical period may occur right after you have your baby, especially if you and your child leave hospital care quickly. Around-the-clock new baby care disrupts sleep. You must recover from labor and delivery, with all the stresses and new TrPs that may have resulted. Your hormones are fluctuating and your usual routines are disrupted. It is no surprise that many deliveries are followed by a flare response.

Because a new baby is usually a study in sleep deprivation in real-time for the mother, it may be difficult for a mother with FMS/MPS to breast-feed. *All* the usual FMS/MPS medications get into breast milk.

Note: If you are breast-feeding your infant, before resuming any medications after delivery, first check with your doctor.

In Conclusion

The impact of FMS and/or MPS on pregnancy has not been studied thoroughly. We hope that women who have these conditions and who have also experienced pregnancy will write to us (in care of the publisher) to help us discover patterns that may shed some light on this important subject.

Part IV

Mind Over Matters

CHAPTER 14

The Body-Mind Connection

There is no question that both the mind and the body are involved in FMS and FMS/MPS Complex. Studies using Magnetic Resonance Imaging (MRI) and newer types of scanning showed that fibromyalgia patients had significant changes in brain tissue (*Fibromyalgia Network Newsletter* January 1995). In addition to chemical factors affecting the brain, FMS/MPS Complex carries with it a number of psychological factors.

This chapter discusses some of the connections between the mind and body in the FMS/MPS Complex.

The Nervous System

The nervous system can seem very complicated. However, like all complex systems, it is easier to understand if you break it into small parts. (Since the minds of fibromites frequently feel broken into small parts, maybe you have a head start!)

There are two major divisions of the "autopilot" part of the nervous system that concern you. These are the parts that work without your conscious direction, automatically.

The sympathetic nervous system causes the body to respond to danger, adversity, stress, anger, and even ecstasy by increasing the heart rate, raising the blood pressure, boosting the air exchange volume of the lungs, and increasing blood flow to all muscles. It prepares you for action, and is regulated by the hypothalamic/pituitary/adrenal (HPA) axis.

The *parasympathetic nervous system* regulates your body functions during rest, sleep, digestion, elimination, and other such mundane affairs.

You must understand this division of the nervous system in order to use your mind to promote your own healing.

The Stress Factor

During periods of extreme emotional stress, the sympathetic nervous system division is activated again and again. If the stress continues long enough, our bodies cannot release all of the accumulated tension and hold on to some of it. The leftover tension mounts until it causes pain. Pain causes more stress, which causes more pain. An ever-increasing spiral develops, and the person with FMS or FMS/MPS Complex is caught right in the middle. Even trigger points (TrPs) are influenced by stress.

Role of the Hypothalmus and the Pituitary and Adrenal Glands (The HPA Axis)

Over 50 years ago, the great endocrinologist, Hans Selye, charted the physiological changes that take place in the hypothalamus, pituitary, and adrenal glands during periods of stress. The following description is a brief synopsis of his findings.

The *hypothalamus* is a small gland in the brain. If it receives enough signals of the right kind, it decides the body is threatened. It then signals the pituitary, which is located close to the hypothalamus in the brain, to prepare the body for action.

The *pituitary* gland is a sort of central control in the body. It is often called the "master gland" of the body because it is so important and regulates so many other glands.

When the pituitary is signaled by the hypothalamus that the body is threatened, it sends a message to the *adrenal glands.* These are a pair of tiny glands perched on top of the kidneys like little triangular caps. They are minuscule but mighty, influencing almost all of the body systems. They produce adrenaline and many other biochemicals that the body uses in stressful situations. The balance and relationship among these three glands is the *hypothalamic/pituitary/adrenal axis.*

Eventually, when the stress or threat is removed, the adrenals signal the pituitary that it's time to relax. Unfortunately, one of the problems in FMS is a disrupted hypothalamic-pituitary-adrenal axis. These glands communicate by way of neurotransmitters, which is to say, in terms of the FMS/MPS Complex, not very well. People with FMS are like the villagers in the town where the boy cried "wolf" one too many times. We have come to alert status too many times. Our "fight-or flight" response system is *always* triggered. The body and mind cannot maintain this state of alert readiness indefinitely, and the system begins to break down.

The "Little Death" of FMS/MPS

A diagnosis of FMS/MPS is what is called in hospice work a "little death." You've lost your old self, and you must learn to deal with the same mental states that are common to those with a terminal illness while you adjust to your condition and learn to evolve a new self.

After the diagnosis, you will probably fight your way through the following stages:

1. Denial/isolation (I don't really have this! Go away, I don't want to talk about it!)

2. Anger (Why me?)

3. Bargaining (Maybe if I do *xyz* it will go away. . . .)

4. Depression (My life isn't worth much.)

5. Acceptance (If I'm fortunate and work hard, I can achieve the positive attitude of: "O.K. I have this, now let's see what I can do about it.")

When faced with a serious loss in life, it is normal to go through these stages as part of a natural grieving process. But after the grieving is over, rather than dwelling on what's been lost, it is very important to focus on optimizing the quality of your life. All of the chapters in Part IV that follow this chapter are intended to help you do just that.

Psychological Aspects of Chronic Pain

Acute pain that diminishes in the course of natural healing is generally manageable psychologically. You know why you hurt, you know what to do about it, and you know it will end.

Recurrent or chronic pain, however, especially pain caused by an undiagnosed, or "invisible" cause, has a destructive effect on one's sense of self. With FMS or FMS/MPS Complex, visit after visit to doctor after doctor often provides no relief. Every doctor seems to arrive at a different diagnosis. Because many of the symptoms of FMS are also symptoms of depression, eventually the doctors begin to urge psychiatric evaluation, which further erodes self-esteem. Frustration mounts, and depression and progressive disability follow.

It is harmful when others, especially physicians and other health care professionals, insist that *you* are somehow to blame for your afflictions. It is also distressing when otherwise well-meaning friends and relatives try to pass your medical problems off as nothing important. "You are young, you shouldn't be using a cane." "My feet hurt too. Get up and move around more. You're just out of shape." "You're just clumsy. If you weren't so preoccupied, you wouldn't knock things over all the time." "It's not as if you had something like cancer" (meaning something real like cancer and not imaginary like your pain). These comments are familiar to many of us.

When patients are told that they must learn to live with their FMS/MPS Complex pain because it is due to arthritis or some other cause, they tend to restrict their physical activity in order to avoid pain. This immobility perpetuates their trigger points, as the muscles start to shorten and eventually form contractures. In addition, these patients are often put on heavy doses of aspirin and other anti-inflammatory medications, which frequently cause digestive problems and further stress.

The Depression Factor

An American College of Rheumatology study by the team of Mason, Silverman, and Simms (1991) indicated that the impact of FMS on our lives is as bad as or worse than having rheumatoid arthritis. According to Mason, a major factor of this negative impact is "clinician bias," which translates as "the doctor thinks it's all in my head."

Note: If the diagnosis of FMS/MPS Complex takes a long time to reach, by the time it is made, you may have cultivated unhealthy behavior patterns that will be difficult (but not impossible) to change.

It's unlikely that a doctor would tell a patient in agony with rheumatoid arthritis to "put on a happy face, ignore the pain, and get on with life, with a little help from weight training exercise and a diet." Yet such things are said to FMS/MPS Complex patients every day, and these statements have enormous negative effects.

You can help yourself by learning positive, life-affirming, peaceful ways to cope with your illness. The following chapters describe many of these techniques and strategies. There is nothing you can do about the poor treatment and cruel comments of the past. You do need to educate others, but you must learn not to take negative talk personally. It's important for you to focus on the present, to work on enhancing your own health, and to take responsibility for your own health care. You can't change other people. You can only change yourself.

Guilt, blame, hurt, anger, fear, and frustration are negative emotions. You wouldn't take that kind of abuse from anyone else, so don't take it from yourself. The world directs more than enough negativity your way. Don't generate any more.

Remember that anything you accomplish is deserving of respect and praise. "Love others as yourself" takes as a truth that you first love yourself. (For more information about self-esteem, see Chapter 15, Taking Control. For more information about depression and changing negative thoughts, see Chapter 16, Coping Day to Day.)

In Conclusion

We hope, that this chapter has helped you to understand a little more about the mind/body connection. In the following chapters you will read about many of the techniques that are available to help you—both your mind and your body. In addition, you may discover techniques and strategies of your own that work well for you. Support groups are excellent places to discuss and share these strategies.

To end this chapter, here's a thought to keep in your mind:

"Life is filled with suffering, but it is also filled with many wonders, like the
blue sky, the sunshine, the eyes of a baby. To suffer is not enough. We must also
be in touch with the wonders of life. They are within us and all around us,
everywhere, any time."

Thich Nhat Hanh, Zen Master

CHAPTER 15

Taking Control

This chapter is about self-empowerment. In this area, your education will be continuously ongoing, for life itself is an educational process. To be truly self-empowered you must learn to educate yourself and talk to your caregivers as peers. By so doing, you will reduce the pain and frustration of not communicating effectively and increase the probability of being completely understood. Good communication can also help to avoid patient and caregiver burnout and hostility, both of which result from misunderstandings.

It's important that you learn to take responsibility for your actions. You can't blame chance, or luck, or God, for the way things are. Consider the following sage reflection: It's a true statement, and if you act on its truth, you will gain a greater measure of control over your life.

"Your mind gives you control, the ability to have any reaction you want."

Deepak Chopra, M.D.

Working with Your Health Care Team

One of the first rules in choosing your health care team is to avoid situations in which the health care providers are a part of the problem—that is, you do not want to work with people who cause you to doubt yourself and who whittle away your self-esteem. For example, some caregivers want you to "keep quiet and just take orders," and they resent any education and/or questioning on your part. You don't need to fight that kind of attitude. You can communicate effectively by following the steps outlined below:

- Tell your team members that you want copies of all their reports.

- Learn to write everything down. Take detailed notes, or carry a tape recorder to your doctor's office and to therapy sessions. That way, you won't forget anything.

- Keep a daily journal. When you write in a journal every day, and read through your entries every few weeks, you will be able to chart patterns and see relationships that might otherwise escape your attention. (See Chapter 17, Keeping a Journal.)

Doctors, nurses, and therapists who are doing their job properly will not feel threatened by your interest and involvement. When you can precisely identify your needs, you have a much better chance of fulfilling those needs.

You'll want a primary care physician you can trust and who trusts you, whether that person is a Doctor of Medicine (M.D.), a Doctor of Osteopathy (D.O.), a Doctor of Chiropractic (D.C.), or a Doctor of Naturopathy (N.D.). You need a primary care doctor who not only believes that FMS, MPS, and FMS/MPS Complex exist, but who is also willing to stay current on new therapies and research, and to share that information with you.

You need a doctor who understands how to treat pain, and a pharmacist to match. If you have a chronic pain condition and no history of drug abuse, there's absolutely no reason you should be denied adequate medication for pain control. Taking medication to control pain does not turn you into a drug addict. If you are in pain, there is no reason to compound it by adding guilt. (See Chapter 9, Chronic Pain States: A Different Animal.)

> I am an M.D., but my primary physician is a chiropractor. I see my Internal Medicine specialist for the medications I need for the FMS/MPS and for advice when chiropractic methods are not enough. I have specialists to consult when needed. We all help each other keep up with new information concerning FMS/MPS Complex.
>
> D.J.S.

Taking Responsibility for Your Own Health

Taking responsibility for managing your own health care doesn't mean assuming the blame for your illness; it means orchestrating the progress you make toward achieving your optimum quality of life. It has been shown repeatedly that those who take charge of their own health care and reach out to others for advice, assistance, and support, are those who achieve the highest levels of wellness.

You have limited control over your external stressors, but you *can* learn to control how you react to stress. You can't control others, but you *can* be in better control of yourself, in spite of FMS, MPS, or FMS/MPS Complex symptoms, which include depression, mood swings, irritability, fatigue, spaciness, and short-term memory loss.

Have a Complete Physical Examination

It's important to have a complete physical evaluation and to address any problems that might be causing or aggravating your symptoms, such as hypothyroidism or anemia. (In this regard, you may wish to review Chapter 6, Coexisting Conditions and Chapter 7, Perpetuating Factors.) Remember, FMS/MPS Complex symptoms can be "triggered" by other physical problems, which your physician can detect and treat.

Educate Yourself

Learn all you can about FMS and FMS/MPS Complex. This will help you to make decisions and solve problems. If you are well-informed, you can ask your health care professionals the right questions. There are a number of resources that are available.

- Search medical libraries in your area. (You may not be able to check books out, but you can certainly review the information in the library. Make photocopies or take notes on the most pertinent information.) Often, if you have the book title and ISBN number, your local librarian can order the book for you through an interlibrary loan; then you can check it out to read at home.

- Attend related support groups, workshops, and conferences.

- Join national organizations so you can receive their newsletters and discover other informational resources. (See Appendix A, Resources.)

- Talk to other people who have FMS or FMS/MPS Complex. Often, they are the best sources for useful information.

If you have access to a computer, connect to the Internet for up-to-date information from all over the country. (See Appendix A, Agency Resources.)

- Consult with a variety of health care professionals who have expertise in working with patients with FMS or FMS/MPS Complex. Ask for advice on treatment scenarios. Explore these options thoroughly. Then, based on what you learn, begin whatever treatment you decide is in your best interest. Know which treatments you would want to begin if your symptoms get much worse. Be prepared to deal effectively with whatever happens.

Set Up an FMS or FMS/MPS Complex File

There is nothing more frustrating than needing a piece of information and not being able to find it. A section of a file drawer or a milk crate and some inexpensive manila folders are all that you need. Make a commitment to file all of the information that you acquire for easy access.

Set Up a Fibromyalgia Support Group

If there is no FMS, MPS, or FMS/MPS Complex support group in your area, consider starting one. (See Chapter 31, Building Your Support Structure.)

Set Up a Support Network

A support network of family members and friends can be invaluable to help you out when the going gets tough. Such a group can enrich your life in many other ways, too. (See Chapter 31, Building Your Support Structure.)

Set Realistic Goals

You can keep your goals realistic by educating yourself, accepting your diagnosis and symptoms, becoming involved, and knowing what your priorities are. Of course, one of the marvelous aspects of human nature is to reach for the stars, and we all should have dreams. Logically, however, you have a much better chance of success if you set out to pick a tomato from your garden.

Offer Alternatives

You have basic rights. Don't give them up. Don't overtax yourself. Some days people will want you to do too much. At such times, give them a choice: For example, "I can either go shopping or cook dinner. Which do you want?" is a perfectly sensible response when you know that too much exertion will drain your energy, cause stress, and possibly aggravate your symptoms.

It can be heartbreaking if you are a grandmother or grandfather, for example, and cannot pick up your little grandchildren. In a situation like this, be honest. Say, "I'm hurting today and can't pick you up. Come over to the sofa and you can sit in my lap. I'll tell you a story." This saves the day, as well as your back.

Avoid Digging Deeper Holes—No Smoking

Don't dig your hole any deeper than it already is. Smoking is a deadly habit, not only for you, but for those around you. Smoking is particularly bad for FMS and FMS/MPS Complex patients. The nicotine in cigarettes causes your blood vessels to constrict and decreases the flow of blood, oxygen, and nutrients to your muscles. This increases pain and muscle tension.

The carbon monoxide that enters your bloodstream via the smoke binds to the hemoglobin in your blood and decreases the amount of oxygen available to your muscles. Less oxygen means more pain. It's as simple as that. Smokers with FMS frequently see an impressive decrease in pain when they stop smoking (Pellegrino 1993).

In Times of Remission

To limit the recurrence of flare symptoms effectively, use the time when you are feeling well to take actions that will improve your chances for successful health care intervention in the future. Although we always hope that our symptoms will never recur, we increase our chances of dealing with them *effectively*, if and when they do recur, by doing some advance planning when our symptoms are in remission and by having our intervention systems in place.

Here are some actions you may be able to do easily during times of remission:

- Have a complete physical evaluation and address any problems that might be causing or aggravating your symptoms, such as hypothyroidism, hypoglycemia, or anemia. (See Chapter 6, Coexisting Conditions and Chapter 7, Perpetuating Factors.) Remember, FMS/MPS symptoms can be aggravated by other physical problems that your physician can detect and treat.

- Consult with a variety of health care professionals who are experienced in working with patients with FMS and FMS/MPS Complex. Ask them for advice on treatment scenarios. Explore these options thoroughly.

- Based on the information you have gathered from working with your health care professionals and your own research and experience, write a plan that describes what you will do if your symptoms get much worse. Update this plan as you obtain new information. Keep it in your FMS/MPS file for easy access.

- Begin attending a FMS/MPS Support Group. As stated earlier, if one does not exist in your area, consider starting one.

- Set up a support network of family members and friends who can help you out if and when the going gets tough.

Work on changing the habits that are not good for your health and on implementing strategies that will contribute to your overall wellness. Here are some of the things you can do:

- Make dietary adjustments (see Chapter 24, on Nutrition: Keep It Natural).

- Set up a regular exercise routine (see Chapter 27, Bodywork You Can Do Yourself).

- Keep a daily journal (see Chapter 16, Coping Day to Day, and Chapter 17, Keeping a Journal).

- Begin a mindwork program (see Chapter 20, Meditation and Mindfulness).

- Learn stress reduction and relaxation techniques (see Chapter 25, Bodywork—Helping Your Body Work).

- Learn to do peer counseling (see Chapter 31, Building Your Support Structure).

- Make needed career changes (see Chapter 33, The Workplace).

- Arrange for support services such as disability payments (see Chapter 34, Disability).

- Start seeing a therapist, if necessary, for advice and support.

- Make a commitment to yourself that you will do whatever you can to prevent a recurrence of flare (see Chapter 12, Flare).

- Write letters to politicians. The Fibromyalgia Network Advocacy Packet contains information about the basics of letter writing: what to say, and how to go about reaching your senators and representatives. Find out who in Congress is involved with the Health and Human Services, and Labor Committees. Write to them. Educate them. When you start out being an advocate for yourself, you end up being an advocate for us all.

The Self-Esteem Issue

How often have you thought, "If only I felt good about myself, I know I would feel so much better"? Low self-esteem and self-confidence are chronic, serious personal problems that exist in epidemic proportions in today's society.

Low self-esteem and lack of self-confidence have a variety of sources. Many of us tend to blame our parents. And, in fact, many parents who never learned good-parenting skills from *their* parents have contributed to this problem. We can all support parenting classes in our schools to help remedy this problem. There are, however, many other sources of low self-esteem in all sectors of our society. Some of these include educational institutions, the media, the workplace, social and religious institutions, peer relationships, personal relationships, and health care facilities. (And that's only a partial list.)

It is very important to recognize that chronic pain conditions also contribute to low self-esteem. Years of pain and fatigue that have obstructed meeting life goals can have a disastrous effect on self-esteem. Other factors that can arise as a direct result of chronic pain will also contribute to low self-esteem. Some of these are as follows:

- Inability to complete educational programs and meet educational goals

- Loss of jobs and career opportunities

- Unstable or failed relationships

- Estrangement from or poor relationships with family members

- Inability to be financially self-supporting

- Inability to take part in community activities

- Cognitive difficulties (fibrofog)

> One of the things I did when I found out that the vice-president of the United States had an e-mail address was to write to him, explaining a little about fibromyalgia and myofascial pain syndrome. I have also written the doctors in control of research monies at the National Institutes of Health. I really feel that we could save millions of taxpayer dollars by educating doctors—and the public—on these two conditions. It's a great project.
>
> D.J.S.

In chronic pain conditions, long-term inability to meet responsibilities worsens low self-esteem, which can lead to *depression*, which, in turn, can become a kind of chronic low-level stress that exacerbates the symptoms of FMS or FMS/MPS Complex.

Pinpointing Sources of Low Self-Esteem

To help pinpoint possible contributors to your feelings about your self-worth, ask yourself these questions:

- Is there anyone in your life right now who is feeding you negative, inappropriate messages about yourself?

- How do these messages make you feel?

- What are you going to do about it?

- What circumstances of your life have lowered your self-esteem and self-confidence?

- How valid were these circumstances as determinants of your worth?

Raising Self-Esteem

No one has the right to offer information or opinions that might have long-term negative impacts on another's self-esteem. Children, however, don't have the ability (or the power) to question the validity of negative, inappropriate messages that they receive about themselves. They tend to believe anything that is said to them, especially by their families and peers.

Raising self-esteem takes a long time and is often a very difficult process. Negative thoughts about ourselves, especially those that originated in childhood and were reinforced by others during adolescence, are deeply ingrained, and hard to dislodge. Nevertheless, the end result is worth any amount of hard work

Note: The methods described here for raising self-esteem and self-confidence are safe for anyone to use. However, to regain a positive sense of their own value, people who have been victims of physical, emotional, or sexual abuse, severe oppression, or violent crime may need the assistance of a counselor, or participation in a program designed for people with post-traumatic stress syndrome.

> I have been working at raising my self-esteem and self-confidence for many years. I find that when I am under a lot of physical and/or emotional stress, my self-esteem drops. I counter these drops in self-esteem by using the activities described in this chapter.
>
> M.E.C.

Achieving a Sense of Personal Worth

Our most difficult problem to overcome is often not pain but negativity. The antidote to a negative self-image is to have a strong sense of individual worth that does not depend on others or society for its existence. As a first step towards achieving a stronger sense of self-worth, ask yourself the following questions:

- How do you feel about yourself right now?

- How self-confident are you?

- How would you *like* to feel about yourself?

So often we tend to give someone else the power to determine how we feel about ourselves. We must not give away our personal power to anyone. We must not let anyone else define who we are. We must, in a very positive way, determine who we are and stick to our definitions.

To optimize the quality of your life, surround yourself with people who will affirm and validate you. They don't have to agree with everything you do, but they must respect your rights. It is often difficult for those with invisible chronic illnesses to find support among their families and friends. They may not believe that you are in pain and will dump guilt on top of your pain, if you permit this. That can lead to deeper feelings of unworthiness.

If people you associate with, including family members, friends, and colleagues, treat you badly, try to correct the situation by explaining the devastating consequences their comments and actions have on you. They may not realize the damage they are causing, and they may be able to change their behavior.

Using Affirmations

Learn to use affirmations, or positive statements. It is an easy way to help you stay on track in your treatment program. Here are some simple sentences that will help you to take control of yourself and your life. Repeat one or more of these affirmations to yourself whenever you need to assert your rights.

You may find it helpful to start each day by repeating one or more of these affirmations several times. You may want to write a few down, to repeat during your lunch hour or break time. They are also helpful to repeat when confronted with a negative influence. Once you get in the habit of using affirmations, they will become automatic.

- I am not a victim.

- I have no duty to be perfect.

- I always have options.

- If I can't decide which of two choices to pick, perhaps my choice should be something else.

- I have a right to make my own choices.

- I have a right to ignore the advice of others, even if I asked for that advice.

- Respecting other people's views doesn't mean I have to agree with them.

- My time is valuable too.

The best antidote to being affected by negative input is to have a clear picture of yourself and to value who you are. A strong self-image will enable you to judge for yourself whether there is any validity to what someone else says about you.

Create your very own affirmation statement. Read it over and over to yourself. Then, whenever you start thinking negative thoughts about yourself, repeat your statement; silently if you are with others, or aloud if you are alone. As you begin to feel better about yourself, you can update this description of your own worth and make it even more positive.

One woman who used to constantly tell herself "I'm no good" now replaces that thought by repeating a list of her good points. When she takes on too much at one time and berates herself because she can't get it all done, she counters her own negativity by doing a *little* of something each day.

The thought "I have no time to do anything I want" is countered with actually taking time out each day to do something she enjoys doing. The pleasure she takes in crafts, reading, or watching television, helps her to reinforce her own positive self-image.

Techniques for Improving Self-Esteem

There are other techniques you can use to reinforce positive thoughts and increase your self-esteem. Some of these are as follows:

- **Thought Stopping:** Every time a negative perception comes up, say to yourself, in a firm voice (or say it in your mind if you are with others) "cancel," "stop," "delete" or "go away"—use whatever phrase works best for you.

- **Meditation:** Relax your body using progressive relaxation techniques. Then repeat the positive thoughts while you are in this relaxed state. (See Chapter 20, Meditation and Mindfulness.)

- **Visualization:** Picture yourself feeling relaxed and happy. In your mind, run barefoot through a sunlit meadow. Laugh at the butterflies on the bright flowers. Form your own images and enjoy.

- **Journal Writing:** Use your journal as the place to change negative thoughts to positive ones. (See Chapter 17, Keeping a Journal.)

- **Signs:** Make signs to post around your home that display positive statements you have developed. (Paper stick-on signs are fine.) Read these aloud each time that you see them. If you stop "seeing" them, the way we all stop "seeing" the furniture and pictures that we live with, put up new signs.

- **Peer Counseling:** Get together with a friend you trust and describe the positive changes you are achieving. Then, give your friend a turn to describe the changes she or he is attempting to accomplish.

- **Counseling:** Regular meetings with a counselor you trust can help you raise your self-esteem and self-confidence, and strengthen your self-image in positive, life-affirming ways.

Note: Many of us find that when we articulate positive thoughts about ourselves, it brings up a great deal of emotion that requires an emotional release, usually crying. Expressing the emotion—such as allowing yourself to cry as much as you need to—will help to reinforce your positive thoughts.

Activities for Enhancing Your Self-Esteem

Use the following activities to give your self-esteem a boost. Incorporate one or several of these exercises into your daily schedule. They are particularly useful at those times when you are feeling very low or down on yourself.

- **Do something you enjoy.** Something that you know makes you feel better about yourself. (For example, fix something, clean your home, paint a picture, take a walk, play a musical instrument, sing, read a light novel, or go to a good movie.)

- **Do something that makes you laugh.** For example, watch a sitcom on TV, watch a funny video, read a comedy, get together with a friend who has a good sense of humor, and so on.

- **Do something nice for yourself.** For example, buy yourself some flowers. Light a candle. Give yourself a massage. Take an afternoon off to read a good book. Allow yourself time to watch a gorgeous sunset.

- **Do something special for someone else.** Read a child a story, shop for a sick friend, send an "I'm Thinking About You Card" to someone special, buy a friend an unexpected gift, or volunteer at the local hospital.

- **Pretend you are giving advice to your own best friend.** And take that advice yourself. Take better care of yourself, eat right, do something just for fun, give your body needed nourishment and care. You may even want to write a letter to yourself and tell yourself that you are a great person and you love yourself.

- **Make a list of your accomplishments in your journal.** List these accomplishments for a day, a week, a month, or your whole life. Don't leave things out and give yourself credit for whatever you have done. *Do not compare yourself to anyone else.*

- **Ask yourself what you need and figure out how you are going to get it.** Is it a better housing situation, better treatment on the job, help with chores from fa'mily members, more and better attention from health care professionals?

- **Learn to ask for what you want and need for yourself.** Advocate for yourself. Don't allow anyone to treat you badly. Don't allow yourself to be a victim!

- **Use subliminal tapes**. People with FMS or FMS/MPS Complex often respond to subliminal tapes. There are many helpful ones such as: "Positive Thinking," "Freedom from Guilt," "Stress Reduction," "Self-Confidence," "Dealing with Anger," and other related topics. (See Appendix A, Resources.)

In Conclusion

Like most learning processes, educating yourself about FMS and FMS/MPS Complex is an ongoing project. The more you know about your own health issues and the more control that you can exercise, the more your health care practitioners will be able to help you.

CHAPTER 16

Coping Day to Day

Do you ever feel that this is just a test life? If it were a *real* life, surely you would have been issued a lifetime-guaranteed working body and instructions on how to use it. At times, every day may seem to you to be an obstacle course—a perverse game you play where the rules keep changing and no one can tell you what they are.

One of your first tasks in learning how to cope on a day-to-day basis is to accept the fact that you have FMS and/or MPS. This is a major loss. Life as you once knew it is over—but a new one is beginning. In many ways, you can mold that life to be just as good as or even better than what you had. Here is a thought to consider: It is not enough to find enlightenment. When you find it, you must use it. This works for meditation. It works for life.

Rather than dwell on what has been lost, focus on optimizing the quality of your life. Learn to live in the present. Sir William Osler, one of my favorite quotable doctors in history, said that the best way to live to a healthy old age is to get a chronic disease and take care of it. Well, you've already done the first part, so let's get to work and tackle the second.

In this chapter you'll find some ideas to help you change your life and guide you along the way.

Minimizing Negative Influences in Day-to-Day Life

The natural grieving process will re-appear now and then, and you can expect occasional bouts with grief and frustration. But you can minimize negative influences by spacing and pacing. Space your tasks carefully, and pace yourself. Learn how to be a good manager of your daily activities. In this way you gain some measure of control over your life again.

Some days the constant grind of chronic pain will really get you down. You can take some small comfort in knowing that you're not alone. When you feel so low you could walk under a duck, be assured that there are many other people with FMS and FMS/MPS Complex right down there with you. When times are tough, be gentle with yourself.

Accept that whatever you can accomplish is deserving of recognition and praise. Those of us who have already run the first stages of the obstacle course are here to help you. This section will supply you with some tools to help remove some of the obstacles, minimize some others, and help you over the rest.

The Invisibility Issue

People with FMS/MPS usually do not appear to be ill. Their illness is "invisible." Others cannot recognize the pain you feel. One of the "fibropoets" on the Internet, Rita, has asked:

> "How many times have we faced the mirror, unable to fully comprehend how much our bodies have changed on the inside, since all outward appearances seem the same. . . . Perhaps, for that very reason, we continue to push, straining to accomplish the same tasks that were easily done five years, three, or even one year ago.
>
> "If our legs were twisted, our muscle bulk gravely diminished, or we were forced to use canes or wheelchairs, would we not be kinder, more understanding of our limitations? Certainly, those around us would be."

You may often find yourself angered because there is no way for others to know how much you are hurting, but you may also be failing to recognize (and honor) your own limits.

Coping with Mornings

Like most people with FMS/MPS, you probably have problems with mornings. "Fibrofog" envelops you. You can't remember things. Items you think you have a firm grip on go flying across the room. You may always have been a "morning person," but now your body and mind seem to be feuding, and every day you need to negotiate a truce before you can begin to function.

Some Simple Steps to Take the Night Before

You can make things easier for yourself in the morning by taking few simple steps:

- Start your morning the night before. Try to make a list of those things you want to accomplish the next day. Then, even if you're foggy in the morning, you can usually start in on something right away and give your mind a chance to catch up.

- Some days the best thing to do first is to go through the list and figure out what you can put off until another day!

- Set out your medications for the next day, especially vitamins. Put them in separate little containers—perhaps for morning, noon, and night. That way you'll never have to scramble under the bed for dropped pills, and you'll have to deal with only one set of pills in the morning.

- Set out your clothes the night before. That saves a lot of time because it's one less decision to make in the morning. You might want to put out one set of clothes and have an alternate set nearby in case you swell a size or two overnight or spill something on the first set.

- Prepare as much as possible for the next day so you can live that day as well as possible.

> I try to wear an old lab coat over my clothes when I eat, but sometimes I forget, and often I spill things more than once.
>
> D.J.S.

Starting the Day

As your day begins, survey what lies before you. Think of all the good things that can happen. Then do everything in your power to make them happen.

Plan on eating breakfast, and keep it simple. It is hard enough to move in the morning. Preparing a meal first thing may be more than you can handle. It could start your day off on a bad note. Collect easy, one-dish recipes.

Helping Yourself Through the Day

You'll encounter numerous obstacles during a normal day. Here are some things you can do about them:

- If you're feeling irritable, tackle a small task, or a portion of a task, that can be accomplished easily. Reaching the goal will cheer you up.

- Time, or your sense of it, is often one of your biggest stressors. Your hours are precious, but you may forget to use them as treasures. There will be days when you feel as if someone is behind you cracking a whip. Too often, the culprit is *you,* so scale down your expectations.

- Live in the present. The past is gone. You don't know what the future holds. Arrange priorities, simplify, delegate, delete. Allow time for *being* rather than *doing.* Don't live *for* today; just *live* today.

- Take a soothing bath.

- Call a friend you haven't seen for a while. Find a reason to laugh together.

- Schedule blocks of rest time for yourself. Acknowledge your limits. If at all possible, lie down for a few minutes at intervals throughout the day. Your muscles are constantly working to hold your head up, among other things; they deserve a rest.

- Go for a walk with a friend.

- At the end of the day, review what you have accomplished. Resting, physical therapy, and exercise are noteworthy accomplishments.

Handling Negative Events

If a negative event occurs during the course of the day, ask yourself some questions to help avoid these situations in the future:

- How could it have been prevented?

- Could it have been handled better?

- What positive way could it have happened?

- Try to visualize the event, but this time, modify the ending. Perhaps that's the way it will happen the next time.

Becoming Proactive

Become proactive, not reactive. Learn to use two hands to carry things. Don't carry heavy things. Be prepared for lots of spills. When your muscles frustrate you, don't dwell on it. Move on. Don't berate yourself for something you can't help. Your worst enemy isn't pain, and it isn't muscle weakness; it's negativity. Cultivate a sense of humor. Wear printed fabrics. (They don't show spills as much as solids do.) Use straws.

Vary your tasks so that you use different muscle groups. Slow your working pace. Listen to your body. Rest often. Cultivate a rhythm of movement. If you can, listen to music while you're at work. Don't fight your body, work with it.

Don't sit too long in any one position. When you drive, pull off the road every hour and walk around the car. Stretch. At home, use a rocker to prevent your muscles from building up electrical "load." When you must lift something, keep the load close to your body, and look up just before you lift. This tightens the long spinal muscles and prepares your back to lift.

When confronted by an annoying recurring task, stop and ask yourself these questions:

- Must it be done?

- If so, must *you* do it?

- If your answer to the preceding question is "yes," then ask: "Is there an easier way to do it?" If you can't think of any easier way, ask your friends, your family, or your support group. Someone will find a way.

Fine-Tuning Your Lifestyle: Turning Things Around

When you feel irritable and out of sorts with the world, you may have a tendency to blame FMS or FMS/MPS Complex for all the negativity that comes your way. You forget to explore the more mundane aspects of your life, your daily living habits, and ordinary activities.

People who have improved the quality of their lives while coping with FMS or FMS/MPS Complex have done so by taking a really close look at the way they live. Then, they directed their efforts to fine-tuning the details.

One of our local support group members had a rough time with the quality of medical support—or lack of same—that she was receiving. She successfully battled for Social Security Disability (no mean feat), found a medical team capable of giving her the care she needed and deserved, and worked on every aspect of her life to improve its quality. She is now the facilitator of an FMS Support Group. She isn't well enough to work, but she does help on a local hot line. She has also supplied a valuable "reality check" for this book. Clearly, this woman's life has value and meaning for her and for others.

> Since I have come to realize that every aspect of my existence affects my physical and mental vitality, and my ability to deal with my limits, the positive changes in my life have been amazing.
>
> M.E.C.

Another woman in the group was depressed because she was no longer well enough to do holiday baking for her family. But she took her depression and turned it around. She wrote out her cherished recipes, made copies, and made a family heirloom holiday present. Now, her offspring can bake family favorites for her.

We have group members who run in marathons and do downhill skiing. We have others who need canes to get around some of the time, but they get around all the same. They have all improved their quality of life.

Dr. Janet Travell described one patient in her autobiography, *Office Hours Day and Night* (1968), whose example may be useful to many of us. Dr. Travell had successfully treated the worst trigger points (TrPs) that had been afflicting this man, but a short time later he appeared at her office with another list of medical complaints. She asked him why these symptoms hadn't been mentioned with the previous ones, as they were not new. His response was that he "had raised his standards of comfort." Janet Travell asks those of us with FMS/MPS to do the same. For those of us with MPS, she and her partner, David Simons, have made this task possible.

Take time during the day to involve yourself in activities you enjoy. These are the activities in which you become so engaged that you can think of nothing else. Be careful not to forget how good doing them makes you feel. There is always something you can do to allow yourself to feel better. Here's a list of suggested activities:

- Gaze at a pleasant view.

- Read a joke book or a good novel.

- Garden.

- Work with clay.

- Work with wood.

- Write.

- Visit art galleries or museums.

- Play with children.

- Play with pets.

- Cook.

- Play games.

- Watch videos.

Doing things that you love to do helps to prevent those episodes of FMS/MPS called flares, when all your symptoms get worse.

Spend some time thinking about the activities that you enjoy doing. You may want to discuss this with a friend or family members who can help you recall things you enjoyed doing in the past that you may have forgotten. At the same time, be mindful of your limits. Although it is good to stretch your limits periodically, don't set yourself up for activities that are beyond your functioning *today*. You may be able to enjoy them in the future.

Cultivating a Sense Of Humor

Researchers have found that one of the least expensive treatments for pent-up anxiety, fear, and frustration is a hearty laugh. Laughter affects the respiratory system, filling the lungs with air over and over and providing pulmonary ventilation. It also has cardiac effects, increasing the heart rate in direct proportion to the duration of the laughter. The heart rate then drops below the level of the pre-laughter period. Initially, laughter increases both the systolic and the diastolic blood pressure, but afterwards, there is a drop in pressure below the pre-laughter levels. A hearty belly laugh results in almost total body relaxation.

A sense of humor is an invaluable survival trait. The fibrom-l Internet support group is rich with humor. It's hard to tell the feelings behind the electronic words, so we often use "smilies," those little sideways smile faces to indicate that the words are said in jest:

:-)

There are many kinds of smilies. To indicate we are LOL (laughing out loud) we use this:

:-D

Lynn Johnston, creator of the wonderful Canadian comic strip, *For Better or Worse*, spoke through her characters to remark, "If life's a journey, the bags sure get heavy sometimes! Ah—but laughter's the porter who helps us to carry them." Well said.

> I found that there were activities I had stopped doing long ago, such as playing the piano and sewing, that really make me feel good. In the "busyness" of life, including raising children and developing a career, those activities had been forgotten. Now, they are now part of my wellness toolbox. If I am sad or stressed, perhaps experiencing early warning signs of an approaching flare, I make sure to spend some time involved in such an activity. It makes me feel better and my life feels enriched.
>
> M.E.C.

Study volunteers overwhelmingly concurred that laughter makes them feel better. Sometimes finding something to laugh about is difficult. Some of their laugh instigators include: comic strips, jokes, puns, certain movies and videos, and good comedians.

Water

Many community-based recreational centers, motels, and Y's allow easy, inexpensive access to water facilities. Check area pools for temperature. (Note that a cool pool can cause cramping in MPS.) A range of 88 to 94 degrees is optimum for people with FMS or FMS/MPS Complex. Avoid doing the breaststroke and the crawl, as they tend to load the muscles. Repetitious laps may not be best for you. Start slowly, for brief periods of time, and build up gradually.

You don't have to go to a pool or buy a spa membership to enjoy the benefits of water. Your own bath tub or shower can suffice. Inexpensive whirlpool units can give you a sense of luxury and provide plenty of relaxation in your own tub.

Note: Like many people with FMS or FMS/MPS Complex, you may have been told to take a hot bath when you were feeling agitated or achy. However, studies have shown that long baths and very hot baths can have a negative effect on some people with FMS/MPS. You may feel totally exhausted after a long bath, in which case try limiting your bath to 20 minutes or less. Water has a calming, relaxing quality, but each of us has to find out what duration works best. Also, using Epsom salts in the bath may help relieve some of the swollen feeling we sometimes have.

> Whenever I see a comic strip that provokes a good laugh, I cut it out. I have a huge notebook of comics and jokes, waiting for me whenever I'm feeling down. I make it a point to watch several British comedies on television. I get at least several good laughs out of them. The comic strips *Calvin and Hobbes*, *For Better or Worse*, and *Doonesbury* tickle my laughter palate.
>
> D.J.S.

Color

Many people with FMS/MPS find that the colors they use when decorating their homes, choosing the clothes they wear, and arranging the things they look at, have a strong effect on their moods. Our heightened sensitivity can work for us.

Choices of color are very personal. Some days you may be able to wear certain colors, and other days you may feel uncomfortable in them.

When you are buying yourself new clothes, focus on the colors that make you feel good. They are your "comfort" colors. If you are having a day when you feel down, wear these colors. It will help perk you up. Every time you look in the mirror, it will give you a lift.

When decorating your own space, use your comfort colors. If you are living in a space where the colors make you feel down, and you can't afford to redecorate, try some inexpensive alternatives. A can of paint for a wall or two, or a coverlet from a rummage sale, can make a big

> I know that a very light shade of pink, almost a white with just a little red coloring added to it, has a very soothing effect on me. I painted all the walls this color in an apartment I rented. It felt great and it had a positive effect on my moods.
>
> M.E.C.

difference. If your workspace is being redecorated, make your color preferences known. Let your employer know the colors that make you feel best.

Music

Most of us find music relaxing. Of course, which kind of music varies according to personal preference. Music is evocative. It touches your feelings, and can change your mood. Use this to your advantage. Whatever the music, it needs to be something you like. If you don't like it, it can increase tension and stress.

Listen to soft, gentle, soothing but upbeat music when times are tough. Avoid "heavy" music with depressing themes. (This also goes for books, videos, and guests.)

Ask yourself what kinds of music please you. Go through your album collection and make a note of those pieces that make you feel more relaxed and peaceful. You may want to combine these selections on one tape for use when you are feeling down or stressed.

Keeping a Journal

People have kept diaries and written accounts of activities, events, and feelings since writing was invented. Recently, the power of this tool has become evident for dealing with various kinds of chronic pain conditions. You have only to look to the popularity of workbook-style self-help books to become aware of the value of writing for releasing pent up emotions and for helping people find solutions to their problems. Because keeping a journal is such an important tool, we have devoted all of Chapter 17 to this subject.

In Conclusion

The challenges of day-to-day life can seem to be insurmountable if you have FMS, MPS, or FMS/MPS Complex. By planning ahead to pace yourself and by adding healing elements to your daily routine—color, water, music, journal-writing—you can cut the problems of everyday living down to size.

CHAPTER 17

Keeping a Journal

Keeping a journal is a way for those who find it difficult to talk to others to create a dialogue with themselves. Too often people with chronic invisible illnesses are misunderstood and/or not believed by others; this failure of communication is a form of invalidation. We suffer not only from loss of self-esteem but also from loss of our sense of "self."

To block the hurts, we not only become progressively numb, we also erect walls in self-defense. These walls become effective barriers to communication, keeping out all others. In time, the walls become thick enough and strong enough to keep out even ourselves.

The Value of Journal Keeping

Keeping a journal is a way of regaining contact with our inner selves. In addition, many people find when they began putting their thoughts down on paper, that communication of other kinds becomes easier.

Writing your thoughts and organizing them can bring order out of confusion or chaos. When your thoughts are constantly racing around in your head and the same negative ideas are repeating over and over, like a record stuck in the same groove, you get the most devastating type of negative reinforcement. You become your own worst enemy.

You will find that putting your thoughts down on paper will enable you to sort and examine your ideas and feelings, and to put a little distance between them and yourself. Doing this can help silence the inner negative dialogue and give you a greater measure of control over your life. The power of the written word should never be underestimated. When you write, you use your eyes and your sense of touch to create another way to get to know yourself.

Once you have written out what you are thinking, you can more easily arrive at new and more positive conclusions. The deep inner exploration and evaluation that keeping a journal encourages can be an invaluable asset for coping with FMS or FMS/MPS Complex in positive ways.

The Value of a Record

Furthermore, when you keep a journal, it provides a record of your daily life that can be useful when you want to search for behavior patterns that may have contributed to stress. For, as you know, stress is a major factor in FMS/MPS flares. Sometimes, in the "dailiness" of life, we fail to see what our obvious patterns are until we reread a week's, a month's, or a year's worth of journal entries.

Note: It is a good idea to reread your journal entries at least once every few months and to think about what you wrote. You get a chance to experience detachment from your emotions, and you can gain a new perspective that only the passage of time allows.

Dealing with Negative Emotions

Deepak Chopra says that an intimate relationship is one that allows you to be yourself. The most intimate relationship you can have is with yourself. A journal is a safe place. Think of it as a completely trusted friend. It offers a safe way to deal with negative emotions. The pain, rage, or fear that you might be unable to express to another human being can be expressed on paper, and the act of writing can have various effects.

For example, you may find the act of writing cathartic and, somehow, when you have finished writing, the negative emotions may have lost some of their intensity and some of their ability to make you unhappy may be diminished. Or you may be able to think more clearly, or to think new thoughts, and you may gain a broader perspective. You may also find that solutions for problems that once seemed insoluble will present themselves in the course of keeping a journal.

All of us have old emotional wounds that seem to have healed over, but internally infections may be festering, keeping the process of grieving from ending. A journal can be like a drain in an infected wound, allowing the negative emotions of the past to seep away, so that the true healing can begin.

You may find that you are keeping only a record of symptoms, medications, therapies, and so forth, but that record may be of great value to you some time down the road, especially if you are searching for patterns that may have contributed to stress or flare.

Keeping a journal is also a safe place to record your hopes, dreams, and ambitions. Ideas that might seem too silly, or daring, or ambitious to speak out loud can all be entered safely in a journal and, sometimes, when they are written down they begin to seem possible. Then, ways to turn them into reality may occur to you, and you can begin to make plans for turning dreams into facts.

If you haven't already started a journal, you may want to start one soon. If you are unsure where to start, you can begin with a simple record of symptoms, medications, treatments, and therapies. Write down what works for you, and what doesn't. Tell your journal which treatment elements affect what symptoms. It is also a good place to record and store any notes you take at your support groups.

What Journal Writers Have to Say

Here is what some journal writers have to say about the value of keeping a journal:

- "Journal writing leaves a trail of my thinking/reflections for me to return to."

- "My journal has helped me get over my addiction to food. When I feel like munching and I know I have had plenty to eat, I write in my journal instead of eating."

- "My journal is safe place to let go of feelings I can't vent in other ways."

- "I use journal writing in my wellness program. It allows me to let go of the day's stresses. I begin by writing whatever thought comes first, and then I write how I feel. Not just about the thought, but how I *feel* about how I feel. I go on from there, writing everything that comes to my head."

If You Already Keep a Journal

It may be that you already keep a journal. If so, examining your past experiences in keeping your journal can help you decide what kinds of things you should record. You may want to change its focus, or modify it to include more of your impressions. You may want to keep two journals. One could be more like a daybook to record medications and symptoms, and the other could be more like a diary of feelings.

What You Need to Begin Keeping a Journal

One person said about keeping a journal, "It's the cheapest kind of therapy. All you need is paper and something to write with, and a place to keep your journal (a safe, private space—like the bottom of your underwear drawer or a high shelf that is inaccessible to others in your household.). Other people in your household should respect your right to a private journal."

If you live alone, you may want to keep your journal on your nightstand for easy accessibility for those times when you wake in the middle of the night and want to record your dreams or night thoughts. You might want to record any thoughts that may be contributing to your wakefulness.

I have kept an ongoing journal since I was a child. I have written on everything from the back of junk mail to lovely, clothbound diaries. My journal is my best friend. It has seen me through the worst and the best of times.

Most of my recent writings are on the computer. I print them out and keep them in a folder. My "journals" are stacked on a shelf in my closet. Sometimes I write daily. At other times, I take a vacation of several months from journal writing. When I feel drawn to my journal, I pick up the pen again (or I sit down at the computer) and begin. At 53, I look back, impressed with all the writing I have done and how my life has changed over the years, and I realize how important this tool is to me.

M.E.C.

> I have often kept my journal beside my bed. Sometimes, when I can't sleep I write in it. I wake up during the night and write and write. Soon I get tired and go back to sleep. In the years that I've done this, I've worked through some very important issues. It has been a very effective tool for healing myself.
>
> M.E.C.

If the privacy of your journal cannot be assured, you may want a trusted friend to keep your journal for you. If it is stored elsewhere, a three-ring binder might work best. Keep a supply of paper on hand and write when you feel like it; then take the pages to your friend at another time.

In terms of the paper you use, use whatever is available and feels right to you. Choices range from the backs of old envelopes and mail to simple pads of paper, to computer paper, to spiral notebooks, to bound journals with fancy covers. (Many people like to honor their journal keeping by purchasing a specially made bound notebook with an attractive cover.)

You may have trigger points (TrPs) (see Chapter 3, Myofascial Trigger Points) that make writing painful and/or difficult. Talk to your physical therapist and doctor about relieving this problem. Often, a spiral notebook and a soft (No. 2) pencil or a felt-tipped pen make writing physically easier.

Rules for Journal Keeping

Journal keeping rules are easy. *There are none.* All you need to do is get some paper and a writing tool and start to write. Write anything you want; anything you feel. It doesn't have to make sense. It doesn't even have to be real. It doesn't need to be interesting. It's all right to repeat yourself over and over. Whatever is written is for your eyes and your use only. This is yours. This is your private kingdom.

Deepak Chopra says to accept what comes to you totally and completely, so that you can appreciate it, learn from it, and then let it go. He was talking about meditation, but, in a way, keeping a journal is a form of meditation.

Many journal keepers have said something along these lines: "I can express any emotion I want while writing, without being criticized or judged. I can rant and rave and carry on like a two-year-old child having a tantrum if I feel like it, or I can express hopes and desires that I wouldn't dare share with anyone else."

> I have a fantasy of a very large journal, perhaps three-feet high and two-feet long, in which I could write to my heart's content while lying on my belly on the floor.
>
> M.E.C.

You don't have to worry about punctuation, grammar, spelling, penmanship, neatness, or staying on the lines. (You don't even have to used lined paper if you don't want to.) You can scribble all over the page if that makes you feel better. (Ferocious scribbling can be a wonderful way to get rid of tension.)

The privacy of the journal should not be violated. Choosing to share your writings is a personal choice. You don't have to share what you have written with anyone unless you want to. Some people find it helpful and feel comfortable sharing some of their journal entries with family members, friends, or health care professionals. Other people never let anyone see a line they have written. Again, this is your personal choice. You have the right to change your mind anytime you wish.

The Time to Write

For some of us, it helps to set aside a time every day for journal keeping, for instance, early in the morning or before going to sleep at night, but it is not necessary. Spend as little or as much time writing as you want. Some people even like to set a timer. It is easy to get lost in your journal, but that's OK, too.

You can make entries in your journal at any time—daily, several times a day, weekly, before you go to bed, when you wake up, after supper, whenever you feel like it—the choice is yours.

You don't have to make a commitment to keeping a journal for the rest of your life—just when you feel like it.

You can write at any speed you want, fast or slow. You can write as much or as little as you want.

You can write poems, paragraphs, comic verses, novels, novellas, political rants, your autobiography, someone else's biography, wishes, letters, fantasies, dreams, beliefs, loves, and hates. Your entries can be similar each time, or they can be very different.

Suggestions for Keeping a Journal

Although there are no rules to follow, here are some suggestions to help you on your way.

- Write your name, address, and phone number inside the front cover if you plan to carry your journal with you. Add a statement, something like this: "This contains private information. Please do not read it without my permission. Thank you!"

- Some people like to take a quiet moment to ground themselves before starting to write. You can do this by taking several deep breaths and then focusing on something pleasant for a moment or two, such as a flower, a pet, or the view outside your window. You might want to take a warm bath or go for a short walk—whatever quiets you down. You might wish to note what you used for this "centering," or have a page in the beginning of the journal that lists your favorite methods of grounding or centering your focus before you begin to write in your journal.

- Claim a quiet space to do your journal writing. Turn off the phone, and ask others to respect your need for quiet and privacy. Parents may choose to make journal entries

> Writing is very painful for me. Using the computer is somewhat better. It isn't that much less painful, but it is much more legible. I find that both are made easier by the use of Hand-eze hand supports and frequent breaks.
>
> I use a notebook for passing thoughts and impressions and the computer for longer journal entries—like the letters I write that I don't intend to mail. I have written to God, long-dead relatives and friends, and to famous people (living or dead) with whom I will never have an opportunity to converse. I get a chance to tell my story, and everyone needs that.
>
> D.J.S.

when the baby is napping, the children are in school, or after the children have gone to bed.

- You can choose a special place in your home that you decorate the way you like and reserve for journal writing. Lighting candles may feel good. Writing outside sitting under a big special tree or on the beach in the warm sunshine also feels good, and can be liberating.

- Consider journal writing while you are listening to your favorite music.

- Date your entries if you wish. Dated entries do help to keep things in perspective when you review what you have written over time, and they also help to pinpoint patterns if you are looking for them.

- Don't fix your mistakes. Just keep writing. Remember, spelling, grammar, handwriting, and style do not matter.

- Draw or paste pictures or words into your journal. Doodle. Making images can be very helpful for loosening up when you are feeling stressed.

- Don't think too much about what you are writing; just let the writing flow.

Goals for Keeping Journals

If you are thinking about using a journal as one of your strategies for staying well, you may want to write down some goals to get started. This could be done in your first journal-keeping session.

There are many, many reasons to keep a journal. Here are some possibilities:

- To understand why you go into flare

- To track treatment effects and mood changes

- To work on issues that have been getting in the way of healing

- To help understand life issues that affect your health

- To guide you on a journey to wellness

- To enhance your understanding of yourself

- To help in achieving life goals

- To get to know yourself better

- To write your own personal history

- To keep a record of counseling, peer counseling sessions, or other activities

> I choose to keep my journal writings. Many people do. Others discard them. I have a friend who burned all her old journals because she said she needed to start anew.
>
> M.E.C.

- To improve your relationships

- To get over a failed relationship

- To grieve a loss

- To assist in problem solving

- To develop spontaneity

- To gain a deeper understanding of issues

- To gain a deeper understanding of others

- To explore dreams

- To pinpoint and address stressors

- To get in touch with feelings

- To become more comfortable communicating

- To explore different aspects of your personality—different parts of yourself

- To discover the good things in your life

- To keep track of life changes and growth

- To tie up loose ends

- To work through feelings safely

- To explore creativity and enhance creativity

- To re-evaluate beliefs and behaviors

Getting Started on Your Journal

If you are still having a hard time starting to keep a journal, some of these suggestions may be helpful:

1. Write a letter to someone you would like to call names but it would not be a wise thing to do. Do the same for someone who is not available or deceased.

2. Write a letter to yourself, pretending you are your own best friend, and tell yourself why you like yourself so much. Mention how your day went, and what tomorrow holds for you.

3. List the best things that have happened this day (month, year) in your life.

4. Describe the worst thing that ever happened to you.

5. Make a list of all the reasons that cause you to want to be alive. Include the little things, as well as the large things, that make your life worth living.

6. Write five things you need to do today (or tomorrow if you write at night) and how you feel about doing them.

7. Take an inventory of your life.

8. Write your own prayer.

9. Write yourself a question and then answer it.

10. Describe your ideal place to live or work.

11. Describe what you would do if you had one day left to live.

12. Describe yourself.

13. Describe someone else.

14. Describe a special moment.

15. Write a dialogue with another person, event, or thing.

16. Have a dialogue with a part of your body.

17. Have a dialogue with a famous person.

18. Make lists: things you want to do in your life, why you like yourself, why you like someone else, why you feel stressed, what you fear, reasons to stay with your partner, reasons to have a child, reasons not to have a child, what have you lost, things to do when in flare, things you would never do again, what makes you laugh, what makes you cry, what makes you happy, what makes you sad, who are your favorite people.

In Conclusion

Keeping a journal provides you with an excellent opportunity to learn more about yourself and also helps you to communicate better with others. Your journal can take any form you wish, and there are no limits to what you can record there. If you define some goals before starting a journal, they will guide you along the way.

CHAPTER 18

Fibrofog and Other Absurdities

FMS/MPS Complex has been described as the "irritable everything" syndrome. However, one of the most frustrating, and possibly the most disabling, of the many symptoms of FMS/MPS Complex is a cognitive deficit we have aptly, but not affectionately, termed *fibrofog*.

What Is Fibrofog?

Perhaps you psych yourself up to go to the grocery and arrive only to discover you've forgotten your wallet. You return home, retrieve the wallet, and set out again. After you reach the store, you realize you've left your shopping list and coupons at home. Once again, you return home, all the while berating yourself for your forgetfulness and stupidity. You search and search, but no list can be found. By now, you're too exhausted to shop. Tomorrow, you probably will find the list under the car seat, or used as a bookmark.

Steam irons get stored in the refrigerator. Freshly made milk drinks go on a shelf, where they silently turn into a dismal green mold. You transpose letters when you write and you do the same with figures when you are trying to balance your checkbook. Some days, you can't even put a coherent sentence together. The words rattle around in your mouth and don't seem to connect coherently to the ideas in your head.

This mental state of utter confusion can last for hours, weeks, or, especially in a period of magnified symptoms called a *flare,* even for months. Fibrofog is a condition way beyond any usual confused states of mind or any other cognitive impairments. Many people have lost their jobs or have had to drop out of school because of the extreme nature of the flare/fibrofog combination. It is one of the least recognized and most serious symptoms of FMS or FMS/MPS Complex.

I've gotten lost in my own house. Our home is small, and most of it is one large room used as the combined kitchen, dining, and living area. There is only one bedroom and one bath.

I am a member of Mensa, which means that my IQ places me in the top two percent of the nation's intelligent folks. But life sure gets complicated when the fog rolls in, and it doesn't matter how small the house is or how smart I am, I can still get lost. And I feel pretty stupid about it.

D.J.S.

Sometimes getting up is just the first obstacle of the day. It's not unusual for people with FMS/MPS Complex to fall down when trying to take their first steps in the morning. If the dizziness doesn't get to you, the foot pain, buckling knee, weak ankle, or *something* will. And all of these symptoms are compounded and magnified by fibrofog. Worst of all is that often you forget to do the things you normally do to minimize the physical symptoms, and that plus the additional stress brought about by fibrofog can lead to a flare.

Fibrofog frustration is compounded by the fact that when you're experiencing it, you can't express yourself well. However eloquent you are at other times, you may be incapable of putting together a coherent sentence. You can even stutter as you vainly grasp for the right words.

You are left vulnerable by your scrambled psyche, and the slings and arrows of an uncaring world zip right through your crumbling defenses. You have lost control, and you can't explain why. Often, people experiencing fibrofog take a hefty amount of unintentional abuse from other people who are unaware of their confused state of mind and/or the reason behind it.

One of the Internet "FMily" describes fibrofog this way: "It's like walking down the hall of my mind, on my way to retrieve a piece of information. I know I have to go to a certain room in the house of my mind. But when I get into the room, either the box with the information is not there or I have forgotten which box I was looking for. So I wander around looking for it in the other rooms, until I get tired and give up."

Another person described it this way: "Why isn't whatever I'm looking for where I thought I put it? My scientific brain calls it the time when all constants become variables. With fibrofog you're in a game where the rules keep changing, and nobody tells you what they are. Life is passing you by, you have your nose pressed to the window, you look in with longing but you are unable to join in the action."

You may find that these mental aspects of FMS/MPS Complex are the most disruptive of all the symptoms. Perhaps you can deal with the pain effectively, but you want your brain back.

One person wrote, "Sometimes I feel like my body is just a shell, and I'm only dust inside. And I can't get out." That's heavy-duty fibrofog. (See the section "Depression" in Chapter 19, Positive Change, for some ideas on what to do when fibrofog gets to be this stressful.)

One of the most frustrating aspects of fibrofog is that it often drifts in slowly. It creeps up on little cat feet, and you may be too fog-benumbed to be aware that you are in the fog state of confusion. (That can also happen with flare, too. It can sneak up on you.)

Note: If fog and flare have ever combined to cause a condition in which you are not capable of making decisions for yourself, you need to be prepared for such an event recurring. See Chapter 12, Flare, for some ideas on preparing for such an occurrence.

Fog Formation

There are probably many factors that contribute to the symptoms of fibrofog. In the July 1995 edition of the *Fibromyalgia Network Newsletter*, Drs. Daniel Clauw and Jay Goldstein reported that cognitive symptoms generally parallel other symptoms in severity. During flare, the fibrofog may be extreme. Increased sleeplessness caused by increased pain may result in more "fog."

There is a fairly new bit of electromagnetic technology called a *SPECT scan*. It has been reported that SPECT scans show that people with FMS have a decreased blood flow in the right caudate nucleus of the brain, as well as in the left and right thalami (*Fibromyalgia Network Newsletter* January 1995). This decreased blood flow could be caused by neurotransmitter dysfunction, or by a problem in the equivalent of myofascia in that area of the brain. This equivalent is called the glial cell.

Fibrofog and Yeast

There have been many instances where fibrofog has been brought on by water retention. One of the worst culprits in this matter is yeast (and the sugar that feeds it). Dr. Wayne London (1994) has described the mood swings, irritability, poor concentration, spaciness, and forgetfulness that can be caused by a yeast overload. He also mentions fatigue, muscle weakness, intestinal symptoms, immune dysfunction, and menstrual irregularities that can be brought about by yeast. (See the section on the "yeast beast" later in this chapter.)

If you keep a journal, it may give you some clues to the origin of your fibrofog. If you are undergoing a period of extreme stress, examine the possibility that your confusion is caused by stress, depression (see Chapter 19, Positive Change), lack of sleep (see Chapter 10, Sleep), or approaching flare (see Chapter 12, Flare).

> There are days when I have to read a paragraph several times before I can remember it, and even then it won't stay in my mind. Sometimes, I can't tell if a book is one that I've already read or not. The good librarians at Brooks Memorial Library know the sound of my voice. I swear there must be an alarm that sounds whenever I get near the Reference Librarian's desk. The library is used to my odd requests, especially when I'm researching science fiction, and they are aware that I am sometimes in a fog. (This is a common occurrence with many writers, though, so they may not attribute it to the FMS/MPS Complex.)
>
> D.J.S.

Cutting Through the Fog

Try creating a greater degree of organization in your life; although it won't eliminate the problem, it will help you to navigate through the fog. It's a good idea to use lists a lot. For example, instead of suffering through the expense of forgetting something important on a business trip, you can make lists of the things you need to take with you and tape those lists to the back of the office and/or bathroom door. (Then, the trick is to remember to check the lists!)

There is some thought (admittedly, mostly by me) that the glial cells of the nervous system could be involved the same way the myofascial cells are in MPS or FMS/MPS Complex. Glial cells form a tough support, and they maintain the elastic framework of the nervous tissue, much in the way the myofascia does for the muscles (Juhan 1987). (Note that this connection is purely speculative.)

D.J.S.

You can train yourself to stop and review what you have to do and where you have to go before you leave home. That way you sometimes can remember anything you might have forgotten.

Try going through files, drawers, and closets regularly to get rid of unneeded clutter that just frustrates you, with the goal of keeping things simple and pared down to essentials.

Things to Do for Fibrofog

You can take some immediate steps to avoid repeating fog-induced misery. For example, if you are always losing your personal phone book, try using a hole punch and hanging up the book near the phone. If you forget your coupons, salvage some of your annoying junk mail—the reply envelopes. Then write the shopping list on the outside of the envelope, and put a large paper clip to hold a pencil and the coupons inside the envelope. You use the pencil to strike out the items as you pick them up. That way, you won't forget to buy what you need. Mostly. . . .

If you're in a severe fog, don't drive. Keep extra food and other necessities in the basement or another safe place. Make plans for a "foggy" day, as well as for a rainy day. When you know you are going to be overstressing your body, keep a careful watch on your limits. Schedule extra mind and bodywork when you know you will experience a great deal of stress.

Perhaps you've discovered that you can no longer trust yourself to write checks. For example, you may forget to enter checks that you wrote into your checkbook ledger, or you may enter them in the ledger and then forget to write them, or to send them. If you are working with figures, be sure to recheck your calculations several times. Even if you use a calculator, you may sometimes reverse numbers when you're entering them. If you can afford it, consider hiring a bookkeeper to handle your financial record-keeping. If your resources are limited, perhaps you can work out a trade with a family member or a friend—a pot of soup, a loaf of bread, or a few hours of childcare in exchange for bookkeeping services.

Try to minimize tasks that can be affected by fibrofog. For example, buy many pairs of identical socks to go with your clothes. They will be easy to match and they will last longer. When one wears out, the mate can be matched with another lonely sock. (Better yet, suggest to family or friends that such socks would make perfect birthday or holiday gifts for you.)

To avoid spelling problems, make good use of the spell checker on your computer, if you have one. If you are using a typewriter, ask a family member or friend to proofread important documents.

My dog, who travels with me locally, understands that once I have him loaded in the car, I am going to go back inside at least once before we finally leave.

M.E.C.

At times, you may need to decrease your sensory input (noise, lights, interruptions) and give your body/mind system a chance to restore communications links. Sometimes decreasing sensory input helps. That's one of the reasons we often need to turn off the radio in a car. It's easier to concentrate on our driving with less distraction.

> I have a self-imposed rule. Anything I buy at a garage sale must be matched by something I take to the garage sale from my own things. This kind of exchange helps to keep the clutter down, and allows life to be more manageable, even during foggy times.
>
> D.J. S.

Singing in the Rain, Laughing in the Fog

It can be a great challenge to keep your sense of humor during episodes of fibrofog. On the Internet, the fibrom-l family delights in sharing fog stories. Here is one of them:

I was going through a massive fog and I was in flare, and, as usual in such times, all the electromagnetic devices in our home went berserk as soon as I approached them. This included our trusty Gateway computer, 'The Millennium Grosbeak.' It decided I shouldn't access the support group during my time of need, and I was challenging that decision.

My friend and fellow writer and FMily member, Miryam, was helping me to regain access. I sent a message to the group: "'This is a test message.' Or so I thought."

At this time, unbeknownst to me, the FMily had been having a discussion on fibrocystic breasts and FMS. Everyone knew I was having problems with flare and with the computer. So when Miryam returned my message as I'd actually written it—'This is a teat message'—and explained the recent topic on the Internet, I laughed so hard I cried. Seeing the unintentional humor in the mistake really helped me get through that stressful time.

Another typical fibrom-l (Internet) exchange concerned a serious topic between one of our laypeople and a medical team member:

Medical team member: "It is possible to have permanent damage if you let it go on too long."

Layperson: "What should I do about it?"

Medical team member: "You should see a neurologist."

Layperson: "I'm sorry. I know this is serious, but the thought of looking at a neurologist and it helping just made me chuckle. I knew looks can kill, but now looks can heal?"

Another story concerns a man who was having vision problems. He mentioned to a friend that everywhere he looked, he saw spots. The friend asked, "Did you see a doctor?"

"No, only spots," the man replied.

We laugh a lot on the fibrom-l and in the local support group. It's a survival trait.

The Yeast Beast

Many people with FMS are beset by the "yeast beast." Women and men can be attacked by one candida infection after another. Many of these people crave sugar and retain water, which compounds their yeast misery.

At one time, it was not unusual for me to drop ten pounds in a few days on an anti-yeast regimen. When I am on a systemic antifungal medication and low carbohydrate diet, my kidneys can excrete the excess water from my body. This decreases brain cellular swelling, and the fog clears. If I have been subjected to a lot of mold, I can often react with fibrofog. An allergy shot will often clear the fog for me.

D.J. S.

Taking a course of antibiotics is begging the yeast beast to come for a visit. This can be prevented by using antibiotics only when absolutely necessary, and taking the antifungal medication, Nystatin, along with the antibiotics. Nystatin is a prescription medication that kills yeast only in the gastrointestinal tract. That means that it won't do anything for an established systemic yeast infection, but it will usually prevent a yeast infection from beginning in your intestines. A yeast infection usually spreads to the vaginal and anal areas from the intestines.

For more about this nasty beastie, let's turn to Camilla Cracciolo, R.N., one of our medical team FMily members on the Internet, who kindly provided the following information.

Signs of the Yeast Beast

The symptoms that can indicate a yeast problem include water retention, throat irritation, tingling of fingers, irritated bladder and bowel, bloating and gas, body thermostat dysfunction, swollen (crowded) glands, itching and discharge, and muscle pain. Yeast also increases irritable bladder complaints.

The yeast normally found in the vagina is *candida albicans*, once called monilia. Yeast overgrowth causes vaginal discharge, itching and burning, although pain can often be the sign of bacterial infection. Yeast overgrowth often comes from using antibiotic therapy, which kills the good bacteria in the gut, as well as the bad. The good bacteria, among other things, keep the yeast in check.

Birth control pills can also enhance yeast production. Sexual intercourse can cause mild abrasions, which give the yeast easy access. Your spouse or significant other can be carrying yeast and reinfecting you.

If you have the symptoms described here, check with your doctor to have diabetes and HIV ruled out. These conditions both favor the development of yeast. Then treat your partner and yourself.

It is important to be sure of the diagnosis. There is a painful condition called vulvar vestibulitis syndrome. This causes severe pain in the vulva, the external part of the vaginal opening. This can be mistaken for a yeast infection and anti-fungal treatments may worsen that condition. Corticosteroids cause yeast to spread rapidly.

Fighting Off the Yeast Beast

Here are some steps you can take to avoid being overtaken by yeast infections:

1. Take acidophilus. You can find it at health food stores and some groceries.

2. Shower rather than bathe. If you must bathe, use vinegar in the bath, and dry yourself with a hair dryer rather than a towel

3. Wear cotton underpants, and iron them after washing. The heat of the iron is sufficient to kill the yeast.

4. You can insert plain yogurt culture or other live lactobacillus into the vagina. Live lactobacillus cultures can be found in many health food stores.

5. You may want to go without underpants, at home, at night.

6. Avoid tight clothing, such as panty hose and girdles.

7. Avoid routine douching—it isn't necessary.

8. Use a water-based lubricant during sex.

If the yeast is deeply rooted in the vaginal wall, or elsewhere in the body, it may be time for a systemic anti-yeast regimen. Fluconazole (Diflucan) is a prescription drug and it is expensive but it is safer than other alternatives. You may find that fibrofog clears and water weight drops when you take this medication. This is a message from your body that it's time to watch your diet better than you have been doing.

Dr. London recommends following these practices for an effective anti-yeast diet. Avoid sugar, avoid or limit (at least temporarily) aged or fermented foods (mold-aged cheese, alcohol, vinegar, tofu) and foods that contain yeast or molds. He says of the latter, "The yeast in bread is dead, but the immune system can still react to yeast as an antigen, just as it does to pollen." He also says that drinking a lot of milk seems to encourage yeast growth.

Note: You may get the impression that taking Diflucan makes you feel much worse. This is called the *yeast die-off phenomenon.* When you have a heavy yeast overgrowth, your body has often adjusted to the burden. When the yeast starts to die in response to the Diflucan, the dead yeast clogs your lymph system and releases toxins into your body. Your body then starts working overtime to rid itself of the dead and dying yeast, and you may feel as if you're coming down with the flu. It isn't the Diflucan. It's the last revenge of the yeast beast.

Myth of the FMS Personality

There's been some talk on the Internet and in the popular press about the so-called "FMS Personality." Studies have shown that this theory has much in common with a certain animal by-product. The animal by-product is useful, however, because you can compost it and put it on your roses. The "FMS Personality" theory has no such redeeming quality.

The theory is part of a dangerous misconception—the "it's all in your head" slander discussed in Part I of this book. You are not to blame for your illness. The "FMS Personality" myth holds that people with FMS set too high standards for themselves. They are supposed to be caring, honest, tidy, committed, moral, industrious, and virtuous to a fault. They take pride in earning their way. This, in some unfathomable way, causes them to get FMS. It's their fault. Right.

The best evaluation of this "personality" was stated by David Nye, a neurologist at a sleep center. He said, "Persons with the 'personality profile' are no more likely to have FMS; they just have what it takes to keep going from doctor to doctor until they are finally diagnosed."

In Conclusion

Fibrofog can disrupt your life in many ways. Recognizing the symptoms and making plans to compensate for them can make things a lot easier.

If you are prone to yeast infections, the suggestions in this chapter can help you to keep such infections at a minimum. And if anyone ever accuses you of having the "FMS Personality," tell that person there's no such thing.

CHAPTER 19

Positive Change

People with FMS and/or FMS/MPS Complex share many things: We are all "in the same boat" in life. But it's your choice how you handle this situation. You can strive to become an expert sailor, or you can spend your entire life being sick over the side of the boat.

Depression

People who are living with constant chronic pain that is sometimes so acute as to be unbearable, pain that forces them to give up or to limit many of their former activities (like making love, hiking, working in the garden, knitting, and so on) have sufficient cause to be depressed.

Then, when they are told by their doctors that they are not *really* sick (as many people with FMS/MPS are told), that they should "just put up with it," that "it's all their own fault," or that "it's because you haven't exercised enough, dear,"—"insult" is really added to the "injury" and is further reason to become even more depressed.

When neurotransmitter dysfunction, which is already indicated as a cause of depression, is added to the scenario just described, we have a prescription for depression that is practically a disaster.

Being depressed is like being in the bottom of a deep dark hole; the whole world is bleak and cold. You don't want to do anything, you don't want to be active in any way, you don't even want to move. All the energy has left your body.

Your body aches and you feel ugly and agitated. Despair, pessimism, and hopelessness fill your life. You may hide out, take the phone off the hook, read and watch sad stories. Or perhaps all you do is cry, or you are unable to hold conversations, do chores, pay bills, or keep appointments.

You feel that there is no hope, and that nothing will ever change. You feel worthless and you may believe that the way you feel is all your own fault; you think that your life is over, and you just want to sleep forever and maybe to die.

Signs of Depression

The Diagnostic and Statistical Manual of Mental Disorders (1987) developed by the American Psychiatric Association, has delineated the major signs of depression as follows:

1. Depressed mood most of the day, almost every day

2. Diminished interest or lack of pleasure in almost all activities of the day, nearly every day

3. Unexplained significant weight loss or gain, and decreased or increased appetite nearly every day

4. Insomnia or hypersomnia (excessive sleep) nearly every day

5. Abnormal restlessness or a drop in physical activity nearly every day

6. Fatigue or loss of energy nearly every day

7. Feeling worthless or excessive or inappropriate guilt nearly every day

8. Diminished ability to think, concentrate, or make decisions nearly every day

9. Recurrent thoughts of death, or recurrent suicidal thoughts without a specific plan; or a suicide attempt; or a specific plan for committing suicide.

If you have these symptoms, you're having more than just a bad day, you are *depressed*. Depression is dangerous. Suicide is too often the tragic outcome. If you are depressed, get competent professional help immediately, before your symptoms worsen.

The first thing you need to do is have a complete physical examination. Although FMS or FMS/MPS Complex is reason enough to be depressed, many other medical conditions can cause or worsen depression. If other medical causes are ruled out, ask your physician to work with you to plan a course of treatment. This may include the use of medications, counseling, lifestyle changes, or referral to a psychologist, psychiatrist, or other mental health specialist.

If you decide to use medications to treat the depression, see Chapter 21, Fibromyalgia/Myofascial Pain Syndrome Medications and Chapter 22, Enhancing Your Medications. If you decide to see a counselor (many people take medications and also see a counselor), make sure the counselor validates your experience of FMS/MPS Complex, encourages and supports you, and does not criticize you, blame you, or try to control your life.

While you are reaching out to others to get help in dealing with depression, the basic responsibility for alleviating these persistent symptoms, as with all of your symptoms, is up to you. You can take and keep control over your own life by setting up a monitoring system that alerts you to the early warning signs of depression, and helps you to respond to these warning signs before the depression deepens and becomes more difficult to treat.

Seasonal Affective Disorder

If you live in a northern climate, observe whether you exhibit any of the symptoms listed below as the days become shorter and winter approaches. You may have a form of depression called Seasonal Affective Disorder (SAD) as well as FMS, MPS, or FMS/MPS Complex.

- a drop in energy level

- a decrease in productivity

- difficulty getting motivated

- difficulty concentrating and focusing

- impatience with yourself and others

- difficulty getting out of bed in the morning

- a craving for sweets and junk food

- a diminished sex drive

Researchers (Copeland 1994) have found that consistent daily visual exposure to bright light reduces or eliminates symptoms of SAD for most people. It is not clear why bright light works in this way, but it is thought it has to do with production of the hormone, melatonin, which takes place in the pineal gland.

Some researchers believe that SAD sufferers are either too sensitive to dim light and manufacture too much of the hormone or are oversensitive to the usual amount of the hormone that is produced (Copeland 1994). Dopamine, a neurotransmitter that carries signals between the nerves in body and the brain cells, may also play a role in SAD. Also, it is thought that depletion of the neurotransmitter, serotonin, may be responsible for the carbohydrate cravings that often accompany SAD.

For most of human history, the focus of daily activity was outdoors. People worked outdoors, and traveled in open carriages, or walked. Even going to the bathroom involved a trek to an outhouse. Today, many of us get in our cars before daylight, spend the day working in an artificially lit office with no windows, and come home after dark.

A simple program that increases the amount of natural or bright light taken in through our eyes often helps to reduce or completely eliminate SAD symptoms. If you think you may have SAD, contact a physician in your area who has expertise in prescribing light therapy. (This involves spending some time each day sitting near a specially constructed device called a light box.)

Some people report almost immediate relief of symptoms when they begin light therapy. For most, though, it takes from four to five days to work. For others, may take up to two weeks.

Light therapy is very well tolerated by most people, with minimal side effects. If you have mild side effects such as headaches; eyestrain; irritability; overactivity; insomnia; fatigue; dry eyes, nasal passages, and sinuses; or sunburn types of skin reactions, decrease your exposure to the lights, use sun blocking screens, and contact your health care professional for further advice. There have been no reports of eye problems due to light therapy. However, regular eye checkups are suggested for anyone using light therapy.

If you are taking certain photosensitizing medications or have a condition such as lupus, which causes extreme skin sensitivity to sunlight, a health care professional is *essential* to help you develop a treatment process.

Of course, you can also get light through outdoor activity. Supplement your light therapy by going outside for part of each day. Gazing at the sky helps, but never look directly at sun.

Keep your living space well lit at all times. Windows should be uncovered during the daylight hours to let daylight and sunlight in. If you work inside, work as close to a window as possible.

Exercise

Exercise is the cheapest and most easily available anti-depressant. It is also very effective. Exercising daily for at least 20 minutes each day is essential to maintaining well-being. In addition to the numerous physiological benefits of exercise, Dr. Edmund Bourne (1995) reports the following psychological benefits:

- Increased feeling of well-being

- Reduced dependence on alcohol and drugs

- Reduced insomnia

- Improved concentration and memory

- Alleviation of symptoms of depression

- Greater control over feelings of anxiety

- Increased self-esteem

Exercise, however, is often very difficult for people with FMS/MPS Complex. Your body may be stiff and achy and exercise may increase the pain for several days or even longer. Often your pain is so severe that you cannot tolerate any kind of strenuous exercise. Do the best you can. Be gentle with yourself, but move whatever part of your body you can move without causing pain.

Many people have found that exercising in a heated pool that is kept at 88 to 94 degrees Fahrenheit works well. If such a pool is available to you, take advantage of it. (See Chapter 25, Bodywork—Helping Your Body Work and Chapter 27, Bodywork You Can Do Yourself, for more suggestions on exercise that is tailored to your ability.)

Note: Many people with FMS, MPS, or FMS/MPS Complex experience severe cramping when they exercise in water below 88 degrees Fahrenheit.

Remember that with FMS, your exercise "sense of time" is not always reliable, and it is easy to overdo. Set a timer or exercise with a friend who will help you to keep track of the time.

Sleep

We have found that a good night's sleep is absolutely essential to avoid depression. Again, FMS/MPS Complex with its inherent sleep problems makes this a real challenge.

It's important to understand that:

- Lack of sleep can worsen depression.

- Too much sleep worsens depression.

- Most people need to go to bed at the same time every night and get up at the same time every morning.

- Even when you don't get to sleep at your regular time, you will still feel much better if you get up at your usual time.

- It helps to eat on a regular schedule. Avoid eating a heavy meal before bedtime.

- Strict weight-loss food plans may cause you to wake up hungry during the night. Distribute your calorie intake throughout the day.

- It helps to have a daily routine so your body knows when it is time to go to sleep.

- Following a prebedtime ritual, such as washing up, getting into night clothes, or reading a chapter from a book, tells your body when it's time to go to bed.

- Sex before bedtime is relaxing for many people and helps them get to sleep.

- You need a sleeping space that is not too noisy or too light.

(See Chapter 10, Sleep, to learn more about healthy habits that may help you get a good night's sleep.)

Living Space

Your living space significantly affects the way you feel. When you have both depression and FMS/MPS Complex, you need to give special attention to your surroundings.

If you live with others, do you have a space in your home that is your private space to decorate to suit yourself, where you can keep your things and they will not be disturbed, and where you can spend time by yourself involved in your own activities?

Is your living space comfortable and easy to clean and keep neat? If cleaning is a problem for you, think about getting a family member or friend to take over your heavy cleaning chores. If possible, hire someone to clean.

Dispose of things you don't need. Lots of "stuff" around makes a living space difficult to keep clean and attractive, and a messy living space usually increases stress if only because it makes it harder to find the things you want.

Changing Negative Dialogue—Cognitive Therapy

All too often, you are your own worst enemy. Almost unconsciously, you berate yourself over and over. When you drop things, often because of trigger points (TrPs), you may call yourself clumsy and klutzy. Yet, the fact that you function at all with FMS, MPS, or FMS/MPS Complex is often a miracle. When you forget things, you may tell yourself you are stupid. Yet, in spite of neurotransmitter dysfunction and "fibrofog," you often are able to navigate through the chaos of life with surprising insight and humor.

How many times do you say negative phrases such as, "How could I be so dumb?" to yourself? This is a dangerous practice, because your subconscious believes everything you say to it, and your own constant reinforcement of negativity can be a considerable obstacle in your journey toward healing. Negativity adds stress to your life. Fortunately, it is in your power to change this destructive habit of reinforcing your negative thinking.

Your moods and emotional states are strongly influenced by what you tell yourself, how you think, and the ways you interpret situations. If your personal viewpoints habitually take the form of self-doubt, generalized fears, and specific phobias, you can use *cognitive therapy*—a method of changing your thought patterns—to improve your life.

Identifying Your Fears

The first step in eliminating self-doubt, fears, and phobias is to identify them. In many cases these fears have become so habitual that this may be a difficult process.

Using your journal, you can identify the following habitual thoughts that create negative thinking patterns:

- Identify self-doubts, such as "I will never be able to learn to drive a car," "No one would ever like a person like me," and "I am not smart enough to be a good parent."

- Identify fears such as, "If I drive I will be in an accident," "If I leave my house, I will be robbed," "I think I have cancer," and "I will never be well again."

- Identify phobias, such as bugs, snakes, darkness, heights, deep water, elevators, and going outside.

Identifying Destructive Thinking Patterns

There is a certain way of thinking that can be extremely self-destructive. This manner of thinking can cause you to have a distorted, rather than rational, perception of different situations. The following section lists some of these ways of thinking and suggests ways in which you can counteract them with positive thoughts.

Filtering

Filtering is a way of looking at one part of the situation to the exclusion of everything else.

Example: "The holidays are going to be terrible. I will never get my cards sent out on time. That will ruin everything."

Rational comeback: "Even though I probably won't get my cards out, I can still have a great time."

Overgeneralization

Overgeneralization means reaching a broad, generalized conclusion based on just one piece of evidence.

Example: "Jane rejected me. Therefore, I am not worthy of anyone."

Rational comeback: "Just because one friend has rejected me, doesn't mean that no one will ever love me. It just means that one person has rejected me."

Control Fallacies

Having *control fallacies* means feeling that you are in some way responsible for everything that goes wrong.

Example: "My son fell off a chair after we argued, and it was my fault that he broke his leg."

Rational comeback: "The chair was wobbly and an insufficient support. That's why my son fell."

Fallacy of Change

The *fallacy of change* is the assumption that other people will change to suit you if you pressure them enough, and that your happiness depends on the actions of others.

Example: "If I insist that my husband come home at 5:30 every day, and he does, then everything will be great."

Rational comeback: "Pressuring my husband to come home every day at 5:30 is not going to help, will probably irritate him, and will not make everything great. It would be more appropriate for me to tell him what time I'd like to have dinner or I will have dinner ready and ask him to call me if he is going to be more than 15 minutes late, so I can plan accordingly. One little change seldom makes everything great."

Global Labeling

Global labeling means making a broad judgment based on little evidence.

Example: "I bought one batch of carrots at the store which was rotten; therefore the store is no good."

Rational comeback: "Just because I got one batch of bad carrots does not mean the store is no good. It just means that there was one batch of rotten carrots."

Blaming

Blaming is a way of making someone else responsible for situations that you are responsible for.

Example: "I am overweight because my mother makes too many good desserts."

Rational comeback: "I am overweight because I eat too much of the good desserts that my mother makes."

Shoulds

Having *shoulds* means operating from a rigid set of indisputable rules about how everyone, including yourself, should act.

Example: "I should be warm and friendly to my neighbor. I should never feel jealous. I should always work hard. I should never get tired."

Rational comeback: "I will try to be warm and friendly to my neighbor. Most people get jealous sometimes. I can work hard sometimes, but at other times I can take things more easily. Everyone gets tired."

A Four-Step Process for Eliminating Distorted Thoughts

You can use the four-step process presented in this section to change your distorted thoughts.

1. **Identify the emotion you are feeling.** For example: "I am feeling angry, tense, and anxious."

2. **Describe in detail the event or situation causing the emotion.** For example: "I went to my friend Peter's house at 4:00 o'clock as previously arranged, to go for a walk and have dinner together. He was not at home when I got there."

3. **Describe the distortion in your thought processes.** For example: "Because he was not there, I decided he really didn't want to spend the time with me, that he really didn't like me, and that he didn't have respect for my feelings."

4. **Eliminate the distortions.** For example: "There was only one piece of evidence, his not being there when I arrived, that caused my distortion. The truth is, we have been close friends for a long time. All evidence indicates that he likes me a lot. An emergency may have come up. He may have gone to do an errand that took longer than anticipated. He may have misunderstood the plan we made. He may have forgotten that we made a plan. The best course of action for me would be to wait on his porch (doing relaxation exercises) until his return, or leave him a note asking him to call me when he gets back."

Eliminating Inappropriate and Irrational Beliefs

Throughout our lives we are all taught by our families, friends, religious, educational, and social institutions, as well as by society in general, various "truths" that may be causing stress and worsening our symptoms. These "truths" vary from person to person and family to family. By examining them, you will discover that many of these "truths" are not true at all, and, in fact, that they are inappropriate or irrational.

One "truth" that you may have learned very early was that if you are not doing something productive, such as cleaning the house, cooking, washing clothes, weeding the garden, or mowing the lawn, you are lazy (a terrible thing to be).

You were led to believe that every waking hour must be spent in some kind of constructive work activity. When you take the time to sit down and relax, spend time chatting with a friend, watch a video, or engage in some other leisurely activity, you may find yourself feeling guilty and unable to enjoy yourself.

Another example of an inappropriate or irrational "truth" is perfectionism. Perhaps you have always felt that you must do everything perfectly, and you aren't satisfied with anything less. You may always think you could have done any job better than you actually did it. Or you may feel that you have to be a perfect parent, perfect partner, perfect housewife, or perfect teacher. Since this is, by definition, impossible, you are, in a very real way, robbing yourself of the joy of life.

To counteract beliefs like these, make a list of your inappropriate expectations and beliefs. The easiest way to discover your inappropriate ideas is to think of situations where you felt very uncomfortable, anxious, or bad about yourself, and study them to get to the root of your feelings. Keep a record in your journal of everything that flows through your mind in stressful situations. This will help you to keep track of your thoughts and assist you in becoming more positive. You will also be able to review your work and see your progress more easily.

Affirmations

Affirmations are short, positive statements that describe how you want to feel, and what you would like your life to be like. It's easy to get into the habit of saying affirmations to yourself to fill empty spaces of time. For example, they can be repeated while waiting for a street light, or washing dishes, upon awakening, at bedtime, and during meditations. This stops any negative self-dialogue you might have.

Development and regular repetition of affirmations seems like a simplistic concept, but many people who are challenged by the negativity of chronic pain use this technique successfully. It is the reverse of negative self-dialogue, and it is noninvasive. It costs nothing and is well worth a try.

Some people carry lists of affirmations in their pockets or purse or tape them to the refrigerator door until they form the positive habit of repeating their affirmations. It is a good practice to start and end your day with affirmations. Make them part of your life, and you will fulfill their prophecies.

Examples of Positive Affirmations

Here are some simple sentences that will help you achieve control of yourself and your life. Repeat one or more to yourself whenever you need to assert your rights.

- I am not a victim.

- I have no duty to be perfect.

- If I can't decide which of two choices to pick, perhaps my choice should be something else.

- I have a right to make up my own mind.

- I have a right to ignore the advice of others, even if I asked for that advice.

- Respecting other people's views doesn't mean I have to agree.

- My time is valuable, too.

- I deserve the time and space to heal.

- I am a very valuable person.

See Chapter 15, Taking Control, for more affirmations that may be helpful.

The best antidote to being affected by negative input is to have a clear picture of yourself and who you are, and being able to judge for yourself whether or not there is any validity to what anyone says about you.

In Conclusion

Negativity often strikes people with FMS or FMS/MPS Complex. If you suffer from negativity, you may need to seek professional counseling. You can also take steps on your own to minimize or even eliminate negativity. Cognitive therapy is an excellent tool for creating a positive outlook on life.

PART V

HEALING TOOLS

CHAPTER 20

Meditation and Mindfulness

In Chapter 21, you will learn what medications are available to take the edge off your symptoms. In this chapter, you will learn about meditation and mindfulness states, which can help achieve the same effect. Too often people believe they are unable to influence their bodies' "automatic" responses. However, it has been well-documented that meditation and mindfulness can produce deep relaxation in the muscles, while thought processes remain clear. These disciplines can induce a generalized hypometabolic state that quiets your body.

This is not the hypometabolism described in medical dictionaries. For people with FMS or FMS/MPS Complex, whose engines idle at 35 m.p.h. instead of the normal 5 m.p.h., our hypometabolic state slows that engine. Maybe only to 20 m.p.h., but that is still a vast improvement. Our hypometabolic state, in turn, slows neurotransmitter actions and decreases muscle lactate production while it increases muscle relaxation. There is a much smaller chance of being hit with "sensory overload" if we meditate.

In the meditative state, breathing slows and deepens, and circulation improves. It has been proven that meditation and other mindwork disciplines can increase blood flow to the muscles (Davis 1995). In fact, the evidence is rapidly mounting that suggests your state of mind, as well as your diet, your environment, and your occupation can affect the state of your physical health profoundly.

What Is Meditation?

Many people are uncomfortable with the idea of meditation, because it's a practice not usually taught in the western world. It isn't difficult to learn, however, and it doesn't require grim training, odd positions, or physical and sensory deprivation. The great Zen master, Thich Nhat

Hanh, defines it in the following way: "Meditation is to be aware of what is going on: in your body, in your feelings, in your mind, and in the world. . . . We have to smile a lot in order to be able to meditate." Meditation offers a way to escape the burden of sensory overload that people with FMS experience, and it requires nothing more than an adventurous mind.

There are many levels and types of meditation. Often, the time just before falling asleep is a good time to meditate and reflect because just then you are in what is called a *hypnogogic* state. In such a state your conscious and subconscious mind become very closely connected. In fact, you have probably practiced a form of meditation without knowing it. It's called *daydreaming*.

To know yourself thoroughly is to embark on a journey, and all journeys, no matter how long, begin with the first small step and then proceed one step at a time. For that reason, it is best to start meditating with a simple form.

Your First Step

To begin a simple meditation, follow the steps below:

1. Find a place where you can be quiet, uninterrupted, and relaxed.

2. Find a comfortable position. It is easiest to start with a sitting meditation. You can sit on a chair or cross-legged on the floor, tailor fashion.

3. Let your body sway slightly from side to side, and then from back to front, until you find your point of balance. It will feel "right" to you. As you become more adept at meditation and at "centering," you will find this point more easily.

4. Breathe in through your nose and out through your mouth. Close your eyes and "observe" your breathing. Make sure you are breathing from your belly, and that your belly is soft, and not guarded. When you inhale, your belly should swell with the incoming air. When you breathe in through your nose, your tongue should touch the roof of your mouth. Exhale through your mouth, expelling all of the stale air.

5. Become aware of your body. How does it feel? Mentally scan your body. Don't visualize it, but try to feel it with your mind. Scan your whole body. Start with the top of your head and work your way down to the soles of your feet. Do any sensations cry out to you? If so, don't dwell on them, just notice them, and move on. When you have finished scanning your body, tell it that you are aware of its problems and that you are doing everything possible to help. Let your body know that things will be getting better.

6. Now, let all thoughts leave your mind. At first, you may find this impossible. Thoughts will intrude. Just make note of them and let them pass. You are not concerned with them today.

   If you find that blanking your mind is difficult, think of one of the affirmations you have chosen, or choose one now. Say it in your mind, not thinking about it, but just letting it rest there in your consciousness. If another thought comes in, note it and then go back to saying your affirmation to yourself.

You might try to just let your mind drift for a while, going in and out with your breath, like a fish riding on the waves. (You become a "human being" instead of a "human doing.") Practice *being* for a while. Like anything new, this may be difficult, but it will become easier with time. When you have drifted for a while, then bring your mind back to focus on your affirmation again. This type of meditation can be a mini-vacation from the stresses of your day.

Types of Meditation

The following section describes a few types of meditations. You may find others appropriate for different times and places.

Walking Meditation

A walking meditation is a good way to start if you have never meditated before. This walking meditation is an easy one, and not rigidly structured like some types of Zen walking meditations; you have to make this one up as you do it.

When times get tough, go for a walk. As you walk, think of a place that you would rather be. It can be a real place or a mythical one—perhaps a world you've read about, or imagined, but make it somewhere you've never been and some place that would be comfortable for you. Then, think of what you'd need to bring from your *present* existence that would make that other world perfect.

It's true there are times when life may seem bleak and unfriendly, but perhaps that's because you're looking at it through a gray filter of pain and frustration. Perhaps it's time to clean away the cobwebs and let in the light. Try a walking meditation alone, or try doing one aloud with others.

Guided Imagery

Guided imagery is a very effective kind of meditation that has been used successfully to deal with a variety of situations, such as enhancing the healing process, and increasing a person's general feeling of well-being. You can use this type of meditation by taping it and playing it back, by having a friend

I discovered the walking meditation one day when I was in flare, feeling achy and confused. I was wandering around the woods on our hill, thinking about how miserable life was at the moment and trying to grasp what Heaven must be like, and suddenly I was in the middle of a meditation. That's how meditation works once you've been doing it for a while. It becomes a very positive force in your life and it is there whenever you need it. I was pretty tired of my existence here, and I was comfortable with the idea of Heaven. Then I decided that Heaven must have McCoun apples, though, because they taste so crisp and crunchy and refreshing; it just couldn't be Heaven without them. Just thinking about the way the apple fragrance blossomed when I bit into one brought a smile to my lips. Then I thought about bittersweet read it, or by reading it over many times until you become familiar with it. It is a way of going on a mind trip; when you can't get away but need to, it can give you the "space" you want.

Here is an example of a guided imagery exercise. It's called *A Walk in the Forest*.

Find a place where you will be undisturbed. Unplug the phone. Turn off the radio or television. Have someone else tend the children. Make yourself as comfortable as you can, either sitting in a comfortable chair or lying down. Loosen any restrictive clothing. Close your eyes. Take five or six deep breaths, releasing the air very slowly. Let your whole body relax completely. Notice any areas of tension and let them relax. You are going on a journey.

Visualize yourself on a glorious, cheerful morning. The sky is soft blue with white, fluffy clouds. You are dressed in comfortable, loose clothes that feel sensual against your skin. You're in a meadow, at the edge of the woods. There is a light pack at your feet. It holds a tasty, nutritious lunch that has no calories. It also holds something special of yours that no one else knows about. Pick up the pack, and begin your journey.

Visualize and feel yourself ambling down a path bordering the wood. Lush ferns line your way. The forest smells green and inviting. The path takes you into the forest. It's pleasantly cool among the trees. Sunlight filters through the leafy canopy. Birds are singing in the trees. A light breeze is blowing through your hair. Your path is relatively flat, with only an occasional gentle rise.

You walk along, at ease with yourself, breathing deeply the fragrance of pine trees. The forest floor cushions your every step. Your walk is steady, and your balance secure.

You come to a clearing and pause, looking over a wide meadow. It is filled with flowers of your favorite colors. A line of trees stands in the distance, and you can hear the sound of a fast running brook just beyond them. Multicolored butterflies dance among the flowers, pausing briefly to drink of their nectar. You take the path through the meadow, stopping now and then to appreciate the sounds and smells. You feel light, oh so light.

Soon you approach the trees. You leave the path for a short distance, walking on the soft grasses. The trees are your friends, and they wave their branches gently in welcome. As you reach them, you notice that some of the trees have holes of different sizes in their trunks. You reach out to touch the closest tree. The ridges of the bark massage your hand as you rub the trunk of the tree, and the tree sighs with pleasure at your touch.

You listen closely and can hear the faint voices of the trees singing softly in the breeze. They offer to take your worries and troubles. There is room for your burdens in the tree holes. There are large holes for great troubles and small ones for lesser worries.

You may find that once you put your troubles in one of the holes, it changes size. Maybe a problem bothers you more than you know. Or maybe what you thought was a large burden becomes much smaller. No matter. You're just letting the trees hold them for a while.

> chocolate butter-creme truffles (yes, I know many of us shouldn't have chocolate!) and decided Heaven needed those too. Heaven wouldn't be perfect without soft, purring cats, either. Then, I remembered how I enjoy taking a walk in the night after a really cold snow, when snow crystals turn to glitter in the moonlight. By the time I finished my walk that day, I remembered that we all have it within ourselves to create a semblance of Heaven on earth.
>
> D.J.S.

Now, you take some time to think of some of those private, special things you brought along with you. You may decide to leave some of those with the trees as well. After you decide what to do with your private, special things, you continue on your way to the stream, feeling lighter, and relieved of your burdens.

The brook calls to you, and you sit on the soft grasses beside it, in the shade of a willow. Violets and emerald mosses edge the brook, and there is a little pool created by stones. The water is slower there, and warmer, although it is pleasantly cooler than the air. Take off your shoes, and dip your feet in the soothing waters of the pool. Feel any remaining tension melt from you, to be carried away by the healing waters.

Take a deep breath. Breathe in gently through your nose, letting your belly swell with air. When you can breathe in no more, exhale slowly through your nose. Breathe all the stale air out, and then take in more of the fresh, healthy air. Enjoy your comfort, be content to be quiet and relaxed.

Turn your attention to your body. Feel the body that is part of you—the body in which you live. Mentally scan your body, noticing all the sensations that are part of you. Observe how the sensations change from place to place and vary in intensity. If you meet with discomfort, pain, or other negative feelings, just observe these feelings. Don't judge them or comment; just note their existence and continue your scan.

Notice whether your body tries to keep your awareness from areas of pain and contraction. Is something holding onto the pain or tightness? Be aware of your natural tendency to linger at areas of pleasant sensations, and to skip the areas of negativity. Examine that resistance. What is its nature? What does it feel like? Is there fear, or anger? Is it dark? What is it that keeps these areas of your body unconnected?

As your awareness begins to encounter areas of discomfort, notice the tight places that are guarding the areas of pain. Gently, let those tight places melt like ice on a summer day. Breathe through the tightness, and when you exhale, notice the softening, the letting go. Allow the sensations to float, weightless. Enter the areas of discomfort, exposing the tender sensations inside. Accept them as part of you, and then move on.

When you have finished your scan, imagine all the other beings elsewhere in the universe experiencing these same kinds of discomfort. Don't take on the pain of others; just link to them and note the connection, and remember that you will never be alone, no matter what your trials. Acknowledge the others, and embrace them for what you share. Then embrace yourself as part of the others, melting resistance with your love and compassion. Allow any residual pain and discomfort to flow down to your feet. Let it be carried away by the gentle stream. If some of it wants to travel upward, let it go. Float it on the breeze to the trees, and let the trees carry it for a while.

Hold on to your connection, but watch the pain drift away. You are part of a vast family of beings, struggling to make the best of life, in spite of many problems. Let your thoughts flow out through the universe, brimming with love and compassion. You feel light, nearly weightless, and nearly floating yourself. Breathe deeply, and know that whenever you feel alone, you can come back to this healing brook.

Now, if you wish, you may savor the delicious food from your pack and drink from the pure, refreshing stream. Linger as long as you like. This is a safe place for you. If you wish, you may return to the trees and resume your burdens. Or you may decide to let the trees hold on to them for now. It is your choice. Just note the size of the holes containing each burden. What does that tell you? Perhaps you will decide to pick up a few of the burdens, or only one, and let the trees keep the others until you can deal with them. You are in control. These are decisions that you can make.

When you are ready to come back from your trip, take another deep breath, and let it out slowly. Move your fingers and toes, and, if you wish, stretch. When you are ready, return to the room and open your eyes.

Using Your Imagination

Ever wish you could leave your stiff and aching body and soar over the land like a bird? Want to see the Alps but a trip to the next town leaves you in pain and exhausted? Besides, all your money goes for medical bills. Maybe it's time you learned how to fly on your own.

Many children fly very well. If you never flew as a child, now is a good time to learn. You are never too old to have a perfect childhood.

Find a quiet place where you will not be disturbed. Imagine you are like a bird, flying. Leave your body behind with its painful trigger points and tender points. Leave all your symptoms behind. Your body will be safe where it is, while the rest of you soars up to the clouds. Be cautious at first, stick to familiar areas.

Is there a special place you always wanted to see? Get a library book, and read all about it. Many libraries have videos of exciting places. Immerse yourself in these places. Then, afterwards, visualize the place you want to see. Think about what it looks like. What it smells like. How it sounds. You can even try this in bed, just before you go to sleep. You might find out that you can program your dreams and visit exotic places in your sleep.

Meditations on Life

Life is a great teacher. Too often you may forget that and become frustrated when your life isn't going the way you think it should. At such times you may find it helpful to think over the event that seems so uncooperative and frustrating and try to figure out what you can learn from it. Here are some examples from the authors' own experiences.

Berry picking: When I first began picking wild berries, I was determined to harvest every berry I saw. Yet the ripest, fattest, most luscious berries often fell off the branches before I could pick them. I saw this as a failure on my part. The very best berries seemed to go to waste, and I contributed directly to this by jiggling the branches in my efforts to reach them.

Now, looking back, I see that the best berries fell as seed berries for the future. Mother Nature is wiser than I am. I have seen our berries get bigger, sweeter, and juicier over the years. As I learned the lesson of the berries, so it is with life. We do not understand all things. Some of the things that we view as losses or failures may contain the seeds of future joy.

The fence: When I was about seven-years old, a fence separated the neighbor's land from our land. The fence was made of about 1-inch diameter metal pipe. It stood about three feet high, with another horizontal bar halfway up. It became my cousin's and my practice to try to walk the fence.

The round pipe was narrow, and balancing on it was difficult for our young legs. It seemed as if we spent months trying to walk the length of that pipe fence. We'd give it up for a while, but we'd always return to the challenge. And, always, there would be the grass and stones below to meet us as we slid off one side or the other. It was really frustrating. Our goal seemed impossible.

But there was a marvelous willow tree beyond the far end of the fence. It seemed fitting that we should approach this great tree by way of a trial. The fence thus became the road of the quest. One day I fell off the pipe one too many times. I became extremely angry and frustrated. That made things even worse. The harder I tried, the faster I fell. I tried to watch carefully where I placed my feet. Nothing helped.

Then, I looked at the tree, and I locked my eyes on my goal. Once my vision locked onto a fixed object, balancing became easy, and I walked the fence at will. It was only when I focused on the object of my desire, ignoring all distractions, that I was able to accomplish my goal.

So it is in life. Often, as you focus on your day-to-day struggles, the harder you strive, the more frustrating they become. But if you focus on that which you desire, your intent becomes clear, and the way is made easy. It is your job to focus on your goal.

Mindfulness

If you're like most people, you go through much of life on autopilot, not consciously aware of how you feel, what is happening, or your surroundings. Mindfulness helps you to simplify your life and to enjoy more of it.

Mindfulness is not really a mind tool—it's a way of life. It means that in each moment you are fully aware of what is happening in the present. Rather than being anxious or worried about the future or regretting the past, you are aware of what is happening in the present—right now—the sights, the sounds, the smells, the feelings, and thoughts of the present moment.

Try it now. Just sit back in your chair and focus on what is happening at this moment. Do it for several minutes. Notice how relaxed you feel.

When your mind is really scattered and you are feeling overwhelmed, one exercise you might like to use is to focus your attention on one thing—a flower, a greeting card picture (you can save your favorites and leave them on the coffee table for this purpose), or a piece of art. Study the object intensely for five or ten minutes. When other thoughts intrude, just send them on their way and return to focusing on and studying the object you chose. You can set a timer to let you know when your time is up.

In the book *Full Catastrophe Living* (Kabat-Zinn 1990), the author describes a mindfulness-meditation program that he teaches to people with chronic pain and other serious illnesses. It contains a series of exercises that will increase your ability to live "in the present moment." It can teach you to live right now, and it can bring a rich new awareness to your life.

There are a number of excellent meditations and exercises in Dr. Kabat-Zinn's book. One exercise called the "Body Scan" seems especially appropriate for people with FMS/MPS Complex. There is one *caution*, however: *don't do the head rolls described in the book*. Tilting the head back and rolling it can really aggravate your trigger points.

Mindfulness is a way to enrich your life. It is also a type of meditation that gives you a new understanding of what life is all about.

Prayer

Although you might not understand how it works, there is healing power in prayer. A recent symposium at Georgetown University School of Medicine held the first conference on "Spiritual Dimensions in Clinical Research." One result was the conclusion that "spirituality is an important medical tool that should be considered when developing a therapeutic regimen for the patient" (Marwick 1995). Other studies have shown that if a degree of "religious coping" is used, a patient with a chronic disabling disorder is less likely to become depressed. Medical science can't explain why this is so. But it is so.

Fortunately, prayer requires faith, not understanding. Consider this analogy: How often have you concerned yourself with the working of electricity? You take it on faith that when you plug in a toaster or the television set, it will work. No matter who you are and what you do in life, you learn to use things you don't understand. There is some comfort in accepting that there are some things you just don't know. Find your own form of spirituality, and discover what works for you. Then try to practice daily.

Connection Meditation

Think about your connection to all creation, and to God, whatever you believe God to be. Consider the unity of all life. Think of the the life force in us all. There is power in the Presence of The Cosmic Force Which Connects. Touch that power. A peace beyond all your understanding is there for you, but it's not a passive gift. Any gift must be taken before you can make it your own. Accept the gift, and give thanks. For you are very special and you are loved. Return that love.

Think of prayer as a form of communication with that Cosmic love. Pray not only for yourself, but for all who are united with you, afflicted with illness and in pain. If you have questions to ask of God, by all means ask them, but allow a time of quiet mindfulness to listen for an answer. Here is a prayer you may find helpful to slow the frantic pace of FMS or FMS/MPS Complex:

"Slow me down, Lord!

Ease the pounding of my heart by the quieting of my mind.

Steady my harried pace with a vision of the eternal reach of time.

Give me, amidst the confusions of my day,

The calmness of the everlasting hills.

Break the tensions of my nerves with the soothing music of the singing streams that live in my memory.

Help me to know the magical restoring power of sleep.

Teach me the art of taking minute vacations of slowing down

    to look at a flower;

    to chat with an old friend or make a new one;

> I am a very New Age Judeo-Christian Mystic. I believe that all mainstream churches should have at least one mystic to keep them honest. I manage to fill this role while being an Episcopal lay minister. Matthew Fox, the great present-day religious teacher, says a mystic is doing a good job if she/he is always in trouble. By all accounts, I'm doing really well.
>
> D.J.S.

to pat a stray dog;

to watch a spider build a web;

to smile at a child;

or read a few lines from a good book.

Remind me each day that the race is not always to the swift;

That there is more to life than increasing its speed.

Let me look upward into the branches of the towering oak and know that it grew great and strong because it grew slowly and well.

Slow me down, Lord, and inspire me to send my roots deep

Into the soil of life's enduring values

That I may grow toward the stars of my greater destiny."

—Wilfred A. Peterson

Distraction—Having Fun!

It has been said that it's pleasure that binds one to existence. To make life more worthwhile, spend more time having fun. Engaging in an activity that makes you happy and keeps you totally focused is an excellent distraction from day-to-day coping with chronic, painful illness.

Comedy tapes and good books are also excellent resources for distraction. Think about it. What do you really enjoy doing? Maybe you haven't done it in a long time—such as reading comic books. Make a list of these things. Attach it to the refrigerator for easy reference. (When you are having a hard time, or in flare, it may not be easy to think of amusing or interesting things to do to distract yourself.)

Have these distractions available so you can do them easily. Buy the paints. Set up the workshop. Start a garden. Plan to have distractions available when you are coping with extra pain or negativity. Be sure, however, that your activity is one that will not present you with an unsurmountable challenge. If you aren't able to do what you want, find a way to modify that desire to fit in with your current limits.

In addition to using these distractions during the hard times, try taking a few minutes *every* day to do something you really enjoy. In the business of daily life, you may forget to do this. But you will feel better if you make a special time for yourself every day. Even a few minutes a day spent in pleasure can make your whole life better.

In Conclusion

By using the tools of mindfulness and meditation you can quiet your mind and deal more effectively with the pain of your symptoms. In addition, if you do something that gives you pleasure on a daily basis, you will not only enrich your life, you will be able to distract yourself from your symptoms when you most need distractions.

CHAPTER 21

Fibromyalgia/Myofascial Pain Syndrome Medications

Until recently, much of the medical world regarded patients with complaints caused by fibromyalgia (FMS) and myofascial pain syndrome (MPS) along the lines of "it's all in their minds." Today, one result of that attitude is that very few drugs are well-established as effective for these conditions.

Finding the Right Medications

You may have to try many medications before you find the ones that work best for you. Each person with FMS or FMS/MPS Complex has a unique combination of neurotransmitter disruption and connective tissue disturbance. What works well for one person can be completely ineffective for another.

For example, a medication that puts one person to sleep may keep someone else awake. There is no "cookbook recipe" for prescribing medications for FMS, MPS, or FMS/MPS Complex. To find what you need, you must first find doctors who are willing to work with you until an acceptable level of symptom relief is reached.

Medications that affect the central nervous system are appropriate for FMS/MPS Complex. These medications target the symptoms of insomnia, muscle rigidity, pain, and fatigue. Pain sensations are amplified by FMS. Furthermore, FMS/MPS Complex patients often react oddly to medications. Discuss your responses with your doctor and your pharmacist, and tell them to keep an open mind.

You may have to try a great many medications in different combinations before you find exactly the right balance. As your health improves, you may have to readjust the amounts and kinds of your medicines. During flares, you probably will have to reduce your stress load and increase your medications.

Medications and Pain

It is the rule rather than the exception that FMS/MPS Complex patients will save strong pain medications that were prescribed for use after surgery or injury for those times when they *really* need painkillers—for times of an FMS/MPS Complex "flare." If you have been forced to follow this practice, read the following quoted material. We hope you will pass it on to your doctor. The quotes are from *PAIN: A Clinical Manual for Nursing Practice* (McCaffrey 1989).

- Health professionals "are often unaware of their lack of knowledge about pain control."

- "The health team's reaction to a patient with chronic nonmalignant pain may present an impossible dilemma for the patient. If the patient expresses his depression, the health team may believe the pain is psychogenic or is largely an emotional problem. If the patient tries to hide the depression by being cheerful, the health team may not believe that pain is a significant problem."

- "Research shows that, unfortunately, as pain continues through the years, the patient's own internal narcotics, the endorphins, decrease and the patient perceives even greater pain from the same stimuli."

- "The person with pain is the only authority about the existence and nature of that pain, since the sensation of pain can be felt only by the person who has it."

- "Having an emotional reaction to pain does not mean that pain is caused by an emotional problem."

- "Pain tolerance is the individual's unique response, varying between patients and varying in the same patient from one situation to another."

- "Respect for the patient's pain tolerance is crucial for adequate pain control."

- "There is not a shred of evidence anywhere to justify using a placebo to diagnose malingering or psychogenic pain."

- "No evidence supports fear of addiction as a reason for withholding narcotics when they are indicated for pain relief. All studies show that regardless of doses or length of time on narcotics, the incidence of addiction is less than 1%."

PAIN: A Clinical Manual for Nursing Practice is very clear in its presentation of facts and it is very well-documented. If you read it, you will have a greater understanding of pain and pain medications, as well as of coping mechanisms. Also, many nonpharmaceutical methods of pain control are thoroughly described.

Types of Medications for Chronic Pain

It's normal to be depressed when you have chronic pain, but that doesn't mean the depression is causing the pain. Maintenance with mild narcotics (Darvocet, Tylenol #3, Vicodin, Lorcet, Lortab) for nonmalignant (noncancerous) chronic pain conditions offers humane alternatives if other reasonable attempts at pain control have failed.

The main problem with raising the dosages of these medications is not only with the narcotic components, per se, but with the aspirin or acetaminophen that is often compounded with them. These NSAIDS (nonsteroidal anti-inflammatory drugs) can create more toxicity and can have more disastrous side effects than the narcotics themselves. Note that neither FMS nor MPS is an inflammatory condition.

Sometimes narcotic analgesics are more easily tolerated than NSAIDs are. Prolonged use of these narcotics may result in physiological changes of tolerance or physical dependence, but these are not the same as psychological dependence. Undertreatment of the chronic pain of FMS/MPS Complex results in worsening contractions of the myofascia, which results in even more pain.

Note: Amitriptyline, ibuprofen, and other medications, as well as FMS itself, can cause water retention.

Psychoactive drugs, that is, medications that affect the mental state such as Atarax, BuSpar, Elavil, and Xanax, influence neurotransmitters. If your doctor prescribes these "anti-anxiety" drugs, it is not an indication that your symptoms are "all in your head." These medications extend the amount of sleep and may ease daytime symptom "flares." They don't, however, stop the alpha-wave intrusion into delta-level sleep. (See Chapter 10, Sleep.)

Many medications are prepared using lactose fillers. This is the case with some over-the-counter drugs, as well as with prescription medications, such as Effexor. If you have lactose intolerance, check with your pharmacist.

Common FMS/MPS Complex Medicines

The list of medications presented here is only a partial listing. Check with your doctor about these medicines and others. Stay tuned to the *FM Network Newsletter* for news of newer medications that may be of use in FMS or FMS/MPS Complex.

Ambien: This is a hypnotic—a sleeping pill for short-term use for insomnia.

Warning: There have been some reports of serious depression when using this medication.

Atarax (hydroxyzine HCl): This suppresses activity in some areas of the central nervous system to produce an antianxiety effect. This antihistamine and anxiety-reliever may be useful when itching is a problem.

Benadryl (diphenhydramine): This is a helpful nonprescription sleep aid/antihistamine that is safe to take during pregnancy. The starting dose is 50 mg, taken 1 hour before bed. The medicine can be increased as tolerated until symptoms are controlled, or to about 300 mg.

About 20 percent of patients react with excitation rather than becoming sedated when taking Benadryl.

BuSpar (buspirone HCl): This drug may improve memory, reduce anxiety, and help regulate body temperature. It is not as sedating as many other antianxiety drugs.

Desyrel (trazodone): This antidepressant helps with sleep problems. Note that it must be taken with food.

Diflucan (fluconazole): This antifungal medication penetrates all of the body's tissues, even the central nervous system. Very short-term use can be considered if cognitive problems and/or depression are present and yeast is suspected. Yeast may also be at the root of irritable bowel syndrome (see Chapter 11), sleep dysfunction (muramyl dipeptides from bowel bacteria induce sleep), and other common FMS problems. Diflucan is very expensive.

Effexor (venlafaxine HCl): This is an antidepressant and serotonin and norepinephrine reuptake inhibitor. The suggested trial dosage is 25 mg, taken in the morning. Food has no effect on its absorption.

Warning: When discontinuing this medication, taper off slowly.

Elavil (amitriptyline): This antidepressant is inexpensive and useful. It often generates a deep stage-four sleep. It can cause photosensitivity and morning grogginess. It often causes weight gain and dry mouth, as well as stopping the normal movements of the intestine. It may cause Restless Leg Syndrome (see Chapter 8). Chromium picolinate (see Chapter 22, Enhancing Your Medications) taken in conjunction with Elavil often relieves "carbocraving" and minimizes weight gain.

EMLA: This prescription-only topical cream may help cutaneous (skin) trigger points (see Chapter 3, Myofascial Trigger Points). It is a mixture of topical anesthetics.

Flexeril (cyclobenzaprine): This tricyclic medication can sometimes stop spasms, twitches, and some tightness of the muscles. It is chemically related to Elavil. It generates stage-four sleep, but it may cause gastric upset and a feeling of detachment from life.

Fluori-Methane: This vapocoolant spray is manufactured by the Gebauer Company for "spray and stretch" treatment (see Chapter 26, Bodyworkers) to inhibit pain impulses and to allow for passive stretching. There are some environmental concerns about the use of fluorocarbons. Doctors and physical therapists can call 1-800-321-9348 for more information.

Guaifenesin: See Chapter 23, Guaifenesin.

Hismanal (astemizole succinate): This is a potent antihistamine often given for allergies.

Warning: Do not take this medication at the same time as ketaconazole, an antifungal medication.

Imitrex (sumatriptan): This medication is available in pill form or in a self-injectable solution. It will not prevent migraines, but in many cases it is effective for migraine pain. Using a different mechanism of action than other migraine medications, it acts directly on specific serotonin receptors, and it constricts specific blood vessels in the brain. Dilation of these blood vessels is often responsible for migraine symptoms. It may provide relief in less than 20 minutes as it alleviates nausea, head pain, and light sensitivity.

Warning: Imitrex should not be used within 24 hours of taking ergot (a common migraine medicine). It may increase blood pressure. It may cause muscle spasms in the jaw, neck, shoulders, and arms. Also reported were tingling sensations, rapid heartbeat, and "the shakes." It is very expensive.

Inderal (propranolol HCl): This medication sometimes helps in the prevention of migraine headaches, although blood pressure may drop with its use.

Warning: Antacids will block its effect and should not be used.

Klonopin (klonazepam): This is not only an antianxiety medication, but also an anti-convulsive/antispasmodic. It is useful in dealing with muscle twitching, Restless Leg Syndrome, and nighttime grinding of teeth (see Chapter 8).

Librax: This medication is often used for irritable bowel syndrome (see Chapter 11). It is a combination of antispasmodic plus tranquilizer that helps to modulate bowel action.

Pamelor (nortriptyline HCl): This tricyclic antidepressant is used to help those with insomnia problems fall asleep. Note that some people find it stimulating and must take it in the morning. Others can use it before bedtime.

Warning: There have been some reports of depression with its use.

Paxil (paroxetine HCl): This serotonin and norepinephrine reuptake inhibitor may also reduce pain.

Warning: Paxil should not be used with other medications that also increase brain serotonin. Suggested dosage is 10 mg (half of a scored tablet). It may need to be taken in the morning, as sometimes it causes insomnia if taken before bed.

Potaba (aminobenzoate potassium): This is a member of the B-vitamin complex. It is used to diminish fibrotic tissue. Travell and Simons (1992) p. 278, recommend it for stubborn cases of myofascial pain syndrome.

Warning: Do not use Potaba with sulfa drugs. The suggested dosage is 500 mg three times a day for five months.

Procaine injection for trigger points: This is to be used as a last resort. Trigger Point Injection protocols can be found in Travell and Simons' Trigger Point Manual (1983). Note that this procaine injection is not as effective for people with FMS/MPS Complex as it is for those with MPS only.

Prozac (fluoxetine HCl): This SSRI (Specific Serotonin Re-uptake Inhibitor) antidepressant increases the availability of serotonin. It is useful for those patients who sleep excessively, have severe depression, and overwhelming fatigue. It may cause insomnia. It has a relatively slow elimination (two to three days). It may be taken with or without food and is metabolized in the liver.

Warning: FMS patients sometimes become worse on Prozac, because it disrupts stage-four delta sleep.

Quotane: This topical prescription ointment is helpful for trigger point relief in close-to-the-surface areas not reachable by stretching. Trigger points that refer burning, prickling, or lightning-like jabs of pain are likely to be found in cutaneous scars (those on the skin).

Relafen (nabumetone): This is a nonsteroidal anti-inflammatory drug that is often well-tolerated because it is absorbed in the intestine, thus sparing the stomach.

Sinequan (doxepin HCl): This tricyclic antidepressant and antihistamine combination can produce marked sedation effects. It may enhance Klonopin but it can also reduce muscle twitching by itself.

Soma (carisoprodol): This central nervous system "muffler" is greatly underutilized. It acts on the nervous system to relax muscles, not on the muscles themselves. It works rapidly, and the effects last from four to six hours. Except for the extremely rare patient with sensitivity to it, it is well-tolerated. It helps patients to detach themselves from their pain and modulates erratic neurotransmitter traffic, damping the sensory overload of FMS. It should first be tried in a half-pill dose. When taking this medication, some people feel as if they are in a meditative state. Soma raises the seizure threshold. It may cause drowsiness.

Warning: Soma may cause drowsiness and raises the seizure threshold. It is not recommended for children under 12-years old.

Tagamet (cimetidine), Zantac (ranitidine HCl): These medications are often used to counter esophageal reflux (see Chapter 8). Tagamet may increase stage-four sleep and enhance Elavil.

Ultram (tramadol HCl): This medication for moderate to severe pain acts on the central nervous system. It is one of a new class of analgesics called CABAs (Centrally Acting Binary Agents). It has a "low-abuse potential," so doctors may prescribe it more liberally than other strong painkillers.

Warning: Frequent side effects of Ultram are constipation, nausea, dizziness, headaches, weariness, tightening of jaw and neck muscles, and vomiting.

More than one Internet doctor has switched all FMS patients to Ultram. One doctor reported that 70 percent of those taking Ultram gained enough control over the pain they experienced so that they resumed more active lifestyles. Ultram is not a controlled substance.

Reports say it doesn't work well on an "as needed" basis—you have to take it regularly for best benefits. Many people said it brought more alertness for longer times and less "fibro-fumble" of the fingers. It has also been reported to have success as a migraine treatment.

Warning: One case of seizures has been reported with its use. This medication can lower the seizure threshold.

Wellbutrin (bupropion HCl): This weak Specific Serotonin Re-uptake Inhibitor (SSRI) and antidepressant is sometimes used in FMS/MPS in place of Elavil.

Warning: Wellbutrin can promote seizures.

Xanax (alprazolam): This anti-anxiety medication may be enhanced by ibuprofen. It enhances the formation of blood platelets, which store serotonin, and also raises the seizure threshold.

Warnings: **(1)** When stopping Xanax medication, you must taper off it very gradually. **(2)** Xanax must **not** be used during pregnancy.

Zoloft (sertraline HCl): This is an SSRI and antidepressant. It is commonly used to help with sleep problems.

Most people who find Benedryl stimulating rather than sedating will have the same response to Pamelor, Paxil, and Ultram.

In Conclusion

Because physicians' understanding of FMS, MPS, and FMS/MPS Complex has been so slow and is still so incomplete, information about effective medications is also incomplete. It is essential to find a physician who understands that your pain is real and should be addressed with appropriate medications. Every patient's medications must be tailored to that person's specific symptoms, and must also be monitored to meet that person's changing needs.

CHAPTER 22

Enhancing Your Medications

Chapter 21 described a number of medications that have been found useful in treating the symptoms of FMS and FMS/MPS Complex. It is important to remember, however, that people with FMS or FMS/MPS Complex often have odd reactions to medications. For example, a little bit of a normally calming medicine may put you out for 24 hours or keep you awake for days. In addition, a medication appropriate for FMS may be inappropriate for MPS.

It is always wise to take as little medication as possible. You should also learn to do whatever you can to enhance the actions of the medications you do take, and to try whatever nonmedical regimens might work to ease your symptoms.

Guidelines for Taking Medications

The guidelines presented in this section will help you to stay in control of your medications. In addition, use the references referred to in this chapter, as well as any other sources you have discovered, to gather information you need. Keep your mind open to a variety of viewpoints.

Before you start any medication or treatment plan, be sure your prescribing doctor has all of the following information:

- The names of all the medications and treatments you take, including over-the-counter medications such as vitamins.

- If you are pregnant, could become pregnant, or are planning a pregnancy in the near future. Are you or will you be breast-feeding?

- Any allergies or sensitivities you have.

- Any other illness or medical condition you have.

- Whether you need any change in normal medication routines, such as the addition of an antiyeast medication whenever you take antibiotics.

If you need to discontinue or change your medication, make sure you discuss the following items with your doctor and pharmacist:

- Whether your medications require periodic blood tests. If so, ask about testing frequency.

- Any physical or emotional side effect that can occur.

- Any possible food or drug interaction.

If you plan to add another medication to your regimen, ask about the following:

- The advisability of filling only part of a new prescription to see if you can tolerate it.

- Is there any need to inform your other doctors, dentists, therapists, etc. of your new medication?

Ask about:

- Any planned vacations, and any extra medications or medical needs you might have to ensure your traveling and vacationing comfort.

- Any vacations your doctor has planned. Be sure you know who will be covering for him/her.

Be sure to follow the advice below:

- Store your medications in a dry, room-temperature place.

- Don't ever share your medications. Don't take medications prescribed for others.

- The first time you take a medication, alert someone nearby that you are taking it. If possible, have someone else in the house. Side effects happen.

- Always keep a medication in its original container.

- If your medication is outdated, throw it away.

- Don't mix medications in one container.

- Store medications high up to avoid having to use childproof caps. (The road to Hell is paved with pain medications in childproof caps.)

- Ensure adequate water intake with your medications. If capsules dissolve in your throat, you might get a cough reaction that could send burning powder to your lungs, throat, and esophagus.

- Remember that a treatment for FMS may be contra-indicated for MPS.

- Use room-temperature water to take your medications. Studies on the availability of medication, as it breaks down in the stomach, are done with room-temperature water to dilute them. You may get unusual reactions if you take your meds with hot or cold liquid. Some medications are rendered unusable if you take them with milk, and taking timed-release medications with hot liquid may negate the timed-release factor.

Trying to treat a patient with body-wide trigger points and severe FMS may frustrate doctors. Remind your doctor that it's frustrating for you, too; and ask for support. You may have to try a great many medications in different combinations before you find the right balance. If your health improves, you may have to adjust your medicines. During flares, you may have to reduce your stress load and increase your medications.

If you've been on a medication for a while, it may seem as though its effects aren't lasting as long as they did previously. Perhaps your liver enzyme system simply has become more adept at breaking the medication down. Discuss this with your doctor and/or pharmacist. Ask for advice.

Be completely honest with your physician. If you forgot to take your medication several times or didn't renew your prescription on time, tell your physician to ensure accurate assessment of the effects of the medication. Sometimes, taking medications becomes so routine, you may lose track of what you have and haven't taken. Set up a system to keep track of your medications.

Tracking Your Medications

One tracking method is to use an egg carton, each seven compartments for eggs labeled for each day of the week. Place the medications for each day in the appropriate container. A quick glance at the egg carton will tell you whether you've taken your medications for that day. You can also use cups to separate morning medications from those that must be taken in the afternoon and evening. Your pharmacist may have other devices for proper pill distribution. Set things up the night before, since you probably won't be up to chasing bouncing pills in the morning.

If you need to take a medication at a certain time each day, a watch with a timer signal or a small inexpensive timer can be a helpful reminder. Be kind to yourself if you forget to take your medications. Everyone forgets—especially people in fibrofog! Just be sure to let your physician know. Consider using a chart or other record to track your medications. A simple check mark on a daily chart or a note in a journal (or a separate daybook for medications) provides an accurate long-term record of medication use and its relationship to symptoms.

Pharmacies and Pharmacists

Have all of your prescriptions filled at one pharmacy so the pharmacist can also warn you of any possible medical interactions, no matter how many doctors you have. Your pharmacist can become a great ally and teacher. It's important to learn everything you can about your medications.

Pharmacists are experts on medications. They have easy access to the answers to your questions. It's important for you to know, for example, that amitriptyline, ibuprofen, and other medications, as well as FMS itself, can cause water retention.

Side Effects

If you develop side effects from any medication you're taking, it's important to know the difference between minor and major side effects. The following medical side effects are *serious* or *dangerous* and must be reported to your physician or to a qualified medical professional immediately. Don't wait.

- blurred vision

- rapid or irregular heartbeat

- rash or hives

- sore throat or fever

- wanting to sleep all the time

- restlessness

- lack of coordination

- confusion

- giddiness

- fainting or seizures

- hallucinations

- numbness or swelling in your hands or feet

- nausea and/or vomiting

- slurred speech

- stomach pain

- stumbling

- jerking of the arms and legs

- ringing in the ears

- large increase/decrease in urination

- infection

- changes in your sex drive/impotence

- changes in your menstrual cycle

Managing Side Effects

You can take steps to reduce or eliminate side effects that are not serious but that may be uncomfortable or difficult to endure. A lifestyle that includes a nutritious diet, plenty of liquids, daily exercise, adequate rest, the regular use of stress-reduction techniques, and a general sense of well-being reduces the incidence and severity of medication side effects in many cases. When life begins to get out of control, side effects tend to worsen.

Many side effects are most severe when you first start taking the medication and your body is still adjusting to it. After a week or two, the side effects may diminish or disappear. Ask your physician if this is to be expected with the medication you are taking.

Worksheet for Recording Medication Information

1. Generic name _____

2. Product name _____

3. What are the risks associated with taking this medication?

_____

_____

4. Why am I taking this medication?

_____

5. What short-term side effects does this medication have?

_____

_____

6. What long-term side effects does this medication have?

_____

_____

7. What symptoms indicate that the dosage should be changed or the medication stopped?

_____

_____

8. Is there any way to minimize the chances of experiencing side effects? _____ If so, what are they?

_____

_____

9. What dietary and/or lifestyle restrictions will I have on this medication?

_____

_____

10. What medications might interact with this one?

_____

_____

11. If blood tests or other tests are used to monitor the medication, how often will I need them?

_____

_____

12. What tests do I need prior to taking the medication?

_____

_____

13. What information is available about the medication?

_____

_____

_____

Other Options—Some Helpful Nonprescription Medications

As part of the job of taking control over your own health, investigate alternative health aids. There are over-the-counter (OTC), or nonprescription, medications you can take. You may need less prescription medication if you take OTCs. Note that the side effects and bioequivalency of OTC medications and health food nutrients often have not been studied as extensively as FDA-approved medications. Be sure to check with your doctor or pharmacist before you use them with your prescription medications.

Vitamin C

The body eliminates vitamin C, even in large doses, in 12 hours. Time-release vitamin C is eliminated in 16 hours. For these reasons it is better to take 2 doses of 500 mg vitamin C, 12 hours apart, than to take one 1000 mg tablet.

CoQ10

CoQ10 is a bioenzyme. Its proper name is Coenzyme Q10, and it is available in many health food stores and drug stores. It may help clear the cognitive (fibrofog) difficulties during a flare. Effective dosage varies.

Note: CoQ10's use is still experimental.

Chromium Picolinate

This mineral supplement is often effective in decreasing the "carbo-craving" some fibromites experience. It seems to improve the efficiency of insulin in the body. Dosage varies (Anderson 1987).

> I've found that a regimen of high-B complex, timed-release vitamin C, timed-release niacin in 250 mg or less a day (no-flush niacin doesn't work as well for opening peripheral circulation), multi-minerals, and anti-oxidants eases the fatigue and the "leaky gut syndrome" often present in FMS and FMS/MPS Complex.
>
> D.J.S.

Melatonin

Melatonin is a neurotransmitter secreted by the pineal gland, which is located in the center of the brain. It is eventually changed in the body to serotonin, another neurotransmitter. Studies on melatonin have just begun. A potent antioxidant and possible age-retarder, it also triggers sleep (Raloff 1995). It is nontoxic, and may make Elavil more active or effective. In normal individuals, melatonin induces sleepiness, decreases alertness, and slows reaction time.

Warning: As many as one-third of those who try melatonin become depressed. If depression occurs, stop taking it.

Seasonal Affective Disorder (SAD) (winter depression) is thought to be due to an overabundance of melatonin that *does not vary* with the daily cycle. It is this lack of variety, according to Lynne August, M.D., that is responsible (1995). She has found that SAD patients often need extra melatonin at night to provide the difference in the sleep/wake cycle. Melatonin is sometimes helpful in resetting the sleep/wake cycle after a time change, or for shift workers. Melatonin secretion in humans can be acutely suppressed by light if the light is of sufficient intensity.

Research on the Internet indicates there is a wide variety of melatonin among brands.

Note: Synthesized melatonin seems more likely to cause depression and often does not help with sleep problems.

> Since the FMS/MPS Complex dragon came to roost, I have been taking raw thymus fairly regularly. Those times when I don't take one thymus capsule every day, I can expect to catch about one cold a month. When I take it faithfully, I catch only a few colds a year.
>
> D.J.S.

Raw Thymus

The thymus gland governs the body's immune system, which is the system that decides what is "self" and what is "invader." It is a spongy, pinkish-gray gland located behind the breastbone. At one time, not many years ago, doctors thought that the thymus gland was a useless relic. Today, we know that it is the "master gland" of the immune system.

It is present at birth, and continues to grow until puberty. It produces the hormone, thymoxin, which activates T-cells that protect us from invading substances. When you reach adulthood, the thymus shrinks and no longer produces T-cells, although it is believed to secrete hormones that keep the T-cells working.

Premier Labs produces a thymus extract made from animals that are fed without antibiotics, hormones, or food supplements. It has been helpful for AIDS patients and for patients with FMS or CFS (Chronic Fatigue Syndrome)—all patients who have impaired immune systems.

L-Threonine

Several people on the Internet have reported that L-Threonine, an amino acid, helps with the Restless Legs Syndrome. Dosage and types available vary.

Calms Forte

Calms Forte is a mix of herbs, calcium, and magnesium phosphates, available over the counter in many health food and drug stores. It may be effective as an alternative medicine to take to promote sleep before going to bed.

Peppermint Oil

This oil, in enteric-coated capsules, often helps Irritable Bowel Syndrome (IBS) (see Chapter 11). If broken down in the stomach, however, it causes flatulence, and you don't need to add more gas to your gut. Look for the brand "Peppermint Plus."

Phazyme

Phazyme and other brands of simethicone may be useful when bloating is a problem. Try taking it before eating foods that normally cause extra bloating.

Salt Water

Using warm salt water for nose drops before going to bed can decrease nocturnal post-nasal drip. It can also stop morning sore throats and aggravated neck trigger points.

In Conclusion

For people with FMS and FMS/MPS Complex, finding the best medications can be a difficult task. Once you've established what works for you, though, you can take steps to maximize the medications' intended effects and minimize their side effects.

CHAPTER 23

Guaifenesin

Due to the experimental nature of guaifenesin (pronounced "gwhy-fen-es-in") in the treatment of fibromyalgia (FMS)and myofascial pain syndrome (MPS), and the fact that this medication is found in most commercially manufactured expectorants, even those sold for children, this chapter is a departure from the typical format of this book.

Many of you may remember studying about the discovery of small pox vaccinations, penicillin, and other such medical milestones when you were in school. Such discoveries are still being made today. What has always been required to make such discoveries is education, an observant and inquiring mind, and a certain amount of courage.

How It Was Discovered

More than 30 years ago, R. Paul St. Amand, an endocrinologist, observed an unusual event. He watched a patient on gout medication scraping tooth tartar off with a fingernail. This patient also had "rheumatism," which improved. (St. Amand 1994). Tooth tartar is a form of calcium phosphate deposit known as "apatite," and he wondered if the hard nodules and lumps in his "rheumatism" patients' bodies might be made of a similar material. If so, perhaps those lumps could be removed if these patients took the same medication. At that time, the medications he used for gout patients were probenecid (Benemid) and sulfinpyrazole (Anturane). Not only did St. Amand have the qualifications for the discovery described above, he also had "rheumatism" himself. So he started taking the gout medication himself.

At first, his "rheumatism" symptoms "flared," and then began to ease. He noticed the cyclic nature of the treatment, which caused periods of flare and then "good days." Soon he noticed that during the good days in the cycle, other kinds of symptoms that had once bothered him were gone. Then, the good days began to cluster, and he began to experience symptom remission.

His results were such that his "rheumatism" patients were also offered the same medication. Although the tooth-tartar experience was rare, the lumps and bumps of the "rheumatism" patients began to disappear, and they began to feel better.

He discovered that uric acid—the problem in gout—was not the problem in "rheumatism," i.e., fibromyalgia (or FMS/MPS Complex). Some gout medications that prevented the formation of uric acid had no effect on fibromyalgia. He tested the urine of his patients on the medications, and found that they were urinating large quantities of phosphoric acid. By then, he had also noticed an obvious family clustering of fibromyalgia cases, and he began to suspect that an inherited defect in phosphate metabolism was the basis of at least some of the fibromyalgia problem.

There were problems with the gout medications. They had side effects, and some people couldn't tolerate them. He still didn't know why they worked the way they did, but he began searching for a kinder, gentler alternative.

When he found that guaifenesin, an over-the-counter (OTC) medicine generally used as an expectorant to loosen phlegm and mucus in the lungs, also had the ability to remove excess uric acid, he tried it. Although he had been taking the gout medication for his "rheumatism" (fibromyalgia), he quickly found out that he still had excess phosphorus remaining in his body. The guaifenesin did an even better job than the gout medication at ridding his body of the phosphorus (St. Amand 1993).

St. Amand uses as his working hypotheses the notion that in fibromyalgia, the mitochondria (our cells' energy factories), are affected. This is the possible cause of the decrease in the body's main fuel, adenosine triphosphate (ATP), in the muscles. This decrease has often been noted in fibromyalgia (*Fibromyalgia Network Newsletter* April 1994).

Increased amounts of inorganic phosphates in the mitochondria depress the formation of ATP. The phosphates remain in solution, but in excess amounts. Areas with the greatest need for ATP, the brain and the muscles, would be most severely affected. (St. Amand, personal communication, Nov. 28, 1995). And excess phosphates would enter various cells of the body.

Note: Guaifenesin is the active ingredient in many cough medication/expectorants. Unfortunately, most of these same medications also contain large amounts of sugar and alcohol, and often other medications such as pseudoephredine. For a reason known only to the Food and Drug Administration, the pill form is available only by prescription.

Mucus Secretions and Guaifenesin

As a rule, fibromites produce unusually thick mucus secretions. If they wear glasses, their lenses may become gunked up from nasal secretions when they blow their noses. They may need more toilet paper or wet wipes than most to cleanse themselves of extra heavy vaginal or anal secretions. Guaifenesin thins all of these thick, sticky secretions.

Guaifenesin Treatment

Guaifenesin treatment for fibromyalgia is not simple. *Doctors can't just prescribe the medication and expect symptom remission.* St. Amand begins treatment by taking a careful medical history of the patient, noting when the symptoms first appeared. He examines the patient for tender points and nodules, which he maps on a chart. He notes the degree of soreness, and the shape and size of the area. He has found that as patients progress, the symptoms tend to disappear in the reverse order in which they first appeared (St. Amand 1994).

His patients keep a careful record of their symptoms, including emotional ones. During treatment with guaifenesin, their symptoms are often more intense than the original ones, but they occur for briefer spans of time. He has found that two months at the *proper* dosage reverses about one year of symptoms. He also checks his patients for reactive hypoglycemia, which is a perpetuating factor discussed in Chapter 24, Nutrition: Keeping It Natural.

No salicyclates may be taken during the course of guaifenesin therapy. Salicylates are chemicals found in some medications, such as aspirin, and in some herbs. (See "Salicylates and Other Concerns" later in this chapter.) Also, St. Amand warns people that guaifenesin therapy is not for the faint of heart. When the excess materials are liberated, the patient may experience a number of unpleasant symptoms. (See the section "Symptoms You May Experience during Guaifenesin Treatment" later in this chapter.)

Sometimes guaifenesin works on *feeder deposits*. These feeder deposits, in my opinion, are large lumps of biochemical debris trapped in myofascial trigger points (TrPs). Over time, these trapped waste materials can become quite toxic. I feel that some of the myofascial TrP structure is formed of the excess phosphates. As the guaifenesin releases some of the phosphates, the matrix loosens and the toxic wastes are released into the bloodstream. Because the liver and kidneys can process only a limited amount of wastes at one time, some of the material redeposits, temporarily. Sometimes these transient deposits even form on the teeth, until eventually the liver and kidneys can catch up with the elimination process. Whether this is the mechanism or not, expect plateaus in the reversal process. Don't become discouraged. We are all different. Allow your body to find the best pace for your own healing.

Dosage

St. Amand has found three subsets of patients in his clinic practice. One subset, about 20 percent of all patients, goes through FMS reversal relatively quickly at 300 mg twice a day.

When I first read about guaifenesin, I wanted to know more. Thus began a long correspondence and friendship with Dr. St. Amand and Claudia Potter, one of his nurses. Early in the correspondence, I began guaifenesin therapy. I have also had the good fortune to discuss guaifenesin and fibromyalgia with Dr. St. Amand in person.

I believe that toxic substances as well as metabolic byproducts and excess materials can become trapped in thickened myofascial nodules and bands of MPS and/or FMS/MPS Complex. This would explain the toxic feeling during the cycles, elevated liver enzymes during some guaifenesin therapy and/or bodywork, and the presence of toxic signs found by acupuncture specialists, homeopaths, naturopaths, Native American Healers, and other health practitioners. I have had severe FMS/MPS Complex for a long time, and I have a lot of perpetuating factors— some of which I can do nothing about. I know it's a long, tough road ahead of me, but I know it's the right one. In two years on guaifenesin (and a lot of bodywork, mind-work, and attention to perpetuating factors), I'm a lot better. Without guaifenesin therapy, I could not have endured writing this book.

D.J.S.

If the "cyclic process" hasn't started in two weeks, the patients are raised to 600 mg twice a day. Fifty percent of all patients experience reversal on 600 mg twice a day. Another 20 percent need 1800 mg a day. The final 10 percent requires 2400 mg or more of guaifenesin per day.

When the first cycle begins, there is usually a period of flu-like fatigue as stored toxins and excess phosphates start releasing. Sleep as much as you can. Your liver and kidneys are working hard to process toxins and excess materials so that they can be excreted. You may have to cut back on bodywork during this time, as this also breaks up TrP material.

For the first few months on guaifenesin, expect to be spitting out mucus that has been clogging your airways. (It's a wonder any of us get enough oxygen.)

Headaches are very common. You may find some "ouch spots" on the back of your neck, or on your hairline, that hurt even with moderate pressure. Putting ice on these spots some-times helps people to endure the first cycle.

Symptoms You May Experience during Guaifenesin Treatment

Among the symptoms you may experience are nausea, fatigue, increased aches, eye irritation, abnormal sensations and abnormal taste sensations (foul or metallic).

Odd skin rashes can be common during the reversal period. These can be scaly rashes, such as eczema, blistering, adult acne, or skin cracking. St. Amand has found that at some time after the adequate dosage for reversal has been reached, the patient may lose a large amount of "inferiorly formed" hair that is replaced with healthy hair. Significant hair-loss appears to be rare.

When I saw Dr. St. Amand, he warned me that my hardest job would be encouraging people to continue guaifenesin therapy through the first cycle. He was right.

D.J.S.

You may also have a burnt taste in your mouth, pimples, gunky eyes, an acidy smelling perspiration unique to guaifene-sin reversal (fortunately), burning on urination (excess phos-phates are excreted as phosphoric acid), bladder infections, and very strong smelling urine. Your urine may become very dark—deep yellow, or even brown. Vaginal secretions also turn acidy. Women may get rashes and burning sensations in the vaginal area. Male partners sometimes also feel the effects. You may experience soreness in the crease between your buttocks. "Bag Balm" or another protective ointment is helpful.

With most people, guaifenesin therapy seems to result in remission of symptoms. When your symptoms are in remis-sion and you have resumed activities, it is time to try cutting down or stopping your other medications one at a time. Try this only after discussing it with your doctor. When you are symptom-free and medication-free, slowly start to taper off the guaifenesin. At some point your symptoms may reappear. You may need a maintenance dose of guaifenesin, as some diabetics need insulin, to help you eliminate excess phosphates. Otherwise they will start to build up again.

It is important to remember that the signs and symptoms described here are *not* side effects of guaifenesin. They are from the toxins and excesses being released by the guaifenesin and are a *good* sign, although it won't feel like it at the time. At least you'll understand why you often felt "toxic." You were.

A Theory

Knowing that guaifenesin thins secretions and works at a cellular level, I believe, at least in part, that guaifenesin may work mechanically, cleaning off gummy cellular membranes. It may be that the nature of one's reversal depends on the nature of one's deposits: how many, how dense they are, how much and what kind of tissue is displaced, and how good one's body is at detoxifying.

Guidelines for Taking Guaifenesin

You can do a number of things to make taking guaifenesin safer and more effective for yourself. Here are some guidelines:

- Drink a lot of water with the guaifenesin. You may feel very thirsty all the time and choose to carry some water around with you.

- As described above, keep the dosage of guaifenesin low at first. It may cause stomach upset or nausea, which will probably disappear in a few days, as your body adjusts to it.

- Store guaifenesin in an environment between 59 and 86 degrees Fahrenheit, not in the refrigerator, nor in a very warm room.

- During guaifenesin therapy, avoid adding phosphoric acid to your body. Cola drinks, for instance, are loaded with it. It makes no sense to add phosphoric acid to your metabolism when your body is already working hard to get rid of its excess. Read your labels.

- Get plenty of rest.

- Eat healthy food, but not too much of it.

- Pay attention to your posture, and stretch when you can.

- Keep a positive attitude.

- Take 15- to 20-minute warm baths (not hot).

- Allow enough time between bodywork sessions to recover from one before the next one begins.

- Allow some time for your body to adjust to healing. It will be finding a new balance every day.

- Remember, you are under stress and going through the trauma of change and rebalancing. Your biochemistry is changing. Baby yourself.

Salicylates and Other Concerns

Salicylates are compounds found in medications such as aspirin, some sunscreens, aloe, Pepto-Bismol, wart and callus removers, Listerine, some Alka-Seltzers, and some muscle rubs. Salicylates block the body's efforts to excrete the excess phosphates.

Mentholatum, found in many menthol-containing OTC topical medications, contains many ingredients, but one of the major ones is methyl-salicylate. If salicylates are taken during guaifenesin therapy, the body's toxins will be liberated from the myofascia but will circulate in the blood without being excreted. Ask your pharmacist to help you find nonsalicylate alternatives.

Salicylic acid is currently being added to some ultrasound and galvanic stimulator physical therapy mineral gels and electrode gels. Some of these gels may contain aloe, which will also block the guaifenesin action. Note also that the presence of aloe can be difficult to ascertain, because it is in so many cosmetics. Again, read your labels.

Avoid large quantities of herbs and herbal teas, since many are rich in salicylates, unless you can be sure the herbs have none. Many herbal medications, such as pycnogenol, contain large amounts of salicylates. Small amounts of herbs for seasoning are acceptable.

St. Amand has found that food materials, with the exception of herbs, do not block the guaifenesin action.

Note: It is interesting that in addition to its expectorant qualities, guaifenesin has been used to help women become pregnant. It thins the cervical secretions, which makes it easier for the sperm to penetrate the egg.

Guaifenesin seems to have a strange side effect. A few of the women trying guaifenesin therapy had had previous breast implants. Every one of them had previously developed hard shell-like capsules around the implants. Guaifenesin therapy eliminated, or at least minimized, these shell-like capsules.

In Conclusion

The only double-blind study attempted on the FMS guaifenesin therapy was seriously flawed. It was started before the effect of salicylates was known, and before the need for varying dosages was discovered. This is not uncommon when attempting to design experiments for old medications with new uses. We are breaking new trails here, and discovering more about guaifenesin and FMS/MPS as we travel.

Guaifenesin is not a cure, but it is a hope. It is not for everyone, as some people cannot tolerate the reversal symptoms. There are, however, people in our local support group who are back to work full-time thanks to guaifenesin therapy. There are many more who are now able to take part in activities they have long been denied due to FMS or FMS/MPS Complex. Others have enjoyed periods of symptom remission, and they look forward to even better health in the future. If you wish to learn more about guaifenesin, information is available. Dr. St. Amand's lecture and question and answer session, plus a testimony by Nancy Medeiros (one of our Internet FMily members) is available as a 2 hr and 30 minute video, for $20. A guaifenesin survey poster chart is also available. Contact Nancy Medeiros, P.O. Box 461377, Escondido, CA 92046-1377, email nancym@owl.csusm.edu.

CHAPTER 24

Nutrition: Keep It Natural

Even very healthy people have problems meeting the precise nutritional needs of their bodies, even if they are intelligent and aware of these needs and want to satisfy them. So, of course, for the person with FMS or FMS/MPS Complex, the proper nutritional balancing act is even more difficult to achieve.

Nutrients

There are three basic types of nutrients:

- proteins, such as beef, fish, and poultry

- fats, such as butter, cream, and vegetable oils

- carbohydrates, such as vegetables, fruits, grains, pastas, and cereals

Lately, the current trend for a healthier diet has caused many people to eat high carbohydrate and low-fat diets. The problem with this kind of diet for people with FMS, especially for those who have reactive hypoglycemia as well, is that they have a problem metabolizing carbohydrates. This can lead to overweight and an inability to lose the extra weight, fatigue, carbohydrate craving, and worsening of many other FMS symptoms. (Fibromites often develop a fat pad in front of their bellies that refuses to go away, no matter what they do.)

The Carbohydrate Connection

Carbohydrates come from plants. High-protein foods such as beef, pork, poultry, fish, cottage cheese, and tofu have negligible amounts of carbohydrates. The important and often overlooked problem with carbohydrate metabolism is that carbohydrates also stimulate insulin production.

Carbohydrates and Insulin Production

Insulin enables blood sugar to move to our biochemical "factories" in the cells, where it is either burned as fuel, or stored for later use. If there is an excess of insulin *and* an excess of carbohydrate, the insulin allows this excess carbohydrate to be stored as fatty acids in fat cells. The excess insulin also prevents the carbohydrate from being used. This means that you not only gain weight as fat, you are also prevented from losing this fat because of the availability of excess carbohydrates.

Symptoms of Excess Carbohydrate Consumption

Lynne August, M.D., is the Director and Nutritional Counselor at Health Equations in Vermont (see Appendix A, Resources). She has studied the intricate relationships between FMS, nutrition, and electrolytic imbalance, and has successfully brought her own FMS into remission. Dr. August believes that a 30/30/40 ratio of carbohydrate, fat, and protein enables people with FMS/MPS to reach their optimum weight with the maximum health benefit (1995). (See "Carbohydrate, Fat, and Protein Ratios" below.)

Dr. August lists the following as common symptoms of excess carbohydrate consumption: carbohydrate craving, excess body fat, high triglycerides/cholesterol, fluid retention, dry skin, brittle hair/nails, dry small stools, decreased memory and ability to concentrate, fatigue or dips in energy, grogginess when waking, headaches, mood swings/irritability, and sleep disturbances. She has also found that a high-carbohydrate diet can contribute to allergies and to many disease processes.

Here are four things you can do that can change this situation:

1. Eat moderate amounts of fat. Fat with your meals will decrease the flow of carbohydrates into the bloodstream and decrease your "carbo craving."

2. Cut down on the amount of carbohydrates you eat.

3. Eat protein as part of your meals. It helps use up the fat stored in your body.

4. Exercise regularly, to decrease the amount of insulin in your blood.

Refined Salt and Electrolyte Balance

Ionized salts (sodium, potassium, and so on) in solution are called *electrolytes.* The correctly balanced exchange of electrolytic ions is what creates energy and allows information to flow properly between the body and mind.

Your electrolytes must be in an ionized state to work for you, since charge exchange is how the body "conducts" its business. Refined salt—the type most people use—has had all of its trace minerals removed. Even sea salt is refined and devalued and skews your biochemistry. Dr. August recommends a special salt called Celtic Salt, which contains needed trace minerals. (See Appendix C, Suppliers of Health Care Items.)

Refined salt, including what is sold as "sea salt," is fairly purified sodium chloride. It is manufactured this way for the use of its main consumer, the chemical industry. Humanity evolved with the true sea salt, and all of its wondrous minerals are still needed by our bodies (de Langre 1994).

When all is in harmony, your body is your best doctor—once you are in balance it will tell you a great deal—if you listen. The more your biochemistry is out of balance, however, the more you cannot trust the messages your body sends, including cravings for a particular type of food. For instance, if you can't tolerate dairy, that may be caused by an electrolytic imbalance, but you may receive messages telling you to eat more dairy. People often crave what they shouldn't eat.

Carbohydrate, Fat, and Protein Ratios

Dr. August recommends a book called *The Zone* (Sears and Lawren 1995). It explains in detail why a ratio of 30/30/40 (the ratio of protein to fat to carbohydrate) is the healthiest way for the majority of people to eat.

Dr. Sears' work shows that the best ratio for food balancing is 3 grams of protein to 4 grams of carbohydrate. Protein should comprise 30 percent of the diet, fats 30 percent, and carbohydrates 40 percent. Each time you eat either a meal or a snack, your food intake should match the 30/30/40 ratio, because there is a need for a balanced hormonal response every time you eat.

At the same time, you will need to adjust your caloric intake and exercise to meet the needs of your body. Your food cravings will become much less intense, once you are eating the proper balance and amounts of food.

When starting a meal, it is wise to eat some protein first. That allows its products reach your brain first. Learn to eat like a gourmet. Eat slowly, chew thoughtfully, and enjoy each bite. Eat less, but eat mindfully, and you will be satisfied. You may have the bad habits of a lifetime to break, but if you succeed, you will live a longer and healthier life.

> Although my dietary fat percentage seemed to go up on this diet, the results were amazing. After three months on the diet, my triglycerides went from very high to normal. I used to be a carbohydrate "junkie," but I'm not anymore.
>
> D.J.S.

Food Allergy/Intolerance

Food allergies and sensitivities differ in many ways from typical allergens that are inhaled into the respiratory system. Food allergies produce a wider range of symptoms, and some of these are emotional. Many of the common FMS symptoms—headaches, fatigue, "fibrofog," mood swings, weight fluctuation, and insomnia, to name a few—can be caused or worsened by foods (*Fibromyalgia Network Newsletter* July 1995).

These days, foods are mostly *not* seasonal. Long ago, when certain foods were available only at specific times of the year, adverse reactions were more obvious. Now, food sensitivities may remain unsuspected and undetected, because we get little doses of the problem foods more often. People with food allergies frequently have a certain "look." They may have baggy, dark areas under the eyes and a certain set to the face that signals a warning to the alert physician. Good doctors use such clues to aid diagnoses.

Which Foods Are Causing the Allergies?

One of the many good reasons for keeping a journal is that you can easily include a food diary. This should allow you to narrow down the list of suspect foods. With such a list you can eliminate suspect foods from your diet for a week or two. Later, return them to your diet, slowly, one at a time. If the symptom that you suspect may be caused by a food allergy *recurs* after you have first eliminated and then reintroduced a particular food, you have found your culprit.

You may have a problem with more than one food. It is common to crave foods to which you are allergic or sensitive. The most common food allergies and sensitivities occur with corn, wheat, fish, milk, nuts, and eggs. Also high on this list are alcohol, berries, cane sugar, chocolate, coconut, coffee, mustard, citrus, peanut butter, peas, pork, potatoes, soy products, tomatoes, and yeast.

If you are intolerant of a food, you can usually eat a small amount without experiencing a reaction. If you are allergic to a food, even a tiny amount will usually trigger allergy symptoms.

If you are prone to headaches, avoid red wine, beer, caffeine, aged cheese, nuts, chocolate, and foods that are fermented, pickled, aged, or marinated. These foods all cause blood vessels in the head to dilate. MSG, sodium nitrates (found in bacon, cold cuts, hot dogs and smoked foods), tyramine (found in aged cheese, chicken liver, fava beans, overripe bananas, and avocados) are also common headache activators.

Five of the most likely food-sensitivity triggers are:

- cereals made of wheat and corn

- dairy products

- caffeine

- yeast

- citrus

The top gas producers are milk and beans. Leading the list for heartburn are chocolate, fats, peppermint, garlic, onions, orange juice, hot sauce, tomatoes, coffee, and alcohol. Read labels. You will be surprised at some of the things found in foods.

To avoid undetected allergies, improve your general health and try to reduce your FMS/MPS Complex symptoms. It is in your own best interests to restrict your diet to fresh, natural food grown without chemicals. Remember, the best way to get yourself out of a hole is to stop digging the hole. Don't add toxins to an already toxic system.

Limit or exclude the following foods from your diet:

- refined sugar

- foods high in saturated fats

- high-calorie, high-fat, low-food-value junk food

- alcohol

- caffeine

Eating Wisely

Today, we are finding that diet and nutrition influence our state of mind. Even if we choose healthy foods, processing these foods can delete needed vitamins. Nutritionists are learning more and more about the short- and long-term effects of a diet high in refined, processed, and artificial, chemical-laden foods. In addition, several classes of drugs increase our need for vitamins, as does the Leaky Gut Syndrome. (See "The Leaky Gut Syndrome," later in this chapter.)

Many people have used various amino acid and vitamin regimes to improve their general health and to reduce their symptoms. You may wish to develop such a program after consultation with knowledgeable health care professionals, such as nutritionists, chiropractors, and naturopathic physicians.

Other ways that you can assure yourself of an adequate intake of healthy foods include the following:

- Make regular shopping trips a high priority so that you will always have a good supply of healthy foods on hand. Make a food plan with a shopping list, and take the list with you when shopping.

- Take the time to cook good foods for yourself.

- Keep a supply of easy-to-fix, healthy foods on hand for those times when you are too busy to spend a lot of time cooking. When you cook, freeze the leftovers in meal-size containers and microwave as needed.

- Identify several local restaurants where you can enjoy a healthy meal.

- Keep healthy snacks available.

- Avoid buying junk food.

- Avoid using food as a reward.

I have had a hard time sticking to good eating habits, especially when I am working to meet a deadline or preparing for a trip. I have tended to put my good eating habits on the back burner. I didn't take the time to go grocery shopping or to prepare good food for myself. When I was traveling, I found it very difficult, and in some cases impossible, to find well-prepared, reasonably priced healthy food. I ended up snacking on junk foods. I always paid with a general feeling of malaise and a worsening of gastrointestinal problems and chronic pain.

Recently, however, I began working with a nutrition counselor. She took a complete dietary history and a blood analysis. From that information she prescribed a specific diet and food supplements. Although the supplements must be determined on an individual basis, the

If your symptoms are very painful or your schedule is too hectic to shop, ask supporters to pick up groceries for you when they pick up their own. You can return the favor when you're able. If getting out is always difficult for you, contact a home health aid service in your area for grocery delivery service. In some areas, nutritious meals can be delivered to your home. The cost for such services is often small and/or on a sliding scale, depending on your income.

There is a difference between wanting food and being hungry. (That sentence would be a good topic for a meditation.) Explore that difference. People often overeat to relieve stress. Eat when you are hungry, and eat just enough to stop the hunger.

If you have a problem with traditional breakfast foods, try eating a balanced, nutritional nontraditional breakfast of things you like.

You may find that taking a walk before or after a meal aids your digestion and reduces stress.

The Leaky Gut Syndrome

One of the major complicating factors in FMS and FMS/MPS Complex is a common condition called the "Leaky Gut Syndrome." In this syndrome, the small intestine has a hyperpermeable lining. This means that too many things pass through the membrane (the hyperpermeable lining) from the intestine into the body. The membrane's normal function is to act as a filter. When it becomes hyperpermeable, toxic wastes leak through it. This creates an overload of toxins, and the liver's detoxification functioning quickly becomes clogged. According to a clinical immunologist from Cambridge Hospital in England, if the substances that leak through the gut aren't properly and promptly detoxified by the liver, an inflammatory cascade can result (Hunter 1991).

This cascade is like a domino effect, except that rather than one domino setting off another, each domino sets off several, which, in turn, set off several more. The cascade activates immune system and hormonal changes, which, in turn, produce diffuse musculoskeletal and neuromuscular symptoms similar to those seen in FMS and MPS.

A healthy, intact, and functioning gastrointestinal (GI) lining is the body's first line of defense against invasion by the "bad guys" (large toxic waste molecules), and it still permits the "good guys" (nutritional substances) to enter the systemic circulation.

The small intestine is not just a waste conduit. It is a marvel of complex nutrient absorption and waste-stream separation. The mucosal lining can be weakened by stress, chronic dietary deficiencies, and toxins, which, in turn, causes it to become more permeable. Unfortunately for people with FMS/MPS Complex, who already have serious neurotransmitter malfunctioning, the important neurotransmitter, serotonin, is formed mostly in the brain and the gastrointestinal tract. The Leaky Gut Syndrome decreases serotonin formation, which leads to mood swings, sleep disruption, and to the general miseries of FMS/MPS Complex.

NSAIDs and the Leaky Gut Syndrome

There are studies (Leaky Gut Syndrome and Fibromyalgia—What Is the Connection? 1995) indicating that use of nonsteroidal anti-inflammatory drugs (NSAIDs) (see Chapters 21 and 22), may be part of the leaky gut cause. NSAIDs cause widening between the cells of the intestinal lining. When foreign bacterial biochemicals and partially digested food molecules pass through the lining, the body mobilizes its antibody defenses. Antibodies sent to fight these invaders can spark food allergies.

> diet works well for everyone and fits in with the usual dietary guidelines of most nutrition programs. It is the 30/30/40 diet recommended earlier in this chapter in the section called "Carbohydrate, Fat, and Protein Ratios."
>
> On this diet I feel much better and have lost a few extra pounds. The nutritionist also recommended a food bar that meets my dietary requirements. I use it in place of a meal or snack when I am traveling or am too busy to fix something to eat.
>
> M.E.C.

Reactive Hypoglycemia

Several researchers have independently found that a large subset of people with FMS also have *reactive hypoglycemia*—low blood sugar that occurs after eating carbohydrates (August 1995; Wurtman 1989). Reactive hypoglycemia is not the same as fasting hypoglycemia, which is low blood sugar that occurs when you do not eat. For this reason, reactive hypoglycemia is not always picked up on routine medical tests.

Reactive hypoglycemia occurs within two to three hours after a meal, when there is a rapid release of carbohydrates into the small intestine followed by rapid glucose absorption, and then the production of a large amount of insulin.

This happens frequently in people with FMS and FMS/MPS Complex. In FMS, it is caused by dysfunctional neurotransmitter regulation and other systemic mechanisms. With FMS, you crave carbohydrates but cannot make efficient use of them because of an electrolytic imbalance and other biochemical imbalances in your body.

When you consume carbohydrates, your insulin production increases. If you have reactive hypoglycemia, your body overcompensates. This results in low blood sugar.

David Simons, M.D., and Janet Travell, M.D., in the *Trigger Point Manuals* (1983, 1992, mentioned that in cases of chronic MPS, the process of eliminating trigger points is hampered

> I have a theory that this immune cascade may be the reason a significant subset of fibromites start out having FMS with an unidentifiable flu-like illness.
>
> D.J.S.

or even thwarted by the presence of hypoglycemia. Hypoglycemia is a perpetuator of MPS (see Chapter 7, Perpetuating Factors).

R. Paul St. Amand found that there is a subset of fibromites with reactive hypoglycemia. He notes that it can range from very mild to severe. The symptoms he lists are: headaches (usually in the front or top of the head), dizziness, irritability, chronic fatigue, depression, nervousness, difficulty with memory and concentration, nasal congestion, heavy dreaming, palpitations or heart pounding, tremor of the hands (especially if a long time elapses between meals), day or night sweats, anxiety in the pit of the stomach, leg cramps, numbness and tingling in the hands and/or feet, flushing, and craving for carbohydrates and sweets. Fainting occurs, but only rarely. The hunger pangs experienced in reactive hypoglycemia can come in the form of acute stomach pain and nausea.

Most of these symptoms diminish five or ten minutes after eating sugar. In women, symptoms often worsen before menstrual periods and become severe immediately after childbirth.

St. Amand found that people with FMS/MPS Complex have a problem with carbohydrate metabolism. He feels that the standard Glucose Tolerance Test is relatively worthless for determining *reactive* hypoglycemia in the general population, not just in people with FMS or FMS/MPS Complex. Hypoglycemic tendency is inherited, and he has found that with hypoglycemia there is often also a family history of diabetes.

St. Amand also found that hypoglycemia, if occurring in conjunction with FMS, must be treated immediately for guaifenesin and other FMS therapies to be effective. He has found that for reactive hypoglycemics, diet is the treatment that works.

For those with reactive hypoglycemia, St. Amand's dietary restrictions are as follows: no alcohol, sugar (in any form), fruit juice (which contains large amounts of fructose), dried fruit, baked beans, black-eyed peas, lima beans, potatoes, corn/popcorn, bananas, barley, rice, pasta, other heavy starches, or caffeine are permitted.

On this diet, people feel some improvement in seven to ten days. They are, however, seven to ten *very* uncomfortable days. The headache and fatigue can be extreme, and if you are aware that sugar can ease the symptoms in the short term, you will be tempted to cheat. In one month, however, you will see considerable improvement. Within two months, the hypoglycemic symptoms should be gone—if you have adhered to the diet. *Note that St. Amand recommends this diet only for his patients with reactive hypoglycemia, not for people with FMS in general.*

Note: There is a book no longer in print, called *A Taste for Life* by Marcia Grad, with a foreword by St. Amand. It is full of tasty, low-carbohydrate recipes especially designed for people with reactive hypoglycemia. It would be wonderful to see that book back in print.

This is one tough diet, because if you need it, you *really* crave carbohydrates. You have to try it for only a few days and your body informs you, "Yes, this is what you must do," because you are attacked by whopping headaches and extreme fatigue as soon as your body begins its struggle for a new balance. Your excess fat will start to break down, and release large amounts of toxic substances and waste material. It is not fun. But it does work.

In Conclusion

Diet is a crucial factor in treating FMS and FMS/MPS Complex effectively. Improper diet is also implicated in many allergies and diseases. In these days of fast food, sticking to a healthy diet is very hard, but it really pays off in reduction of symptoms, increased vitality, and overall wellness.

Not totally in jest, I refer to this diet as the Inuit/St. Amand diet, because the Inuit eat lots of protein, some fat, and very little carbohydrate. It's what I use.

D.J.S.

CHAPTER 25

Bodywork: Helping Your Body Work

"There is no tissue that is not 'body,' and there is no response that is not 'mind'. . . . There is no local activity which does not affect or is not affected by the entirety of the activities of the organism." (Juhan 1987)

Bodywork is a term used to describe any physical therapy techniques that are used to help your body. You can often perform these techniques yourself, once you learn them. There are other forms of physical therapy that you cannot do by yourself. This doesn't mean, however, that you should view any bodywork simply as a passive process. Your health care team needs your feedback and reinforcement to work at maximum effectiveness with you. Bodywork includes such techniques as massage, craniosacral release, Alexander method, yoga, and acupressure. You will learn more about specific techniques in the next chapter.

It is very important that you and your health care team understand the fundamental concepts of myofascial trigger points (TrPs), chronic myofascial pain syndrome (MPS), and fibromyalgia syndrome (FMS), as they have been described in the first five chapters of Part I. These concepts are the basic building blocks for an understanding of FMS and FMS/MPS Complex. Too often these conditions are lumped together, resulting in inappropriate therapies that hinder rather than help the healing process.

The misunderstandings prevalent among medical practitioners today are due to failure to grasp the basic concepts. In the medical literature, the terms FMS and MPS are not used consistently, and it can be hard to figure out exactly which condition is being discussed. Once the fundamental concepts are clearly understood, however, proper therapeutic interventions can begin.

Bodywork and the Pain Issue

Pain, like all other sensations, is carried along the nerves. Nerves, like muscles and bones, are encased by an elastic framework that supports and connects them. The framework for muscles and bones is the myofascia. In the case of the nerves, this elastic tissue is called the *glial cells.* Glial cells serve the nerves as the myofascia serves the muscles. These cells surround every nerve fiber, group of nerve fibers, and so on, and they provide elasticity and support.

In addition, glial cells form what is called the *ground substance,* which moderates the exchange of gases, fuel, wastes, and other materials to and from the nerve cells.

Membranes of nerves and muscles constantly exchange biochemicals back and forth. They also exchange negative and positive ions—the plus and minus charges that run the bioelectrical functioning of the body. These ions are in the form of certain minerals, such as sodium, potassium, calcium, and phosphorous, which are called *electrolytes.*

When there is a change from a plus to minus charge or a minus to a plus charge, that change releases neurotransmitters and energy. This is what the nerve cells called *neurons* do. They send waves of energy from one place to the next. That's the nuts and bolts of body and mind communications.

For communications to be smooth, there must be a continuous flow of circulating materials in and around each cell. When a part of the nerve is pinched or constricted and the area is obstructed with wastes, sensations and messages become garbled. Some areas may become numb, others may become hypersensitive. "Fibrofog," delayed reactions, and many other symptoms of FMS/MPS Complex develop under these conditions.

There are many levels or layers in the nervous system. One layer, called the *dorsal column,* is coated with insulation. This insulation is called *myelin,* and it gives this part of the nervous system a white color. The dorsal column is like an express train. It crosses few nerve junctions and bridges few gaps, and the myelin insulation allows nerve impulses to travel from 40 to 70 meters per second (Juhan 1987). This is the system that carries sensations of fine pressure, vibrations, and the sensation of body parts in motion.

The "gray matter" of the spinal cord, which has no myelin to color it white, bridges many gaps. This system is called the *spinothalamic* system, and it is the system that carries pain. It also carries messages of heat and cold, itches, tickles, and sexual sensations. Spinothalamic sensations move at one-fifth the speed of dorsal column sensations. This means that you experience a time lag between the stimulus and the sensation. The lag gives you the opportunity to analyze the cause of the feeling, such as pain, before you react.

During the time lag, you have a chance to flood your consciousness with the more rapidly transmitted touch sensations and thus to block some of the pain with the faster-signaling, pleasurable touch sensations (Juhan 1987). That is why bodywork, such as massage, is an important part of any therapy directed at FMS or FMS/MPS Complex symptoms.

How Bodywork Can Help Control Other Symptoms

Bodywork is beneficial for more than just pain relief. For example, in FMS/MPS Complex, the muscles and other parts of the body do not receive sufficient amounts of oxygen. Proper bodywork can result in the slowing and deepening of your respiration, in which case you will take in more oxygen with less effort. Some bodywork will also help break up the tightened myofascia.

Bodywork can help to diminish muscle tension in trigger point (TrP) areas, as well as tension in the entire body. It can improve circulation, which will also help the muscles to receive more fuel and oxygen. With most types of bodywork the resting heart rate will also drop. This means that the heart achieves the same degree of functionality with less effort.

In Chapter 27, Bodywork You Can Do Yourself, you will learn more about respiration and how you can enhance your breathing. But now you must get to the heart of the matter.

Workings of the Heart

Oxygen-rich blood flows into the left atrium of the heart. This oxygenated blood then passes through the mitral valve to the left ventricle. The mitral valve is largely composed of myofascia. This is important, since a condition called *mitral valve prolapse* occurs frequently in FMS. In this condition, the myofascia of the valve loses its elasticity and it no longer functions as well as it should.

The heart has its own blood supply, which is delivered through the coronary arteries. Each pulse, each heartbeat, pushes about two and one-third ounces of blood on its way. The beat rate is determined by the internal generator of the heart, for the heart is also an electrical system—just like the rest of the body.

Your blood pressure and pulse are two reliable and accessible "vital signs" that help your medical team to monitor your health. While you learn about bodywork techniques, become informed about what your blood pressure and pulse readings mean. Understanding these readings will reinforce the importance of bodywork to your health.

Making Progress

As you progress with various physical therapy methods, you will begin to observe changes in your body. In the long-term, the changes will be for the better, but change never comes easily. You might find that the first time you do bodywork, you experience an *increase* in your pain level. You might begin hurting in places you didn't even know you had. That's because bodywork will often activate latent trigger points. This can be discouraging, because, after all, you are doing bodywork to *improve* the quality of your life.

It's also not uncommon to experience nausea, a dramatic increase in headaches, and even complete exhaustion after any bodywork has moved a large amount of toxins and wastes from constricted muscles. You may need to sleep after a session; so, at first, don't schedule anything immediately after your bodywork sessions. The sleepiness is a good sign. Your body is telling you something, so listen to it. The bodywork isn't what causes you to feel awful. The toxins and material released from the myofascia are the real culprits. And your liver and kidneys can handle only so much of the biochemical by-products released during a good bodywork session at one time. Aren't you glad you are getting them out of your system? Take it easy on yourself for a while.

Making Things Easier

You can ease the strain on your body during the course of bodywork by drinking large amounts of water to dilute and flush out the waste materials. You should rest frequently, and enjoy a good book or some other healthy treat.

Avoid strenuous activities (including travel) during the day you have scheduled for bodywork therapy and for several days thereafter. After your TrPs are broken up, your muscles will probably be sore for several days. If you have many TrPs, you may have to take it easy for a full week after each treatment. Allow time for your body to recover between sessions. Avoid perpetuating factors (see Chapter 7), if possible, and learn to respect your muscles. Muscles are supposed to relax, contract, and be mobile. Give them a chance to remember how to do so.

Become more aware of your body and how it communicates. Too often, we are taught to ignore our sensations. This can lead to problems. When TrPs are extremely active, your muscles are overwhelmed by TrP activity and cause you pain even when you are at rest. They are telling you they need to be handled with care. At this point they require gentle passive stretches and hot packs. Trying to force them into action might cause them to contract even more tightly in response. This is called a *rebound contraction.*

As your muscles improve through bodywork, you will be able to recognize and avoid activities that stress them. Your journal (see Chapter 17) should come in handy for this. Decide which aggravating activities are unnecessary and/or modifiable. Write down any activity that causes pain. Then write down how you can avoid or modify that activity to reduce or eliminate the pain.

The best way to treat FMS/MPS Complex is to work from many angles, moving slowly to allow your body to reach new balances. This is the kind of therapy you can expect:

- After your doctor identifies your pain patterns by comparing them to the Travell and Simons illustrations in *The Trigger Point Manuals,* she or he should check for the TrPs that cause those patterns.

- Your doctor, with your help, will attempt to identify any perpetuating factors of these TrPs (see Chapter 7, Perpetuating Factors). Your journal may help with that. Only *after* any perpetuating factors have been identified and treated should you begin specific treatment for your TrPs.

- Your treatment plan will include physical therapy. Different types of physical therapy are explained in the following two chapters. You will be able to do some of this for yourself.

- Your diet and lifestyle may need modification. This is discussed in depth in Chapter 16, Coping Day to Day, and Chapter 24, Nutrition: Keep It Natural.

- Your doctor may recommend, or you may decide, that cognitive therapy, meditation, or some other type of stress reduction or coping skills will help you (see Chapter 20, Meditation and Mindfulness).

In Conclusion

When you begin any form of bodywork, don't expect an overnight cure. Think of how many years it's taken to get your body into the state it's in today. Be gentle with yourself, and give your body and mind a chance to recover. It will take some time, and lots of work. But the results will be worth however much of your time and effort it takes.

CHAPTER 26

Bodyworkers

Bodyworkers are healers who heal through the use of touch and physical contact. Although there are some forms of bodywork that can be self-administered (see Chapter 27, Bodywork You Can Do Yourself), there are special types of bodywork that only professionals can perform. This chapter looks at some of the better-known types of physical therapies that professionals practice. To find out about some of the lesser-known methods, see Chapter 28, Alternatives: Other Cultures, Other Ways.

Medicine has, in recent times, become an electronic technology. Some of this is good, and even necessary. Still, too often, there has been a loss of focus in the healing arts. It is wise for us to return to the roots of medical practice periodically, and to remind ourselves what the art of healing is all about. The following poem, the "Prayer of the Tibetan Physician," is an eloquent reminder.

> "May all living beings be free of suffering . . . May everything that I do
> go to ensure that they be free of suffering and the cause of suffering.
> May all living beings have joy and the cause of joy . . . May I be the one
> to ensure, to remind them that they are in fact living in joy and have the
> causes of joy. May all living beings interrelate fully, lovingly, compassionately
> and joyously with one another, without any discrimination or partiality
> of near and far, of like or dislike. May I be the one that does everything in
> my power to see that they do this. May I be the one to make sure that this
> takes place."

To start you on the road to recovery, this chapter introduces you to some people who will give you a helping hand and a lift along your way.

Your Physical Therapist and You

Some of the most important people in your life are your physical therapists. Yes, some people have more than one, and they receive a different type of bodywork from each therapist; furthermore, there are many different types of physical therapy. It is vital that you find the best and the most appropriate physical therapist for yourself. The proper physical therapy for arthritis, for example, is not applicable to FMS or FMS/MPS Complex.

If you have fibromyalgia (FMS), find a physical therapist who is knowledgeable about it, who is comfortable dealing with it, and who understands your pain. If you have chronic myofascial pain syndrome (MPS), find someone who knows the *Trigger Point Manuals* (Travell and Simons 1992 and 1983). If you have FMS/MPS Complex, it is best to find someone who can provide you with Galvanic Muscle Stimulation (GMS) or ultrasound with electrostimulation therapy, as described later in this chapter.

People with a diagnosis of FMS, but who have undiagnosed tender and sore trigger points (TrPs), should take care not to be treated with inappropriate bodywork therapies. For example, Travell and Simons have made it abundantly clear that weight training and work hardening programs should *not* be used on people with active trigger points.

For people in this situation, their pain and muscle tightness will grow progressively worse as the inappropriate therapy continues. When their grip strength finally gives out, weights may be strapped to their wrists. When the patient refuses (rightfully) to continue the program, the health care team may even blame him or her for being uncooperative. This is truly an intolerable situation.

With MPS, if you have pain from TrPs, even when you are at rest, all that you will be able to tolerate at first is passive stretch work, hot packs, craniosacral and myofascial release, and, perhaps, some sinewave ultrasound with electrostimulation or galvanic muscle stimulation, as described later in this chapter. Note that the same therapies are appropriate for people with FMS who are experiencing a flare, minus the use of the electronics. Electronic stimulation is *only* for treating trigger points.

If you have active TrPs, avoid weight training, repetitive exercises, and cool swimming pools or lakes. If your physical therapist wants to use these in your therapy program, show him or her the information in this chapter.

Chiropractors

Chiropractors are bodyworkers who are also doctors. Their training takes just as long as that of an M.D. who is a general practitioner. (Chiropractors often refer patients to M.D.s, but unfortunately, this process is rarely reversed.)

Often chiropractors can straighten and release extremely tight areas so that your physical therapist has a chance at loosening the myofascia. Chiropractic medicine is based on the fundamental idea that if the structural bones (especially the spinal column) and the muscles of the body are in proper alignment, the inherent recuperative powers of the body will take over, and the body will heal itself.

Your first visit to a chiropractor should include a careful, detailed medical history, a thorough physical examination, and sometimes X-rays. Only then can a treatment plan be formed.

Chiropractors use many methods to coax the bones back into their proper position. They also work on the muscles to ease the tightening that caused the problem in the first place.

Sometimes only a few visits to the chiropractor are needed to realign your body. However, if you have FMS, MPS, or FMS/MPS Complex, after each chiropractic adjustment, your tight muscles will pull your bones slightly out of alignment again. Your body has limited means for restoring function when parts of it are busy fighting other parts. This kind of internal warfare can cause other symptoms to develop throughout your entire body.

Of course, just as in all professions, there are chiropractors and there are chiropractors. When looking for a chiropractor to work with you for treatment of FMS, MPS, or FMS/MPS Complex, ask others at your support group for recommendations. When you find one with a good reputation, try calling. Ask him or her about myofascial trigger points and Drs. Travell's and Simons' work. Most chiropractors are far ahead of M.D.s regarding this area of knowledge. You will even find chiropractors with well-thumbed volumes of the Trigger Point Manual close at hand in their offices.

Spine Manipulation

The central focus of chiropractic medicine is the manipulation of the spine to relieve pain and body imbalances. Manual adjustment (the familiar "cracking") of body manipulation can line up the spine, although this method is not recommended for people with MPS or FMS/MPS Complex. Manual adjustment can cause great pain if there is nerve entrapment, especially with TrPs in the neck (see Chapter 3, Myofascial Trigger Points). Activator methods of chiropractic adjustment usually work very well, however. (See the section on the Activator below.)

Blocking, or straightening out the spine by placing blocks under the hips and coaxing the spine into alignment, is a gentle method that many chiropractors use. Blocking is especially good for those of us with MPS or FMS/MPS Complex. Traction usually doesn't work with MPS or FMS/MPS Complex, since the muscles revert to the same tightness and misalignment after the treatment.

Chiropractors use heat, cold, and other types of bodywork discussed elsewhere in this book. Electrical stimulation is especially effective in eliminating or minimizing TrPs. Many chiropractors can also help with exercises and nutritional advice.

I know exactly where I'd be without chiropractic medicine—in a lot more pain. If I'm going on a trip or planning something that will place unusual stress on my body, I visit my chiropractor before I leave for the trip. I do everything to ensure that I am in the best possible condition *before* I tackle something difficult—chiropractic can be great preventive medicine. I also schedule an appointment following a stressful activity. My body needs that alignment help before it can begin to heal itself.

D.J.S.

Chiropractic treatment can be frustrating at first. Bones are coaxed into alignment, only to have tight and contracting muscles pull them right back out of alignment. Liberated toxins and wastes can cause you to feel toxic and exhausted after a treatment, as do most successful treatments of other kinds of physical therapy. However, the results are worth the effort. It can be an ironic comfort to know that if you are hurting, you are working with someone who is getting you back on the healing path.

The Activator and Other Treatment Methods

One of the kindest innovations in chiropractic medicine is the Activator. The Activator is a small (about the size of a pen), handheld instrument that delivers a low-force tap where directed. It is the most widely used low-force technique in chiropractic practice. Some people have described it as looking like a "mini-pogo stick." (Others think that it looks like a metal hypodermic, without a needle, but with a spring attachment.)

The chiropractor aims one end of the Activator at a vertebra or other misaligned bone, and lightly taps the other end. This engages the spring mechanism, which immediately realigns the bone. When used expertly by a Doctor of Chiropractic, it can realign the skeleton almost instantly. It can be used on all types of patients, and has different settings.

The Activator works faster than the body's ability to tense and resist. It appears that very few people are unable to tolerate Activator adjustment. It is important to remember that it cannot be handled by the patient and should be used *only* by an expert practitioner.

I am exceedingly fortunate to know several excellent chiropractors, and they have made a great difference in the quality of my life. In fact, my chiropractor is my primary care physician. It was my chiropractor who first told me about the work of Drs. Janet Travell and David Simons.

D.J.S.

Massage Therapists

There are many forms of massage, and books have been written about most of them, from aielaia, (an ancient form of massage, practiced with the hands barely touching the body, which works on energy fields) to ancient Zen forms. Massage can be a relaxing, powerful, healing tool, but it must be respected and carefully managed. The wrong kind of massage, too vigorous a massage, or too short a time between massages can be detrimental to your healing.

The type and duration of massage must be decided on a person-to-person basis and is best left to the discretion of a skilled massage therapist and to what feels best and works best for you. *You* must be in control of your healing path, once you are educated in the types of treatment that are possible.

The first few times you experience massage, it may leave you exhausted, and you may feel the need to go home and sleep. This is a common occurrence with FMS, MPS, and FMS/MPS Complex massage patients. It's a sign that toxins and blockages in the body are being released into the bloodstream. Your liver and kidneys will be working overtime, so help them all you can.

Drink plenty of pure water, avoid toxins such as secondhand smoke and alcohol, and eat lightly but nutritiously.

After a massage, just as with any other physical therapy, plan to take it easy for a while. You may have a sore body the day after a massage, especially if you have a lot of TrPs. This soreness should disappear by the following day. If it does not, tell your massage therapist to take things a little easier the next time. Your body needs time to adjust to the new balance it has found.

Some types of deep muscle massage, such as skin-rolling, Rolfing, and Hellerwork, may be beyond your endurance and will usually worsen your symptoms by triggering *rebound contraction*. This causes your muscles to tighten up much worse than they were before the massage, and your condition will continue to deteriorate. Other types of bodywork, such as the Alexander Technique and Bowen therapy, can be extremely gentle and effectively provide some relief from symptoms.

Alexander Technique

The Alexander Technique focuses on correcting body mechanics. It improves posture and movement styles, thus relieving muscle tensions. The patient's thought processes and body movements are both retrained and the patient learns to move with greater ease, avoiding perpetuating factors that can lead to tense muscles and TrPs. It is an exceedingly gentle method of relief for tense muscles.

Alexander Technique practitioners are trained to teach their method to their clients. Their relationship with their clients is that of teacher and student. At first, the teacher may observe the student lying on a table, fully clothed. Then observation takes place as the student stands, walks, and performs daily activities. Lessons are usually on a one-to-one basis, because the teacher must touch and adjust the student's movements, although group classes are becoming more common. Lessons usually run from half an hour to a full hour, once a week, for a minimum of 15 weeks. Generally, the lessons continue for 30 or more weeks.

Bowen Therapy

Bowen therapy is a very gentle, noninvasive form of bodywork that doesn't require a long series of treatments. Some therapists using Bowen therapy treat people only once a week for a month and then once a month for six months. It uses

I went into meditative mode for the Bowen treatment. While some of my muscles were being reset, I felt an immediate release. Other muscles that had been very tight began to twitch—often hours later. I was told to avoid sitting still for more than half an hour before I slept that night. All night, my muscles responded with twitches now and then, although I slept deeply for the first part of the night. (Many local support group members have told me they too slept very well after Bowen treatment.)

I was unable to take many treatments, as Bowen is normally not done in conjunction with other physical therapy and I knew I needed a great deal of galvanic stimulation and acupressure massage to continue writing this book. I would like to try Bowen therapy again when this book is done.

D.J.S.

a light, specific touch with a rolling motion on an out-of-alignment muscle. That touch signals the nerves beneath to signal the brain to move the muscle back to where it belongs, like a reset button. For informaion, call Blue River Institute 413-665-3492.

In Bowen therapy, some of the areas that are worked on are TrP locations, and some are acupressure meridians. It often takes five to ten days for the muscles to respond after a treatment.

Craniosacral Release (CSR)

The craniosacral system is composed of the brain, spinal cord, cerebrospinal fluid, a membrane that separates the brain from the skull, the cranial bones, and the sacrum. (The sacrum is a group of five fused vertebrae at the base of the spinal column, right above the coccyx.) The fluid in this system moves with a rhythm all its own. But the rhythm of any patients with chronic conditions, such as those with FMS/MPS Complex, is often very low and fast. Craniosacral release (CSR) can normalize these rhythms (Upledger 1983).

CSR is based on the premise that the brain expands and contracts with a very gentle pumping that circulates cerebrospinal fluid throughout the brain and spine. This very gentle method of bodywork releases tensions and blocks that have developed in the crainosacral system.

Many people with FMS and FMS/MPS Complex are electromagnetically sensitive because of their dysfunctional neurotransmitters. (See chapter 28.) When the practitioner is also electromagnetically sensitive, even if the practitioner's hands move the patient's skin only fractions of an inch, it can seem to the patient as though the whole of her or his body is moving. That's because the whole of the myofascia is adjusting; and this is what the patient feels. Layer after layer of tightness can be released with the proper application of this bodywork technique.

Often, emotional releases accompany craniosacral work, as well as physical releases. CSR practitioners use the term "energy cysts." These form in the craniosacral system and block energy flow. They are described as emotional blockages that often present an electromagnetic blockade to healing.

Feldenkrais Method

The Feldenkrais method is a bodywork/mindfulness technique that enhances the communication between the body and brain. It is based on movement and postural mechanics and uses movement and structural training through the use of patterning. The movements are very slow and gentle, and the focus is on correcting postural misalignments. The practitioner guides the patient in muscle movement patterns to retrain them.

Jin Shin Do Bodymind Acupressure

Jin Shin Do bodymind accupressure is an integrated healing method that uses gentle, deep finger pressure to liberate physical and emotional tensions. It also employs Taoist breathing techniques.

Manual Lymphatic Drainage

This massage technique "milks" the lymphatic ducts, removing blockages. This reduces tightness and swelling and stimulates lymphatic immune components. Most people performing these procedures are trained massage therapists.

Proprioceptor Neuromuscular Facilitation (PNF)

Proprioceptors are sensory receptors that tell your subconscious mind how your body is moving in relation to its environment. They tell the brain which muscles are contracting, and which ones are relaxed. With FMS or FMS/MPS Complex, because of neurotransmitter dysfunction, proprioceptors often lie. Their information superhighway is cluttered with roadkill, and the messages don't get through or become garbled during the journey.

Proprioceptor neuromuscular facilitation (PNF) can trick the proprioceptors by retraining them. The PNF therapist puts the patient in a comfortable position and then has the patient try to push out of that position. Each time this exercise is repeated, the muscle stretches a little further. Only specially trained massage therapists can perform this technique.

Reiki

Reiki is a Japanese form of one type of chi gung (see Chapter 27, Bodywork You Can Do Yourself). The term "reiki" translates as universal life energy. Reiki method was founded by a Japanese-Christian monk, Mikao Usui, in the mid-1800s. This therapy is founded on the premise that ki (universal life force) energy is everywhere and can be focused, channeled, and applied to others, promoting harmony, balance, and healing. Reiki practitioners are available at several levels. A reiki master can rebalance the universal life force within a patient by the laying on of hands.

Spray and Stretch

In spray and stretch massage, after your massage therapist takes a detailed history and performs an examination to find your trigger points, you learn to release tightened muscles with the use of a vapocoolant spray that cools only the myofascia—not the muscle underneath. The massage therapist sprays the vapocoolant in very precise patterns and directions. This cooling inhibits muscle-tensing reflexes. Then, the practitioner stretches the muscle, a little at a time between specific sprays. The patient must give the practitioner constant feedback since the patient is in control of the treatment, and her or his comfort must be ensured.

This method is explained in detail in the *Trigger Point Manuals* (Travell and Simons 1983 and 1992). There is also an excellent set of tapes on spray and stretch for physical therapists. (See Appendix C, Resources.) The movement of the spray, the timing of the spray, and the stretch of the muscle are critical to the release of the muscle tissue. This method can also use ice, as long as the ice is kept covered and prevented from directly touching the patient's skin. After the muscle has been released, the muscle group is passively stretched several times, through its normal range of motion. The muscle group is then rewarmed.

Strain-Counterstrain

Strain-counterstrain is a form of physical manipulation to relieve tense muscles and the pain caused by that tension. After finding a trigger point, the practitioner moves the patient's body into a position where the pain is relieved. The patient then pushes against the practitioner's hand in the direction of the painful position. The patient relaxes. The patient is then moved slightly toward the uncomfortable position, and the procedure is repeated. Eventually, the trigger point is eased. This treatment is often used in osteopathy and physical therapy.

Electronically Speaking

Since Dr. Willard Travell, Janet Travell's father, discovered that an interrupted rhythmic electrical discharge produces a vigorous exercise of the muscle if it is directed properly, we've known that electromagnetics has a lot to do with the tightness of a muscle.

Alternating muscular contractions and relaxations increase blood flow through the muscles. Sustained contraction decreases blood flow. Thus, it is not unreasonable to expect that muscle stimulation and pulsed ultrasound can help to break up myofascial TrPs.

Warning: Electronic devices should not be used on cancer patients, on patients with heart trouble or seizure disorders, nor used *near* patients who are wearing pacemakers. Electronic equipment should not be used in the lower trunk area of a pregnant woman, nor around the cardiac or carotid artery areas. All manufacturer contraindications and precautions should be followed.

> I've tried all of these, plus some that didn't work. I found GMS to be one of the most reliable. It isn't pleasant, but in the hands of a skilled physical therapist, it can diffuse the most troubling TrPs. It's especially good for deep TrPs. Travell and Simons recommend it especially for pelvic TrPs.
>
> D.J.S.

Electronic devices should be used only by skilled practitioners and those they have trained. Certain areas of the body are hypersensitive to electromagnetic pulses and must be avoided.

Warning: Some gels used with electrical bodywork devices contain salicylate and/or aloe. Do not use these if you are taking guaifenesin! (See Chapter 23, Guaifenesin.)

Galvanic muscle stimulation (GMS), sine wave ultrasound with electrostimulation, and electronic neuromuscular stimulation (EMS) are some of the types of electronic devices used with varying success on FMS/MPS Complex patients.

Trigger Point Muscle Stimulation and Pulsed Ultrasound/GMS

Note: The information in this section is *only* for the use of the bodyworker familiar with electronic muscle stimulation. This section is meant to be used as a guideline for practitioners who are doing trigger point work.

The use of ultrasound (*Trigger Point Manual* Volume I, page 27) and high voltage pulsed galvanic stimulation (*Trigger Point Manual* Volume II, page 128) to break up TrPs has been suggested in the medical literature. Travell and Simons theorized that "rhythmical contractions may increase local blood flow and help equalize sarcomere length," and that the galvanic stimulation may be utilized effectively to interrupt the pain/contraction cycle.

Whatever the exact mechanism, the authors have observed that ultrasound with stimulation can be utilized as a noninvasive way to break up TrPs. One machine combines low-volt AC muscle stimulation (sine wave) with pulsed ultrasound. High-volt DC stimulation is also effective.

In cases of TrPs in localized muscle groups, the treatment regimen is relatively straightforward. Muscle stimulation should be set to patient tolerance. If fibromyalgia symptom amplification is present, patient tolerance may be quite low, so patient input is vital. The clinician must raise the setting slowly, with the gelled probe-face kept *in motion* over the suspected TrP area to avoid overheating the tissue in any one site. (If the probe is kept stationary, heat will build up and may burn the tissues beneath.)

With a prone patient, activity will be first noticed in the indifferent pad, with applicator probe activity following. Craig Anderson has found that TrPs are often responsive to a setting of 1 to 1.5 watts/cm2. GMS or ultrasound with low-volt muscle stimulation can also be used in a diagnostic "search and destroy" mode. Deep TrPs and latent TrPs will respond to this method, and can be located and broken up in this way.

The patient will feel either a "pins and needles" sensation with more superficial TrPs, or feel as of there were a raw sore deep inside the tissue at the site of the TrP when the probe is traveling over it. When there are many deep TrPs, as in the hamstring areas, some of these TrPs respond to the sine wave ultrasound with a prickling feeling.

The eventual relief is worth the discomfort. The "concrete" breaks up, and the patient can start to feel the lumps of myofascial TrPs under the skin. When the TrPs start breaking up, the muscles will need toning—they've been in the TrP "straitjacket" too long. Bony areas of the body can be "defused" by using the stimulator without turning on the ultrasound.

Chronic myofascial pain syndrome (MPS) complicated by long-standing pain/contracture mechanisms and other perpetuating factors poses a greater challenge to the clinician. It is vital to first find and eliminate or minimize TrP perpetuating factors before beginning electronic muscle stimulation therapy.

> When I first came to northern New England, I had already found that sine wave ultrasound with electro-stimulation would relieve the tightness of my trigger points, although I did not know what they were at that time. I had a considerable amount of trouble finding a chiropractor who would try this therapy. Fortunately, I found Dr. Craig Anderson. Over the course of many years, he developed a specific treatment regimen for my TrPs. I am deeply indebted to him, not only for helping to keep me mobile, but also for helping me write this section, as well as the section on chiropractic.
>
> D.J.S.

In MPS, the muscle grouping with the most impact on the patient's quality of life should be the first treated. Note that the primary muscle group is often difficult to pinpoint, as satellite and secondary TrPs may be very active.

Once the pain/contracture cycle is broken, the TrP may shift first to latency, and then break up (Simons 1988 (b)). During the course of treatment, the pain may shift from side to side as more TrPs are revealed under the softening musculature. As the TrPs break up, they release toxins. The patient needs time to detoxify.

If too much therapy is done at one time, nausea and/or low-grade fever and flu-like symptoms may appear. Even a five-minute treatment may leave the especially toxic patient feeling fatigued, and it is prudent to counsel the patient to take it easy for the rest of the day.

Neuromuscular Electronic Stimulator (NEMS)

This method is also called microstim, short for microstimulation. It delivers a very low electrical pulse through electrodes applied to the skin. It is beneficial for relaxing muscle spasms and muscle tightness, increasing circulation, and increasing the range of motion.

NEMS requires a prescription and should be used only under a doctor's guidance. When it is applied to TrPs , it helps to relax the tightness of the myofascia.

Galvanic Muscle Stimulation

Galvanic muscle stimulation (GMS) can turn concrete-like muscles into softer, healthier muscles. It doesn't happen in one treatment, but the myofascial splinting (or rigidity) is eventually broken up. Although the electronics vary, the machine and its uses appear exactly the same to the patient as ultrasound with electrostimulation.

After the treatments are finished, the patient may find that muscle tone is diminished or has disappeared. The patient's muscles may seem as if they have been in a body cast for years. If such is the case, the patient must begin to slowly start strengthening her or his "new," unsplinted muscles.

In Conclusion

Now you know something about some of the most modern and sophisticated tools and techniques available to professional bodyworkers to help you manage the symptoms of FMS and FMS/MPS Complex. In the next chapter you will learn some older, low-tech, but very effective bodywork techniques, some of which you can use by yourself.

CHAPTER 27

Bodywork You Can Do Yourself

This chapter describes a number of commonly used bodywork techniques that you can perform yourself, without the need of a bodyworker. In Chapter 28, Alternatives: Other Cultures, Other Ways, you will find additional suggestions.

Travell and Simons (1983 and 1992) have shown that in muscles with trigger points (TrPs), the muscle surrounding the TrP receives a normal supply of oxygen. The muscle tissue in the center of the TrP does not. Many of the techniques in this chapter are aimed at providing a better oxygen supply to the *entire* muscle.

Note: Be sure to check with your doctor before starting any exercise program, even walking.

Staying Within Your Limits

Staying within your individual limits may be difficult, but it is important to do so in order to feel the best you can. There are many ways to do this. One plan is to make a contract with yourself. This can specify when, how much, and how often you will do specific exercises. Exercise with a friend, or use a timer. And, most importantly, you must learn to listen to your body.

Whatever bodywork program you start, start *slowly*. Add new activities or therapies gradually. Be realistic. The wrong exercise can be every bit as damaging as the wrong medication. Consider all the variables.

Some Guidelines

There are many things you can do for your body through the day that will help lessen your symptoms over the long run. Here are some guidelines to help you on your way:

> I tried water aerobics, thinking that would be easy enough on my body. Wrong. I kept scaling down my idea of "slowly." I couldn't figure out why even the Senior Citizens' water aerobics did so much damage to my body. Then I found out that being in a swimming pool with a temperature outside of the 88- to 94-degree Fahrenheit range can cause long-range worsening of symptoms in myofascial pain syndrome (MPS). Doing the crawl and the breast-stroke can also worsen symptoms.
>
> D.J.S.

- Start only one type of bodywork, self-administered or otherwise, at a time.

- Pay attention to your posture.

- Lie down for at least five minutes a few times a day, if at all possible. If you can, put a cool pack on your neck.

- Use positive imagery and visualization at some time during the day. Visualize yourself looking healthy, doing exercises effortlessly (see Chapter 20, Meditation and Mindfulness).

- Play soothing music while you are doing self-administered bodywork.

- Make every reach a stretch and every movement an exercise.

- Take 15- to 20-minute warm baths, but be sure the water is not too hot.

Self-Massage

You may find that self-massage of your own muscles hurts your hands and arms too much. Try using a light, soft, stroking massage—just a feathery light touch. This can be very effective in releasing tension in the muscles in your face and head. Sometimes this kind of feathery stroke even results in a light myofascial release of muscle tension.

Exercise

When choosing a form of exercise, be sure to pick one you enjoy. Be committed, but not compulsive. Schedule blocks of time for exercise in your daybook (see Chapter 16, Coping Day to Day).

You can do many exercises from a seated position, and there are many types of exercise, such as flexibility exercises, range of motion, strengthening, and balance exercises, that you can try. Proceed slowly and gently. Do not bounce in any of these exercises. (Bouncing can force your muscles to stretch beyond their ability to do so without experiencing damage.)

Exercise each side of your body equally to maintain balance. Proper exercise can reduce your pain load and even help you fall asleep faster at night.

Be cautious when exercising outdoors in hot, humid weather, especially if you are taking decongestants and/or pain relievers. These medications can enhance fluid loss. Drink extra fluids and avoid exercising during the hottest times of the day.

Before you begin any exercise program, you have to learn how to breathe properly, as described in the section on page 259, "Breathing."

The Dangers of Repetitious Exercise

Exercise can be a great help in relieving symptoms, but any type of bodywork you choose should avoid repetitious exercises. Travell and Simons make this danger very plain: "Patients should avoid activities that produce repetitive muscular loads, such as shoveling snow, raking leaves, vacuum cleaning, painting a wall, or unloading a dishwasher. If such tasks must be performed, then the movements should be varied and sides alternated so that muscles on each side of your body are used in turn. The number of repetitions of the movement should not exceed six or seven, with pauses to allow muscles to rest." (*Trigger Point Manual*, Volume I, page 97) This was written about simple TrPs—for patients who don't have the complications of fibromyalgia (FMS) as well as chronic MPS.

You should not do even gentle repetitive activities when your muscles are cold or tired. Even such slight amounts of exercise should be held off until after your TrPs have been broken up.

Studies have also shown that FMS patients don't relax their muscles normally between repetitive motions (Joos 1994). In addition, FMS patients tend to underestimate the amount of exercise they've experienced. That may be caused by the fact that in FMS, exercise causes a *reduction* in body temperature and blood flow to the brain. (That's the opposite of what most people experience when they exercise.)

So, in addition to your normal fibrofog, you may not be able to think clearly enough during exercise to set sensible limits. You may overexert yourself when you feel relatively well. This can lead to rebound pain and to the yo-yo effect. After the exercise—sometimes a few days after—you may wind up feeling as though you've been hit by a truck. So your muscle pain and tightness will force you to abandon exercise until you feel better when, once again, you might overdo.

Clearly, it's important to avoid pushing your muscles to maximum exertion. Exercise when you feel at your best. Often this is between 10 a.m. and 2 p.m. Your schedule may need to be modified during hot weather, to avoid the risk of dehydration. Aerobic exercise, such as walking, swimming, or dancing is great, once your body is ready for it. Aerobics will help to normalize your sleep cycle and will release your body's internal painkillers—the endorphins.

Your muscles are supposed to work together, and they are out of practice. A single muscle by itself can not accomplish anything at all. To function, it requires the rest of its muscle group. Your muscles are going to have to learn coordination. If one muscle is not functioning as it should, then *all* the muscles in that group are not functioning as they should, because other muscles have modified their actions to take up the role of the dysfunctional muscle. Remember, everything in your body is connected through the myofascia. It will take time to coax your muscles back to healthy functioning.

Gentle Stretching

Muscles are either lengthened, contracted, or at rest. Leaving a muscle in a contracted condition for any period of time can activate TrPs, especially if your body has been weakened by illness or some other stressor.

Immobility is a fairly common TrP activator, and it's one of your greatest enemies. If you stay in one position for too long a time, you *stay* in that position. Your body stiffens because the myofascia forms its own kind of "splinting" (see Chapter 2, Myofascia).

Conquering Carpal Tunnel Syndrome and Other Repetitive Strain Injuries, by Sharon J. Butler (1995) is an excellent book to teach yourself "self-myofascial release." The book is well illustrated, easy to understand, and extremely useful for people with TrPs. It is also very helpful for people who have not been exercising and need a gentle way to start moving their bodies in the right direction. For those who already exercise, it discusses ways to prevent muscle tension from building up in the myofascia.

Excellent stretching exercises for a variety of activities can be found in a book called *Stretching,* by Bob Anderson (1980). There is also a video of the same name that is helpful.

When you stretch, if you are feeling pain, don't force your body into extreme stretches either by bouncing or by exaggerating the stretch. This is the only body you get in this life—treat it gently.

Warm-up stretching exercises are essential before any exertion. Muscles are designed to work optimally at a warmer temperature, and warm-up stretching prepares them for exertion. This is true whether you are gardening, hiking, or running the Boston Marathon. (And, yes, there is a woman who has FMS and runs the Boston Marathon.)

There is a good exercise for just about every TrP. The sternalis and pectoral TrPs (see Figures 8-17 and 8-18), for example, are helped by a doorway stretch that is performed as follows:

Doorway Exercise

1. Stand in the doorway with one hand firmly resting on each side of the doorjamb at shoulder height.

2. Take a step forward and feel the stretch across your chest.

3. Try the same motion with your hands held further down on the doorjamb, and then with your hands placed even lower. Do this stretch once or twice a day for each hand height.

Describing stretches for all the various TrPs would take up a whole book itself. So, talk with your physical therapist, and have a stretching regimen designed just to meet the needs of *your* body. All the information you and your physical therapist need to create such a regimen is in the *Trigger Point Manuals* (Travell and Simons 1983 and 1992).

When you exercise, muscles tighten as they are used. You need postexercise stretches to get them to lengthen again, or the exercise may do more harm than good. The postexercise stretches will also help you to avoid injuring any muscle the next time you work out.

Warning: Some people with FMS/MPS Complex have hypermobility—their joints are very loose and pliable. They shouldn't try to lengthen their muscles. And everyone must be careful not to overstretch muscles, because this will lead to rebound contraction.

Rocking Chair Exercise

A rocker can be a marvelous exercise tool. Rocking tenses and relaxes the soleus muscle (see Figure 8-29) in the calf of the leg, which is the secondary pump that helps the heart to circulate blood. Remember John F. Kennedy's rocking chair? In the press, much was made of the fact that he brought his own specially designed rocking chair to the White House. Dr. Travell, who was John F. Kennedy's White House physician during the whole of his tenure, designed many pieces of White House furniture to fit the President including that rocking chair.

Although most people do not have the means to have furniture specifically designed to fit their bodies, Dr. Travell has supplied your medical team with all they need to know to show you how to modify your furniture. It's all in the *Trigger Point Manual* Volume I (Chapter 42, Section 14).

Rocking is a marvelous activity that prevents immobility and gently stimulates the muscles. It is a form of low-impact cardiovascular exercise.

Walking

Walking is another great exercise, and it's free. But, like all things, there is a right and wrong way to do it. Check with your physical therapist. Learn to lift your legs from your hips, not your knees.

Note that TrPs can cause "foot slap" and "foot drop"—which can cause you trip over your own feet because your body doesn't know how high to lift them to clear the ground. TrPs also can cause buckling knees, ankles, and even hips. Find someone to walk with at first, and make sure not to overdo it.

Walking can be helpful to neck TrPs because they are often aggravated by the "head forward" position. You can learn to use a type of stride that will help to correct this. To balance your head, practice the "Native American Lope." described below. It is often used by Native Americans for walking long distances.

1. Shift your weight to the balls of the feet, leaning forward with your head held back for balance.

2. Walk very rapidly, without swinging your arms.

3. Push off each step from the toes, using the calf muscle.

4. Move twice as fast as in a normal walk.

Guidelines for Walking

Following the guidelines described below will help you to protect your body while you build up your walking endurance.

- First and foremost, when you exercise, you increase your air intake. If that air is loaded with pollutants, the exercise may be damaging to your health. If you live in an area of high air pollution, such as Los Angeles or Houston, you may want to confine your walking exercise to an indoor area, with air filters in the cooling/heating system.

- Go easy. If you have TrPs or MPS, make sure that your walking ground is level. That may be an easy condition to meet in Florida or the plains states, but in northern New England, it's nearly impossible. School tracks are good places, when they're available.

- Make sure you have well-fitting shoes with good support and flexible soles. Sneakers and running shoes don't last forever. It's a good idea to check out all your shoes for evidence of wear. If the heels or soles are worn on one side, it's time to get rid of them. The imbalance in your footgear will only worsen your body's imbalances.

- You may be able to manage only a very short walk at first. Relax. If you begin to mouth-breathe and gasp, you're pushing it. Remember, don't overdo it. People with FMS or FMS Complex take much longer to repair damage that results from overdoing exercise. Nonetheless, anything you do at all is a good start. The most complex, elaborate fitness programs begin with a first single step.

Guidelines for Longer Walks

Once you've started walking, you will be able to increase the amount you walk. You would do well to follow the guidelines presented here.

- Do stretching exercises before you begin your walk. There are many excellent books on stretching, including *Stretching,* by Bob Anderson (1980). Check your local library and examine several books. Ask your physical therapist for recommendations of specific stretches that will help your individual problems.

- Begin with a three-minute warm-up. During the warm-up, walk about half as fast as you intend to go.

- Once your walks increase in length, always tell someone where you are going and about when you expect to return.

- Don't hike by yourself if you're going to walk away from populated areas.

- Wear at least one brightly colored article of clothing, so you can be spotted, if need be.

- Always carry water with you.

- Walk during daylight.

- Check out the weather before you start.

- Carry a police whistle.

- Breathe as normally as possible when you walk.

- After your walk, stretch again slowly to cool down.

Note: As with any of the therapeutic methods described in this book, it is important to remember that we are giving guidelines only.

Callanetics

Callanetics is an exercise method you may find helpful. It consists of sets of exercises, each set concentrating on a separate group of muscles. Using very small movements, these exercises can firm and reduce the excess tissue that so many people have in overabundance. It works faster than most other exercise techniques, and you do it indoors. (See Appendix A, Resources, to find out where to order books and tapes to learn how to do this.)

Breathing

Proper breathing is the first requirement for optimum health. Sadly, many people develop bad breathing habits when they are young, and most adults use only a small portion of their lung capacity. Because breathing is an automatic function, we tend to take it for granted. You are breathing well enough to stay alive, but that doesn't mean you are breathing for optimal health.

Take a moment to consider your breathing. Is it deep, rhythmic, and relaxed? Or is it shallow, jerky, and constricted? If it is shallow, jerky, or constricted, you need to learn better breathing habits.

One of the first things that happens when you are frightened or angry is a change in your breathing rhythm. Your body tenses for the "fight or flight" stress reaction. If you have FMS or FMS/MPS Complex, however, you are stuck in that stress reaction much of the time. You have to help your body learn to relax as much as possible. Breathing awareness is the key to body relaxation.

Unfortunately, in this society, packaging is all important. You may pay more attention to—and currency on—the way food is packaged than to the food itself, with the result that advertisers and packagers get the bulk of your money, and the farmers who actually nourish you get very little. So it is with breathing and our bodies. Many people are taught to be fashion conscious. They are told to keep their bellies firm and pulled in and to breathe through the chest.

Unfortunately, this type of breathing, called "paradoxical breathing," worsens TrPs—you can't break the laws of nature without getting caught. If that's how you breathe, you develop a hunger for air that actually causes you to gasp for breath. When you breathe through your mouth, your breath is shallow and rapid. This causes your body to struggle even harder for adequate oxygen. Note that many people are mouth-breathers and don't even know it.

Breathing Correctly

When you breathe in, you must first fill your belly, then your middle chest, and at last fill your upper chest. Sometimes, it is easier to begin breathing properly when you are lying down.

- Lie down on your back, in a comfortable position. Place your hand on your belly, right below your navel, so you can tell what is happening. Take a deep breath in through your nose and hold your breath for a few moments. (If you are wearing constricting garments, you may have to loosen them to take a really deep breath. This alone will show you why constricting clothing can be detrimental to your health.)

- Let your breath out slowly through your nose. When you think all of the stale air has been expelled, open your mouth and breathe the rest of it out. Chances are there will be quite a bit of stagnant air that was not expelled.

I have been studying breathing techniques for 30 years. Still, I have been amazed at how many times I caught myself mouth-breathing just during the time I was writing this book. Even a short walk out to the garden sometimes left me gasping. I knew that my mouth-breathing was a side effect of serratus anterior TrPs, and allergies, and I knew what to do to about them. But I needed to become consciously aware of the problem before I could correct it.

D.J.S.

- Many people fail to use the diaphragm muscle—the main muscle in the body devoted to the breathing process. It forms the base of the chest area and moves up and down with the breath. Not using the diaphragm creates tension in the body, as well as causing shallow breathing.

If your breath is shallow, you aren't using your diaphragm muscle, and you are always keeping some stagnant air in your lungs. Breathing "from the belly," using the diaphragm, supplies your body with more oxygen.

You need oxygen to create energy. Think of a fire. It needs oxygen to burn. So, too, do the energy fires of your body require oxygen to burn the fuel you feed it.

Deep breathing will help to rid your body of waste gases. Breathing correctly also massages some of your organs and improves your mental clarity and focus. By breathing mindfully and consciously, and slowing and deepening your breath, you can relax and ease anxiety and stress.

Posture and Body Mechanics

Your posture is exceedingly important, as is body mechanics. No, we're not talking about people who work in a body shop. Body mechanics is the study of the physics of the body—how you stand, lift, sit, walk, and so forth. It's about how your body finds the correct balance. If your body is out of balance, strain results.

If you are healthy, frequent proper bending actually strengthens back muscles. But if you have FMS or FMS/MPS Complex, never bend, lift, and twist at the same time. If you must bend, first turn your feet in the direction you want to bend. Before lifting, look up. This will help your spinal vertebrae to line up properly.

Anything that throws the body out of balance, either literally, as in a fall, or figuratively, as in surgery or an auto accident, can cause serious problems. Even asymmetrical body parts (as when the right and left sides aren't the same size) can cause problems. For example, many people have one leg shorter than the other. (For more details on structural asymmetry, see Chapter 7, Perpetuating Factors.)

Check your posture during all of your activities, i.e., check your sleeping posture, your reading position, how you sit at the table when eating, and so forth. We've all developed bad habits. Learn to stand with your neck stretched up, *not* with your head thrust forward as so many people do.

There are lots of tricks you can learn about good body mechanics. Consult your physical therapist for details. There are many techniques for learning posture correction. The Alexander method, described in Chapter 26, Bodyworkers, is a form of training to improve posture for the relief of pain. It involves conscious control over learned habits. Feldenkrais, also mentioned in Chapter 26, is another method for learning how to correct poor posture.

Ask your research librarian about these and other methods of posture correction. Before you pick any method to try on your own, check with your doctor and/or physical therapist to ensure that you have no structural problems.

Heat Therapy/Cryotherapy

You can use heat or cold (cryotherapy) to ease muscle tightness and lighten your pain load. These methods of pain relief use what is known as the "Gate Theory," which states that pain impulses can be prevented from reaching the higher levels of the brain through the stimulation of larger nerves, in this case, with heat or cold. You should use these types of therapy, as you would all other types, with care.

Myofascial muscle pain with nerve entrapment responds *unfavorably* to heat. Heat increases circulation, adding more fluids to the area and causing the aggravated nerve to complain even more. If there is no nerve entrapment, however, heat relaxes the muscles and decreases the pain. It will also increase flexibility.

Deep heat sometimes triggers rebound pain and malaise. Too long a time spent in a hot bath or hot tub can cause extreme fatigue. If the tub is not too hot, and you limit your time in it to five to 15 minutes depending on your tolerance, you may find a hot tub relaxing. Saunas may help, or they may result in "sauna hangover," which is the most common FMS presentation in Finland, where saunas are practically the national sport. Each of us is different, and we must experiment to find out what works best for us.

If ice gives you pain relief, this indicates that there is possible nerve entrapment. Ice massage is often helpful, but you must stringently limit the surface area to be treated, and avoid icing the muscle beneath the myofascia. Keep your skin dry with plastic wrap. Go slowly, exposing only one area at a time. Cold can be very helpful in easing the pain in the TrP referral zones. Also, you may find that gel packs are the perfect relief for tight muscles or headaches.

Warning: Cold water on the hands can trigger cardiac arrhythmias in people with FMS. With FMS/MPS Complex, there is always the possibility of heat and/or cold intolerance.

Tennis Ball Acupressure

Tennis ball acupressure is a form of acupressure you can do yourself. You place the tennis ball between the trigger point and an immovable object, such as the floor, a wall, or the sofa. Then you lean into the ball, compressing the TrP, so that many of the liquids in the area are forced out. When the pressure is lifted, then the blood and other body fluids move back in and flush the area. Acupressure, tennis ball acupressure, and shiatsu are all forms of ischemic compression, also called pressure point therapy. (See Chapter 28, Alternatives: Other Cultures, Other Ways, for more information on acupressure and shiatsu.) For those of you who find tennis balls too hard, try using the smaller balls that are used as dog toys.

It is best to start tennis ball acupressure by leaning against the back of a sofa for back TrPs, or lying down on a sofa for belly, back, leg, and arm TrPs. At first, compress the points for a few seconds only. The sofa will "give" a little bit, so the acupressure will be gentler than if you used the floor. Of course, it won't be as effective either. The TrPs are painful to compress, but once you have flushed out some of the irritants, you may be able to "graduate" to the floor:

1. Start by lying on your back with your knees bent, and your feet flat on the floor. Your knees should be separated by about the width of your hips.

2. Raise your hips slightly and slide a tennis ball under one of them.

3. Come back down and rest on the ball. You can roll it around somewhat, once the pain eases.

Both sides of your body should be treated in this fashion, and the sides of your hips and front—especially where your legs join your trunk. This means that you will be rolling over on your side or stomach, with the tennis ball between you and the floor or sofa. This type of treatment on the belly is especially helpful for women who have bloating or pelvic pain. It reduces the congestion and frees the fluid passages

You can even use the tennis ball under your hamstrings when you must sit for a long time, as when traveling, or at a meeting. Move the ball under your leg from time to time, and do both legs. This stretches the hamstrings. It hurts. Keep in mind that you are flushing out the toxins and irritating chemicals in the TrP. Visualization and imagery will help with this body-work (see Chapter 20, Meditation and Mindfulness).

You can also use two tennis balls in the toe of a knee sock, which you knot tightly against the balls. (The two balls can also be taped together.) This is especially good for the spine area.

Warning: Avoid doing the tennis ball acupressure–head exercise if you have had a stroke or a head injury.

1. Recline on your back, on the floor or sofa. If your trigger points are very active, start by lying on the sofa. It is softer and will "give" more.

2. Place the tennis ball sock under your head so that the entire weight of your head rests on the two balls, with your top vertebrae in the space between the balls. Place the balls about midway "up" the back of your head, where there is a depression just above the attachment to the main neck muscles, a little higher than the level of your ear openings. There are tender points and TrPs in this area, so it will be sore. You are controlling the pressure, so start slowly.

3. Rest your head gently on the tennis balls. Relax as much as you can, and breathe deeply. Hold that position for a few minutes. You may shift your position slightly to maintain comfort.

4. Slowly arch your back and allow the tennis balls to roll down your spine, holding for a few seconds at each vertebra. Let the balls roll slowly down to the base of your spine. Note the very sore areas. Be sure to tell your physical therapist about them and be able to pinpoint their locations

Qi Gong

Qi Gong (often called Chi kung in the United States) is discussed in greater depth in the next chapter. It means, in Chinese, "breathing exercise." Once you learn it, it is an excellent exercise to do by and for yourself. There are varied levels of training and proficiency. As with everything else, you get out of it what you put in to it. Even the most handicapped and physically limited person can begin working with Qi gong. These exercises massage the organ systems and can be tailored to affect your specific problem areas.

Tai Chi Chuan

The method of exercise and healing called Tai chi chuan is becoming more common in the United States. It enhances mind/body communication, balance, and harmony. Tai chi involves slow, fluid, circular motions in graceful sequences called "forms." It was first developed as a martial art, for dealing with aggression without using force. Tai chi, pronounced "tie-gee," strengthens muscles, especially lower body muscles, and greatly improves coordination and balance. It increases flexibility, improves posture, and promotes relaxation and focus. It is a wonderful way to defend against the tension of FMS and FMS/MPS Complex. It is a moving meditation, and as much mindwork as bodywork. It needs no equipment. Tai chi balances the internal forces of chi—the universal energy flow—and clears pathways for more effective body/mind communication.

There are many forms of Tai chi. All of them are forms of self-massage—the internal martial arts. Fluid external movements of the body enhance fluid movements within the body. The movements also help you develop a sense of postural awareness. Once you are adept at awareness, you immediately become alert if something is in a strained position.

> Janet Travell says, "The magic never fails." Trigger point work does seem like magic. What has me dumbfounded is how any medical school can graduate a doctor without a thorough grounding in TrPs. TrPs are everywhere, and will remain so until doctors are better educated.
>
> D.J.S.

Yoga

There are many forms of yoga. Kripaulu yoga is a beneficial form combining breath training, meditation, and movement. Prana yoga deals specifically with the breath. Hatha yoga and other types of yoga often require sitting in extreme postures for lengths of time, or putting pressure and strain on joints and muscles. Before beginning a yoga program, talk to your physical therapist about which form would be most suitable for your state of health.

Making a Contract with Yourself

Contracts are often used as a self-management tool. Your contract should be realistic and mindful of the state of your health. Your contract should state your short-term goals, and describe how you plan to meet them. Making contracts can help you to reach your goals and develop healthy habits.

Pick your goal for the next week. It might be to walk a mile every other day. It might be to walk out to the mailbox every day. Take it one step at a time. It is often an excellent idea to specify *when* you will do your bodywork, for how long, and how often.

After a week, evaluate how you did. You might want to modify your plan.

Contract for Implementing Your Bodywork Routine

I,_____ , this day of _____, contract with myself to perform the following bodywork in order to optimize the quality of my life. I realize the importance of bodywork. Next week:

1. I will _____ (what)

2. For _____ (how long)

3. At _____ (when)

4. For _____ (how many days)

5. How certain are you that you will complete your contract? _____ percent

Each day you fulfill the terms of your contract, put a check mark down:

Day	Check	Comments
Sunday	_____	_____
Monday	_____	_____
Tuesday	_____	_____
Wednesday	_____	_____
Thursday	_____	_____
Friday	_____	_____
Saturday	_____	_____

At the end of the week, evaluate how you did. Make adjustments if needed, and write a new contract for the following week.

In Conclusion

FMS and FMS/MPS Complex are just now being recognized as true medical conditions. Be aware that you are blazing trails. Be cautious. Before you try anything, ask around. Find out which forms of exercise and other self-administered bodywork have worked for other people. Consult recognized groups such as the FM Network and the National Foundation for Fibromyalgia (see Appendix A, Resources).

CHAPTER 28

Alternatives: Other Cultures, Other Ways

If you study alternative therapies long enough, you'll discover that Western medicine often doesn't know much about what goes on during the healing process. It makes a great deal of sense to look to other cultures and to other relatively unknown therapies for some new insights. If you think that you always know what to expect, you may miss what should be obvious. Why waste time reinventing the wheel if someone else has already perfected the radial tire?

This chapter may be hazardous to anyone with a narrow mind! If you enjoy the "X Files," however, read on.

Electromagnetic Sensitivity

There is a phenomenon that, although not restricted to those people with fibromyalgia (FMS) or FMS/MPS Complex, I have observed consistently in people with either of these conditions. For want of a better term, I call it electromagnetic (EM) sensitivity. Some of us stop watches. Some can't sleep if there is a full moon. We are "wired" or energized by electrical storms, and the noise of fluorescent lights can drive us up the wall. Some of us are dowsers, or can "feel" electromagnetic fields. Many of us have difficulty with electronic devices. I don't know why, nor do I know whether it is related to neurotransmitter action. I only know I have it to a great degree, and can feel its presence in others. This is a mixed blessing.

There was a study done on EM activity and the "Serotonin Irritation Syndrome" (Giannini 1995). The researchers (all M.D.s) who did this study found that "weather sensitive" people reacted to certain types of winds that were high in EM activity. This included the "føhn" in Central Europe, the "sharav" in Israel, the "sirocco" in Italy, the "mistral" in France, the "Chinook" in the Rockies, and the "Santa Ana" in California.

When I'm in flare, I can turn on the computer from across the room. The phone beeps when I pass it. I affect electronic equipment, not always well, although I was able to get into the hospital earlier this week when the electricity was off and other people were standing around waiting for the emergency generator. Animals are attracted to me—even wild ones. Unfortunately, this includes mosquitoes and black flies. Naturally, I am interested in discovering why this is so.

D.J.S.

Signs and symptoms of these sensitivities were caused by an increase of serotonin brought about by the positively charged winds. The researchers found that high-voltage lines also cause this phenomenon. Since those of us who have FMS have a lack of serotonin, perhaps various atmospheric and other phenomenon supply what we need.

We are like electromagnets, living in a universe of electromagnetism. Solar flares dump quantities of charged particles into the earth's magnetic field. Flashes of lightning release energy bursts. The surface of the earth and the ionosphere act as the charged plates of a condenser, producing another electromagnetic field. We are in between. Potential interactions are staggering. If one nervous system could sense the nervous system of another, would that explain the realm of ESP? This may be why many of us with FMS and FMS/MPS seem to have an empathic sense. We also seem to respond quickly to subliminal tapes.

The earth pulses with a strong EM beat, and some animals can sense changes in the earth *before* earthquakes happen. Who's to say sensitive people, such as those with FMS and FMS/MPS Complex, can't develop this extrasensitivity for good purposes?

Acupuncture

Endorphins are the body's own natural painkillers. They occur naturally in the brain. Acupuncture is a Chinese therapeutic technique that seems to raise endorphin levels by the use of small, solid needles inserted into the skin at different depths. Acupuncture is based on the theory of energy balancing, which attempts to replace imbalances and restore the body's harmony. It has been suggested that acupuncture *meridians* (the imaginary "lines" along which the needles are inserted) are energy paths that signal the brain to send healing to the area of pain. Note that there have been mixed reviews on acupuncture's effectiveness.

Acupuncture has been around for quite a long time. Archaeologists have found acupuncture needles that date from 4000 years ago. Sir William Osler, the great Canadian physician, was using acupuncture for back ailments around 1900.

Norton Maritz Carneiro, M.D., from the Universidade Federal de Santa Caterina/Brasil is the president of the Brazilian Medical Society of Acupuncture. He estimates they have about 2500 physicians and 1000 nonphysicians in the organization.

In Brazil, acupuncture is the treatment of choice for FMS. In Asia, it is successfully used in conjunction with massage and other methods; it is seldom used alone. Shiatsu massage and herbal remedies are frequently used in combination with acupuncture as well as with other types of healing.

Caution: Before beginning any acupuncture treatment, first check to ensure that your practitioner is certified by the National Commission for the Certification of Acupuncturists.

Ayurveda

Ayurvedic medicine originated in ancient India and has been around for thousands of years. It is based on spiritual and physical balancing, and parts of it are somewhat similar to Hatha Yoga. Using a mix of lifestyle changes, diet modifications, purification practices (including purging, enemas, therapeutic vomiting, and bloodletting), and harmonic balancing of the five elements; earth, air, fire, water, and ether, Ayurveda practices aim to harmonize the balance between the body and mind so that healing can be accomplished by patients themselves.

Biofeedback

Biofeedback training, which is taught in hospitals and by some physical therapists and other health care professionals, teaches you to control aspects of your body and mind that you didn't know you could influence. The most common type of biofeedback used in medical settings is electromyographic (EMG) biofeedback.

In this form of therapy, machines that are attached to your body, monitor your blood pressure, skin temperature, other biological markers, and/or neuromuscular activity. You don't feel anything while you are hooked up, but you learn how to influence your blood pressure, temperature, and so on by making changes in your mental and emotional states.

Biofeedback can't reverse muscle contracture, but it may work well for simple muscle tension states. If you have no contractures, check with your physician to locate biofeedback training in your area, or contact the Biofeedback Certification Institute of America (see Appendix A, Resources).

Some people with FMS have found great pain relief in acupuncture. Others have found it to be of no help, and a few have reported it made things worse. Asian acupuncturists have told me that this may be because the chi blockages were not cleared. (Chi, or ki, or prana is the flow of the energy of the life force within the body.) It may also be that the FMS was treated, but not the trigger points.

D.J.S.

Polarity Therapy

Polarity therapy concentrates on balancing energy forces in the body. It is based on the premise that energy fields are everywhere—that the human body has energy fields within itself and also surrounding it. The interrelationship between the human body and the energy fields of the environment is of primary importance. Polarity therapy utilizes a concept analogous to the Asian concepts of chi, ki, and prana—the flow of life force energy in the body. Illness is related to blocked energy flow. Healing takes place when the flow is redirected to find a harmonic balance.

Before I figured out my diagnosis, I was really on the edge. I was working at something that required exceedingly fine handwork and repetition, and I often held my hands in nearly the same positions for long periods of time. I now know that contributed greatly to the steadily worsening quality of my life. But I kept pushing myself, because I "looked just fine." I'd come home from work and cry. Then I'd need to do extra physical therapy. Any leftover energy went into researching my condition.

I became very negative, and I knew I had to do something to turn my attitude around. I played a positive-thinking subliminal tape every day, even though the music in the background sent my conscious mind "up the wall." The analytical part of my mind kept fighting it. This tape, and one on frustration, kept me going until I found the diagnosis and had it confirmed.

D.J.S.

The polarity therapist and the client work together to achieve this balance. The therapist places his or her hands on designated energy centers of the body, one on a positive center and one on a negative center. Then, the therapist's hands redirect the flow of the client's energy, not by physical manipulation, but by harmonizing the energy flow.

Reflexology

Reflexology treats the feet and/or the hands as a way of treating the whole body. Its premise is that there are areas of the feet and hands that correspond to areas of the body, including organ systems. These areas are treated with pressure point therapy to evoke healing in the corresponding body parts.

Reflexology is a form of "touching" therapy that stimulates the organs, glands, and nerves of the body by massage and pressure on the reflex points in the feet. It is often done after soaking the feet in an herbal bath.

Subliminal Tapes

Subliminal tapes can be a very important tool for people with FMS/MPS Complex. Many healthy people are not sufficiently sensitized to respond well to subliminal tapes. But for people with FMS or FMS/MPS Complex, your hypersensitive neurotransmitters and sensory endings can work to your *advantage*, for a change.

You can use this by using subliminal tapes. They come in audio and visual modes, and some can be played while you are doing chores. Often the audio tapes have subliminal messages on one side and the same messages with the audible words on the other side. For those with FMS/MPS who tend to be overly analytical, subliminal tapes can be a way to open your mind to the power of subconscious healing.

Focusing

Focusing is a simple, safe, free, noninvasive, yet powerful self-help technique. The focusing sequence, using a series of well-defined questions or steps, helps you to focus on the "real" issue of most importance at any given time, not what you may think "should" be the real issue. The sequence then connects you with the feelings generated by that issue.

When connection with your feelings is made and explored, positive changes in feeling can be achieved. The result is understanding at a new level that translates into feeling better much of the time.

Some people may find focusing difficult at first. With daily practice it becomes easier. It is also easier if you have a teacher when you are learning this technique. Information on teachers in your area is available through the Focusing Institute of Chicago (see Appendix A, Resources).

One problem that many people have with focusing is differentiating between physical feeling—e.g., a queasy stomach or an aching back—and the physical/emotional "feeling sense" that occurs with a change in their perception or understanding of problems and issues. Again, this becomes easier with practice.

Focusing is something like meditation, but it is not meditation. Meditation is a quieting and healing process in which you clear yourself out, empty yourself, and give yourself a chance to "just be." When "focusing," you respond, feel, and gain insight. The best way to understand focusing is to try it.

Focusing Instructions

Have a person you trust and with whom you feel safe slowly read the following instructions to you, giving you time between each step to follow the instructions in your mind and body. If no one is available, tape record the instructions, again allowing time for action, and play them back to yourself.

1. Do whatever is necessary to make yourself comfortable. Lie down or sit on a comfortable chair. Loosen any clothing that is tight or restrictive. Take several deep breaths and relax fully.

> Focusing therapy was brought to my attention by friends in England. Based on their strong recommendation, I attended a focusing workshop. It was led by Dr. Neil Friedman, a student of Eugene Gendlin, the founder of this method, who teaches and writes on focusing.
>
> Once I had basic instruction in this technique, I began my own regular practice of focusing. Whenever things feel too busy, confused, or hectic, I find myself a comfortable space and go through the steps of a focusing exercise. It helps! Instead of feeling "so scattered," I get a sense of what is really bothering me.
>
> M.E.C.

2. How are you feeling? What's between you and feeling fine? Don't answer: Allow what comes up in your body to do the answering. Several issues may come up. Greet each concern that comes to your mind. Put each aside in your memory, acknowledging but not addressing it. Except for these things, are you fine?

3. Review the list of concerns that stand between you and feeling fine. Which one seems the most important—which has the most effect on how you are feeling? Choose that problem to focus on. What do you sense in your body when you think about all aspects of that problem? Feel *all* of it. Where do you feel it in your body? What does it feel like?

4. What is the quality of that feeling? What one word, phrase, or image describes and fits it best? Take several minutes to explore the possibilities and find the one that feels right.

5. Go back and forth between the word or image and the feeling. Do they match? If they don't quite fit together, explore further until you come up with the right word or image. When it feels as if they match, let your attention go back and forth from the feeling to the word or image several times.

6. Ask yourself, "What is it about the problem that makes me feel so _____ (word or image)?" Let the answer come to you. If an answer doesn't come easily, ask yourself, "What is the worst of this feeling? What's so bad about this? What does it need? What should happen?" Don't answer; wait for the feeling to give you an answer. Now ask, "What would it feel like if it was all OK? What is in the way of feeling that it is all OK?"

7. Feel the change that comes from having this new information. Welcome and feel the feelings and information that come to you. Be glad it spoke. Understand that it is only one step on this problem. Now that you know where it is, you can leave it and come back to it later. Don't analyze it or criticize it.

8. Ask your body if it wants another round of focusing, or is this a good stopping place?

Hypnotherapy

Hypnosis and self-hypnosis are being used more often in the health care field, especially to help overcome habits such as smoking and overeating. These techniques are not about the loss of conscious control, as some may fear. You have complete control at all times. In a special way, all hypnosis is self-hypnosis.

These techniques can help you to focus your energies. You can use them to banish negative thoughts and to enhance your own creativity. You can also use them to assist in healing yourself.

Every time you daydream you are in a self-hypnotic state. Sometimes you hypnotize yourself when reading or watching a movie; you experience accelerated heart-pumping and breathing just as though you were participating in the real events. Studying self-hypnosis will enable you to channel this ability to work for you when you need it.

Before you decide to use hypnotherapy in any form as part of your healing process, learn about it. There are excellent books you can get from your library, either on-site or from interlibrary loan. If you choose to work with a hypnotherapist, choose one that is certified. (See Appendix A, Resources.)

Pet Therapy

A great many people with FMS or FMS/MPS Complex report amazingly positive effects from having a pet in their lives. One person who has a cat and a dog says, "They have taught me a great deal about human intelligence and sensitivity to moods." There can be something incredibly satisfying about being owned by a pet (let's not kid ourselves here). Pets seem to sense it when you are ill, and often cling, offering moral support.

With an animal there is always something to smile about. They can keep you from feeling too grumpy. Dogs can help you stick to your exercise routine by needing (and demanding) to be taken for walks. You may feel safer with a dog when you are out. Pets are always there for you, even when you are in a bad mood and feel as if the rest of the world is against you.

Here are some of the advantages you can expect to reap by inviting a pet to share your home.

- Petting an animal is relaxing.

- Pets are not critical, threatening, or judgmental.

- Pets focus your attention on the positive aspects of life.

- Pets help to reduce tension and stress.

- Pets can improve your state of mind so that when you return to more pressing concerns, you can see your problems in a better perspective and cope more appropriately.

- Pets don't try to change you.

- Pets love to be loved, touched, and held.

- Pets remind you that you are lovable.

- Pets can give life new purpose and meaning.

- Pets encourage play and laughter.

- Pets may even help boost your immunity to illnesses and cause a drop in your blood pressure and other vital signs.

Dogs and cats are the most popular pets. However, guinea pigs (which are very affectionate), will cuddle on your lap all evening, and squeak when you open the refrigerator; rabbits, birds, and fish are also popular. Many people find watching the movements of fish relaxing.

Animal shelters are an inexpensive source of pets, especially dogs and cats. When you get a pet from such a shelter, the

---

I am rather biased on this topic. We presently have four children in the house—Elliot, Jennifur, Tribble, and Ian. All are furkids of the feline variety. If I'm in flare, sometimes the only things that help are cold packs and purrs from the catlets. Two of our cats rarely come out for strangers—unless the strangers have FMS/MPS. Even wild animals seem to sense the electromagnetic fields swirling around at least some of us.

D.J.S.

I never thought a dog would make such a difference in my life. Several years ago I "dog-sat" my daughter's dog while she was traveling. By the time she came home, I knew I had to have a dog.

M.E.C.

animal is usually in good condition, has been carefully checked for medical problems, and has received the necessary shots. The shelter will provide you with information on the animal's care.

Unfortunately, in many rental housing units, tenants are not allowed to keep pets, even though a well-managed and maintained pet is no dirtier or more offensive than your average run-of-the-mill human being. Sometimes, though, a landlord will make an exception to the rules if you have been a good tenant, or will allow a smaller pet such as a guinea pig or a bird.

Caution: Not everyone likes animals or enjoys pets. Don't force yourself or anyone else to get a pet if they are really not comfortable with the idea. Pets need a lot of love and care.

Make sure you can properly take care of a pet before you consider having one. Pets are a lot of extra work, and extra money, and a great deal of responsibility, so be sure you understand what it involves. Once you adopt a pet, it's a 24-hour-a-day, 7-day-a-week contract that you sign. Lives are not disposable, and the pet you contract to care for will depend on you to keep your part of the contract.

Other Mindsets, Other Ways

Sometimes looking at your problems in a whole new way can lead you to some new solutions. This section describes some avenues you might want to explore.

Traditional Japanese Approaches

Some Japanese practitioners feel that the center of the FMS/MPS problem is to be found in "hara." Hara is understood to be the center of body strength—the abdominal area, between the rib cage and the pelvic bone.

This attitude is reflected in the language. "Hara guroi" is a sneaky, dishonest person. "Hara o tateru" is an angry or upset person. "Hara ga aru," to have hara, describes a brave person with energy and spirit. "Hara kiri" means to cut off the hara. Traditional Japanese people who are angry squeeze their hara to express fury and relieve it. The ki energy force comes from the hara. The Japanese "ki" appears to be the same as the Chinese "chi." It is the vital life force flowing through the body. The Japanese use shiatsu, a form of acupressure massage, as one of the main treatments for FMS/MPS Complex.

Native American Approaches

Each Native American tribe is different. Generally, Native American bands treat people with some of the symptoms of FMS/MPS Complex with great respect. They are considered people with a special link to the spirit world, and they are consulted on many manners of importance (personal communication).

In many tribes, illness is not considered a state of being but a process of transformation. The basic attitude is that you must surrender—there is no way out but *through*. Accommodate, and optimize life within your limitations. Use your "down time" wisely. Eventually, you will be restored to harmony. Your passage through the illness will give you a greater understanding of life, and a great deal of wisdom. Concentrate on the discomfort instead of ignoring it, and it will fade faster. The belief is that the body is trying to teach you something. It will keep trying until you learn.

Native Americans emphasize creative dreaming and visualization as forms of healing. If you visualize a situation you usually don't handle well, figure out how you could do better and visualize yourself doing it.

Traditional Chinese Approaches

China is a large country. There are many different peoples, customs, and ways of healing. Many Chinese healers view FMS or FMS/MPS Complex as a disturbance of chi energy. They use herbs, acupuncture, acupressure, and equalization and balance of energies to unblock the flow of chi. Tai chi is recommended as a healing path, and it is becoming more common in the United States.

If you find Tai chi too complicated, or if your movement is severely limited, Qi gong, sometimes called Chi kung in the United States, is a good place to start. It is also an exercise of moving "chi" (which is partially electromagnetic and ties in with neurotransmitter functioning) by performing specific movements in a disciplined manner. One channel of chi flow is opened at a time. The physical martial art form of this is Qi gongfu, or kung fu, as it is known here. Unfortunately, as in many Tai chi schools in the United States, the mental preparation and spiritual work are often minimized.

Chi kung clears electrical channels in the myofascia, and releases constrictions that bind lymph and blood vessels. When the chi is flowing easily, muscles elongate and stabilize. Tendons and ligaments regain flexibility. Chi kung can loosen emotional blocks as well, and this is a greatly desired effect.

Nei gong is the physical and mental exercise of moving the chi with the mind rather than with the breath. It opens all the hundreds of chi channels simultaneously. It is an integration of the chi of mind, body, and spirit.

In FMS and MPS, the chi becomes blocked and "discolored" by pain and by toxic, stagnant wastes in the chi flow. The Chi kung Master teaches the student ways to "clear" and balance the chi, and to encourage a strong downward chi flow with specific movements and body positions, so that the channels re-open. The channels must be properly freed and "insulated" so that the powerful chi current may flow unimpeded. The energy is there for the taking, but there is great danger in taking it before you are ready.

It is possible to find Chi kung, Tai chi, and Reikei instruction in the United States. There are many forms of these healing arts, and many other types of internal martial arts. (See Appendix A, Resources, for the names and addresses of some of these organizations.)

The Native Hawaiian Approach

With respect to health, The Kahunas of Hawaii pay attention to emotions. According to a ho'ola—a healer on the Big Island—FMS/MPS Complex is the self talking to the self. In this system, the mind is not found in the brain, but is the whole body, enlivening energy and correlating functions. The Kahunas use herbs to aid the process of understanding. They believe taste and smell are the most easily conditioned senses, and they often work through these senses for healing. Grief is seen as positive and healthy, and is separated from depression, which is negative and unhealthy.

Laughter is important in healing, as it not only provides a psychological boost but also reduces stress, lowers heart rate, and enhances circulation. They also move energy, which is considered a tangible entity like the Asian chi, or ki, but it is called "mana."

A World of Healing

The practices described in the preceding sections have a lot in common with each other. All of the healers who use these practices expect disruption of normal body processes while healing is taking place. The practitioners of these disciplines believe that TrP blockages are not only in the myofascia, but in other tissues as well. For that reason, they work on every part of your body. And they believe that eating natural foods and vitamins isn't sufficient when your body is clogged with toxic products; more aggressive therapies are called for in such cases.

These healers exhibit many similarities across their disciplines in the advice they give to their patients, as well. They tell their patients to avoid unnecessary changes in their lives while healing, and to simplify things as much as possible. They suggest that their patients should take an inventory of what is important to them, and streamline and simplify their lives.

In addition, in one form or another, they all ask their patients to learn "responsible selfishness"—that is, they ask their patients to take the time to find out what their own needs are and then to meet them. They tell their patients to first find out what is most rewarding and fulfilling in their lives and then to find ways to do those things.

In Conclusion

This chapter has briefly described some forms of bodywork that you may not have been familiar with before reading this book. These disciplines are worth examining. You never know where you'll find some new solutions to the complex problems that accompany FMS and FMS/MPS Complex.

PART VI

LIFE ISSUES

Chapter 29

Advocating for Yourself

Many people with FMS/MPS have often found it difficult to get what they need and deserve in order to deal with their disorder. Sometimes your rights are violated. It is essential to remember that you have a serious, chronic illness that causes severe pain and disability. You have special issues and needs that others do not have and you deserve to get your needs met.

Authority figures and others may say things like this to you: "You look fine. Why can't you work 40 hours a week?" or "Why can't you walk two miles to attend class?" or "Why do you need weekly physical therapy appointments?" or "Why do you need disability payments?" To counteract these hurtful comments and erroneous beliefs, you must be able to advocate successfully for yourself.

Taking Steps Toward Self-Advocacy

This section describes some preliminary steps that you can take to help you advocate for yourself.

Believe in Yourself

You must believe that you are a very special and valuable person. It's very difficult to advocate for yourself if you do not have a basic belief in your own worth.

If you do not believe in yourself, or if you know that you suffer from the low self-esteem that is so common to those with chronic illnesses, you will have to work on changing your attitude about yourself or you will not be able to negotiate for what you must have.

Here are some suggestions that may help you:

- Repeat over and over, "I am a unique and valuable person. I am worth the effort it takes to advocate for myself and protect my rights," or use another statement proclaiming your own worth that feels right to you.

- Ask a trusted friend to spend five or ten minutes telling you all the things that are wonderful and special about you.

- Spend time with people who affirm and validate you. Avoid people who are judgmental and critical.

There are many good resource books available to teach you how to raise your self-esteem. See especially *Self-Esteem* (McKay 1992).

Know Your Rights

Everyone is entitled to equality under the law. Some people with chronic illnesses erroneously believe that they do not have the same rights as others. There are Protection and Advocacy Services in every state. Call them to find out what your rights are. (See Appendix A, Resources, for the names of some Advocacy Services.)

Decide What You Want and Need

Deciding what you want and need helps you to set goals and to be clear in your communications with others.

Your needs may be in the treatment area. This is often the first place where you can gain experience in advocating for yourself. Perhaps you will insist on a complete physical examination from your doctor, or an appropriate accommodation in your workplace. Maybe a flare will force you to demand the sick leave mandated by law for your job, but that your employer doesn't want to grant.

Perhaps your advocacy for yourself will be to contact your state or Congressional legislators about health care programs that do not acknowledge fibromyalgia syndrome (FMS) or myofascial pain syndrome (MPS) in terms of entitling people with FMS, MPS, or FMS/MPS Complex to the same rights as those granted to people with other chronic pain conditions.

Get the Facts

When you advocate for yourself, you need to know what you are talking about. You need to be sure your information is accurate and up-to-date. Here are some things you can do:

- Write down all important information. Everyone forgets things. Writing important information down and keeping it where you can find it helps.

- Develop an FMS/MPS health file and keep it updated and in good order. For instance, when advocating for appropriate physical therapy, go to your appointment prepared with references such as this book, the *Fibromyalgia Network Newsletter*, and so forth, to show to your physician. If you are advocating for sick leave when you are in flare, contact your state agency of protection and advocacy, or your attorney, to find out what your rights are.

- Make phone calls. The Fibromyalgia Network has advocacy material. So does the National Foundation for Fibromyalgia. They are only a phone call or letter away.

Gather Your Support

It's much easier to advocate for yourself when you have the support of others. Nothing helps self-advocacy more than supportive friends. You can build your support by joining a fibromyalgia or chronic pain support group.

Many people with FMS/MPS have found that it increases their credibility when advocating for what they need if they take along a supportive friend to back them up. It's too bad they have to do this, but it helps them get what they need. If necessary, call your local protection and advocacy organization for additional support.

Target Your Efforts

Who is the person, persons, or organization you need to deal with to get action on a particular matter? Talk directly with the person who can best assist you. It may take a few phone calls to discover which organization or person can help, or who is in charge, but it is worth the effort. Keep trying until you find the right person.

Express Yourself Clearly

Good communication skills are vital for effective self-advocacy. Learn effective communication so you can get your message across. It's not difficult. Just remember the following rules:

- Be brief.

- Stick to the point.

- Don't allow yourself to be diverted or to ramble on with unimportant details.

- State your concern, what you want, or how you want things changed.

- Write things out in advance, if you feel that you won't remember what to say.

- If you feel you have a hard time communicating clearly or effectively, practice with a counselor or supporter.

Assert Yourself Calmly

Stay cool. Don't lose your temper and lash out at the person you are dealing with or at the character or organization of that person. This is often very hard for people with FMS/MPS.

Your neurotransmitters are touchy at best, and everyone feels irritable when they hurt. Explain this to the person you are talking to, if you feel it will help.

Speak out, and then listen. Respect the rights of others, but don't let them put you down or walk all over you. Again, taking a supporter with you often helps.

Be Firm and Persistent

Don't give up! Keep after what you want. Always follow through on what you say. Dedicate yourself to getting whatever it is you need for yourself.

Advocating in Person

Speaking to someone in person is the most effective way to advocate for yourself. Here are some guidelines:

- Be sure to make an appointment—don't just show up.

- Bring a tape recorder with you and turn it on. Explain that you need it to help you remember what is said. It is amazing how much more helpful people can be if they know they are being recorded on tape.

- Plan what you are going to say and the points you need to make. Practice with the help of friends, tape recorders, or mirrors if you feel unsure of yourself.

- Dress neatly for the appointment. This gives the person the message that this is an important meeting.

- Always be on time for your meetings. If you are tardy, it gives the impression that this meeting and the issue to be discussed are not important.

- Look the person in the eye and shake hands firmly in greeting. Call the person by name. Use positive body language.

- State your message clearly and simply. *How* you say something often makes a greater impression than *what* you say. Tell the person exactly what it is that you want. Explain why you need it. Tell the person why it is in his or her best interest to respond to your request. Speak loudly enough to be heard without shouting.

- Expect a positive response.

- Listen to what the other person says. If you don't understand something, ask questions for clarification.

- If you feel you are not getting anywhere, tell the other person that you wish to pursue your issues further, and ask to speak to the person's supervisor.

- At the end of the meeting, restate any action that has been decided upon so you both understand each other clearly. For instance, you might say, "As a result of this meeting you are going to order a glucose tolerance test for me." Or, "As a result of this meeting, I understand you are going to change my status to active." Thank the people you met with for their time and assistance.

- Send a follow-up note thanking them for meeting with you and summarizing any agreed upon action. It's a nice gesture. It also acts as a reminder, and provides assurance that you both have the same understanding about the result of the meeting.

Here is a sample thank-you note:

> Dear Ms. Gretsky:
> Thank you for meeting with me last Wednesday morning.
> I appreciate your attention to my housing situation. I look
> forward to hearing from you next week, after you have
> contacted Mr. Shula. Thank you for understanding that I cannot
> climb steps easily, and need a first-floor apartment.
> Very sincerely,
> Jane Drew

Getting Action Through Letter Writing

Writing is a useful way to request information, present facts, express your opinion, or to ask for what you need. Here are some suggestions:

- Make the letter short, simple, and clear. One page is best. Long letters may not be read, and often don't stick to the point.

- It is acceptable to write the letter by hand if you don't have access to a typewriter or computer, but make sure it is readable and legible. You may think it is readable and legible, but you are used to your own style of writing and already know what you are trying to say. You may have to print. Ask a supporter to read your letter and answer whether it is clearly readable, understandable, and legible.

You may have a difficult time writing by hand due to FMS/MPS. In that case, you may find it easier to write using a computer or word processor, because all it takes is a light touch. Alternatively, perhaps a relative or friend could print a letter for you. In addition, typing services are inexpensive and might be worth the cost.

- If appropriate, send copies of your letter to others you want inform such as your legislator or advocacy agency. Put "cc" (which means copies circulated) at the bottom of the letter, with a list of the others to whom you are sending copies.

- Keep a copy of the letter in your file for future reference.

- It's a good idea to follow up a letter with a phone call. That way you make sure the person got the letter, and you can discuss the situation further.

Advocating for Yourself by Phone

You can initiate letters and visits with phone calls if appropriate. The telephone is useful for gathering information, keeping track of what's going on, and letting people know what you want. Before you call, write down the essential points of what you want to say.

When calling, follow these guidelines:

- First identify yourself. Then, ask for the name and position of the person to whom you are speaking.

- *Briefly* describe your situation to the person who answers, and ask if he or she is the right person to deal with such a request. If this is not the right person, ask to be transferred to someone who is more appropriate. If that person is not available, ask that he or she return your call. If you have not had a response by the next day, call back. Don't be put off or give up because your call has not been returned. Keep calling until you reach the person you need.

- Once you have reached the appropriate person, make your request for action brief and clear.

- If the person cannot respond to your request immediately, ask when she or he will get back to you, or by what date you can expect action.

- Thank the person for being helpful, when that's the case.

- In some cases when a person has been particularly helpful, it is a good idea to send a thank-you card. This may help to open the door for further contact on related issues. Everyone appreciates positive feedback.

- Keep a written record of your calls in your file. Include the date of your call, whom you spoke to, issues addressed, and promised action.

- If you are not contacted when a return call is expected, the promised action is not taken, or the situation is not resolved, call the appropriate person or persons back. Persist until you reach the right person, the promised action is taken, or a satisfactory resolution is reached.

In Conclusion

If you have FMS/MPS, you need all the help you can get. If you believe in yourself, believe in the rights you have, and learn to communicate your needs, you have the best chance of receiving the assistance you ask for.

CHAPTER 30

The Home Front

It has been said that home is where the heart is. You may have the grandest estate or the tiniest apartment, but you can still invest it with "heart." Make your home your "safe" place. Have a special area in which you meditate frequently. Put things you love around you. Add personal touches that make it uniquely yours. When you are happy and comfortable at home, that contributes to your overall wellness.

At home, people with fibromyalgia (FMS), or myofascial pain syndrome (MPS), or both (FMS/MPS Complex) have a number of challenges to rise to—the success, or lack thereof—in meeting those challenges, can mean the difference between a secure and happy life in spite of chronic illness or a life of utter misery.

Arranging your daily life to accommodate your needs takes work. Getting along with, and getting help from, family and friends also takes work—and understanding—on both sides. This chapter offers you some ideas to help you accomplish these goals.

Family and Friends

Family dynamics that fail to take the special problems of people with FMS or FMS/MPS Complex into account can certainly add to the normal day-to-day difficulties that all families encounter. For example, when you try to explain your many frustrations to a family member, you may have trouble concentrating, thinking clearly, or remembering what it was you wanted to say. Perhaps you won't even be able to get out the words you want to say.

This can be demoralizing and frightening both to you and the family member with whom you are speaking. At other times, fibrofog may cause you to forget even very familiar surroundings. This can also be frightening to both of you. When it's all "straightened out," you may wind up feeling stupid, which, of course, you are not. And all of this, of course, causes more stress, which ultimately causes you more pain.

Irritability, mental confusion, and mood swings are part of the burden people with FMS/MPS carry, and their families carry these burdens, too. But far too often the people who should be your strongest source of support become the strongest source of your depression.

When your need is greatest and you are beset by self-doubts, you crave the comfort of those closest to you—your family and friends. If you are met with impatience and distrust, however, you may feel shattered. You may withdraw like a wounded animal when people you know well say to you, "You look just fine to me."

There is no way to measure the emotional cost of pain. There is no way to compute the loss of trust. Trust depends on the world staying constant. With FMS or FMS/MPS Complex, all constants have become variables. And any emotional problems in a family's normal interactions tend to become magnified.

Without proper support and treatment, people with FMS frequently experience severe social consequences in addition to their physical and emotional difficulties. Divorce, separation, severed friendships, and social isolation are common. Increased dependence on others and vulnerability to life events can result in severe depression. (Remember, depression is a normal response to pain and loss of control and it should be treated as such.)

Any chronic illness is a family stressor, but FMS/MPS is more than most. Many of our local support group members have seen their marriages or other relationships end because of their condition. Many relationships break up even before a diagnosis is made. To avoid such a devastating turn of events, you may need the services of a marriage or family counselor.

How often have you wished that you had the power to let others feel exactly what you feel, if only for just a few minutes? If the "unbelievers" could get even a five-minute "zap" of FMS/MPS Complex, you would no longer have to worry about support or understanding. Of course this isn't possible, but there are many things you can do to help your family and friends understand your situation. In regard to intimacy, consider this:

"An intimate relationship is one that allows you to be yourself."

Deepak Chopra, M.D.

What Family Members Experience

When one member of a family gets a chronic illness, especially a chronic "invisible" illness, either the whole family "gets the illness," too, that is, the whole family accepts the illness, and the family members become part of a compassionate support structure, or else the family bonds begin to dissolve and family members start to distance themselves from the "afflicted" person.

Members of your family may practice denial when you become ill. Like you, they may have to go through the same stages of grief and denial that you had to endure before they can accept the reality of your illness. They need for you to be well. Because of this, they often make unreasonable demands on you, and you may find it difficult to say "No."

For example, if you are not working, your family's finances can become severely stretched, while your medical costs are skyrocketing. In response, you probably feel guilty, especially if you can't take care of the kids at home, or do household chores.

To make it right with your family, you may tend either to exaggerate your symptoms (to prove they are real), or to cover them up and pretend they aren't real. Both responses are understandable, but they are not good coping mechanisms, and they interfere with creating a new, healthy family dynamic around your illness.

One of the most disruptive aspects of FMS/MPS Complex in terms of family interactions is the lack of control that results from the variable nature of the symptoms. You might make plans for a family trip months ahead of time and then have to cancel at the very last minute; often because what you needed to do to get ready for the trip will have put you into flare.

Communications, Communications, Communications

It can be hard for *you* to understand how FMS or FMS/MPS Complex affects you. It may be even harder for your family to understand. Without communications flowing freely both ways, resentment can and will build. Communication is the glue that holds a family together. With honest and open communication, you can help your family understand what you are experiencing, and also help them to help you more effectively.

> Some days, I have the feeling that all I do is stumble through life, cleaning up one mess after another. Sometimes I am so frustrated that I wonder how much longer I can go on. I need someone to lean on. I know that an illness like FMS/MPS Complex impacts on the whole family, as well as upsetting all the interactions between family members—that balance we call family dynamics.
>
> D.J.S.

Common Courtesy

Too often people forget the use of "Please" and "Thank you" in the home. Common manners are no longer common. It's time for a change. Don't take anything for granted. Write thank-you notes to family members when they do something nice. Use a master family calendar, so you don't forget special events.

Be Open to Receiving Help

One of the hardest things for many people to learn is how to be a cheerful receiver. All of their lives, people are taught to give, and often fibromites give too much. But how can others be givers if there are no receivers? It's time for you to learn how to accept help. And the proper response to kindness is a heartfelt "Thank you." Not guilt. Only joy.

For some people, though, as difficult as *receiving* help may be, it's a cinch compared to *asking* for help. Asking for help is not easy. In fact, it can be extremely difficult. But given the facts of FMS or FMS/MPS Complex, asking for help is a skill you must learn. And it is one well worth learning.

Verbalize Your Thoughts

Healthy relatives often say, "Oh, sure, I ache too. I know what it's like. But I manage OK." Statements like this may cause you to feel growing resentment. Don't hold on to resentments and seethe silently.

If you verbalize your thoughts and allow others to know how things have changed for you, you will give them the information they need to really understand. For example, you might say, "Gee, I really want to look my best for your picnic tomorrow, and I want to wear my new white sneakers, but I'm afraid I won't be able to tie them. My hands aren't working too well. Would you tie them for me?"

Then again, there may be days when you feel like one big exposed nerve spread out and lying on the floor for everyone to step on. You are irritable and angry. You hurt. You can try to hold it all in until you implode or you could let the others know what you are going through.

If you let the others know you're struggling, at least that gives them the opportunity to be understanding. It also gives them fair warning that you need your space today. They are not mind readers. You may still feel like one big exposed nerve, but now it's lying against the wall, safer, where most people probably won't touch it. If they do brush against it, accidentally, there is a good chance both they and you will be forgiving.

A bridge of understanding will have been constructed. Even if others don't cross it, they can smile and wave from the other side; and you will know that if it is needed, the bridge is there.

Use Your Journal

Use your journal to write down family situations that cause you anger or emotional pain. Is one person often involved in these situations? Write that person a letter in your journal. Put it aside for a week. Then read it. Put it aside again. Rewrite it. Later, try to talk with that person. You may need a supporter or mediator with you at this time.

Be Prepared

You may dread the question, "How are you?" If you lie and tell people you feel OK, they will expect you to function normally. After all, you look just fine to them. If you feel awful and tell them so, not only do you feel as if you're always whining and complaining, but they often reply, "But you look just wonderful!" adding insult to injury. You still feel awful, but now you feel guilty about it too. Just what you needed, right? Yet you don't want to compound the problem by adding to the guilt and frustration of those you love.

Your family and close friends are the people most intimately involved with you. Naturally, they are the ones most susceptible to FMS/MPS burnout. Family members and close friends need some consideration and "buffering" from FMS/MPS. They want you to be included in their lives and activities, yet aren't always sure how their requests and needs might impact on your disability.

You, too, may have difficulty finding a balance. You want your relatives and companions to be aware that you are handicapped, but you don't want to have to remind them of it all the time. You also don't want them to become resentful when you can't always do what they expect from you. One thing that will help to "survive" these situations gracefully is to:

Have some honest replies ready that will not sound like complaints, but will inform those who ask that you aren't 100-percent OK, but you're coping. Use this time as an opportunity to educate.

Here are some examples of such replies:

- "I don't know what I'd do without medications on days like today. At least I can function."

- "What you see is proof of the power of positive thinking."

- "I'm auditioning for the slot of FMS/MPS poster child."

- "It's one of those days."

- "Mentally I'm coping, emotionally I'm adjusting, and physically, well, two out of three ain't that bad."

In addition:

- Try to be authentic at all times. Don't hide your pain, and don't exaggerate it. Be the best "you" that you can be.

- Tie up loose ends. Heal the relationships in your life. The best way to lighten your load in life is to ditch those heavy grudges you've been carrying. Remember, you can't change others, you can only change yourself.

- Give the gift of listening. Listen first. Learn how to listen. It is what *you* need, and if you want to be heard, you must learn to listen. There are excellent books on "active listening." Ask your librarian to help you find one.

- Share your feelings. You may think that everyone knows how you feel. Don't be so sure. People who don't listen are hard to get along with, but sometimes it's even tougher to deal with someone who never opens up and shares. Don't be one of those. The lowly oyster can become special because of the pearl within. Open up and let your inner self glow.

- Before you respond to words that hurt, give yourself a moment or two to reflect on what was said. What did he or she mean? Don't be afraid to ask. Repeat the words back. "I think I heard you say, _____. Did you really mean that?"

Language is ambiguous. Words can mean different things to different people. If you say, "Sorry I'm late. I was tied up at the hospital," what does that mean? This statement could be made by a doctor or nurse who had to work late, or it could come from a patient who was literally "tied up" in restraints on a mental ward. Same words, different meanings. Too many hearts have been broken by people jumping to hasty conclusions.

Partner Participation

In this culture, people sometimes deal with their problems by ignoring them. What they don't realize is that they are not just ignoring the problem, they are placing an added burden on the ill spouse. If you have FMS/MPS Complex and your Significant Other refuses to participate in your treatment, you are doubly cursed—you are cut off from one who should be your prime source of encouragement and understanding, and your healthy Significant Other is a part of the problem; not a part of the solution.

In many cases, it is the "healthy" spouse who is handicapped by the lack of his or her ability to nurture. This lack of support can vastly magnify the pain and other symptoms of FMS or FMS/MPS Complex that you are experiencing. One of the best ways to enhance your partner's understanding is to have him or her accompany you to support meetings.

It is an added bonus if your partner learns to help with your therapy. If you can, make your partner a part of your healing. This will give you a chance at closeness you would otherwise miss. You can take walks and talk together. You can exercise together. Eat healthy together.

If you can, teach him or her a way of doing trigger point acupressure on you that won't increase your soreness too much. Teach him or her to gently feel for the trigger points (TrPs). If your muscles are very tight, he or she may not be able to feel the lumps under your "concrete" myofascia. This is probably an indication that you need galvanic muscle stimulation (GMS) or some other type of physical therapy before you can begin acupressure.

In severe cases, a light stroking touch may be all that you can tolerate. Ask your partner to gently brush his or her fingers over the top of your skin, smoothly stroking and hardly touching the surface. This can works soothing wonders on your head and neck.

Don't have your partner use acupressure on the tender points of FMS. (See Chapter 1, Fibromyalgia Syndrome, What It Is and Isn't.) The TrPs of myofascial pain syndrome (see Chapter 3, Trigger Points) respond well to acupressure, but, unfortunately, it is easy to overdo. Have your partner start gently, so that you won't be sore the next day. Find what works for you.

Be sure to return the favor when you feel better, using the very light strokes. It is very relaxing, and mutual massage like this can help the two of you to bond more deeply. Gentle touching is very good for that.

Relinquishment Exercise for Family and Friends

The exercise described in this section is not for you, but for your spouse, partner, close friends, and family members. It will help them understand what you are going through—a sort of "hobble a hundred yards with my cane" approach. The participants will each need ten small pieces of paper, a pencil, an open mind, and some time. Imagination is useful, as well.

These are the instructions you give to participants: "Think of ten things that make you you. What defines "you"? What is most important to your identity? Your job? Your hobbies? Maybe your ability to handcraft items, or your fine singing voice? Your relationship with someone, or with a group? Your keen sense of humor? Whatever. Anything that comes to mind when you think of yourself. Now write each of these ten things on a separate piece of paper."

After everyone is finished writing, instruct the participants as follows: "Take these ten items and assign them a number from one to ten, one being the most important, and ten the least. Consider these things carefully. Visualize yourself involved with each one. Give them shape and substance in your mind. You are now going to lose them.

"One at a time, crumple them up in a ball and *throw them on the floor.* Before you crunch each one, think of what is on the paper and imagine it and your relationship to it. Then imagine never having that again. As you crumple it, know that it is lost for good. The relationship is forever changed. The ability is lost. Do this to each piece of paper, one at a time.

"If you are honest, you may find that some of these things are more important than you thought. If you are really honest, the very idea of losing some of these things may reduce you to tears.

"Once you are done, think about what has happened. Observe your actions. Are the papers only lightly crumpled, or even just folded? What does this tell you? Are the papers shoved aside rather than thrown on the floor?

"It is possible to lose these things. Think how much your person with FMS or FMS/MPS Complex has lost, or has had irrevocably changed. Think about how frightening it must be to lose abilities and control, without knowing why. Think about it."

Significant Others: Sex and the Fibromite

Hans Selye said that one of the best stress relievers for the body and mind is sexual intercourse. This great release is often denied to you if you have FMS/MPS Complex, because of hypersensitivity to touch, fatigue, pelvic TrPs and/or pudendal nerve entrapment. Perhaps you have such hypersensitive skin that even cuddling is denied to you because of pain.

On the Internet, people give and receive electronic hugs, but, clearly, such hugs aren't the hugs of choice. {{ }}. Usually, hugs on the Internet are shown as (( )), but on fibrom-l we use {{ }} to imply gentleness, even electronically.

FMS/MPS can turn what should be a positive stress release into a source of stress for an already strained marriage. Again, open, honest communication is part of the answer. You may need to learn how to talk with your Significant Other about sex. You may need to seek help to open communications channels. There are special seminars for couples, and a Well Spouse Foundation support group (see Appendix A, Resources). Contact the Special Needs Project at 800-333-6867 for a book list including *Enabling Romance: A Guide to Love, Sex, and Relationships for the Disabled and the People Who Care About Them* and *Meeting the Challenge of Disability: A Family Guide.*

Female Problems

"Female problems" often start with pain before and during the menstrual period. Premenstrual syndrome (PMS) may make life difficult for the whole family. There are medications and preventive acupressure and exercises throughout this book that can help you. See Question and Answer No. 19 in Section III in Chapter 8, Common Symptoms and Why They Occur, for specific TrPs that may be implicated in these problems.

Pain with Intercourse

Pain with intercourse can occur to the male or female fibromite, and can be due to a variety of sources. The commonest are achy muscles and trigger point pain. Vaginal dryness may be prevented by a water-based lubrication (ask your pharmacist).

Check for vaginal TrPs and pelvic floor TrPs in case of sharp, radiating pain. For aching discomfort and cramps during sex, check for abdominal and low back TrPs. For sharp stabbing pain, check for piriformis TrPs, which can entrap the pudendal nerve (see Figure 7-2). Piriformis TrPs can also create sciatic radiating pain, lumbago, and low-back pain. Pain from the entrapped nerve may extend down to the sole of the foot. These TrPs respond well to stretching (especially groin stretches), tennis-ball acupressure on the belly points, and craniosacral release.

Impotence

Impotence can be created by piriformis entrapment of the pudendal nerve (see Figure 7-2) This is a cause that is commonly overlooked. Blood vessels may also be entrapped by this small but very busy muscle. Again, stretches, tennis-ball acupressure, and craniosacral release are ways to reduce this problem.

A List of Rights

There is a list of rights, as compared to traditional assumptions, in *The Relaxation & Stress Reduction Workbook* (Davis 1995) that the authors have given us permission to use here. Understanding these rights can help you in dealing with people on a day-to-day basis. Each right would make a good topic for a meditation, and for a discussion. The following list presents each assumption in italics , followed by your actual rights in roman type.

- *It is selfish to put your needs before others.* You have a right to put yourself first.

- *It is shameful to make mistakes. You should have an appropriate response for every occasion.* You have a right to make mistakes.

- *If you can't convince others that your feelings are reasonable, then your feelings must be wrong, or maybe you are going crazy.* You have a right to be the final judge of your feelings and to accept them as legitimate.

- *You should respect the views of others, especially if they are in a position of authority. Keep your differences of opinion to yourself. Listen and learn.* You have a right to have your own opinions and convictions.

- *You should always try to be logical and consistent.* You have a right to change your mind or decide on a different course of action.

- *You should be flexible and adjust. Others have good reasons for their actions, and it's not polite to question them.* You have a right to protest unfair treatment or criticism.

- *You should never interrupt people. Asking questions reveals your stupidity to others.* You have a right to interrupt people in order to ask for clarification.

- *Things could get even worse; don't rock the boat.* You have a right to negotiate for change.

- *You shouldn't take up others' valuable time with your problems.* You have a right to ask for help or emotional support.

- *People don't want to hear that you feel bad, so keep it to yourself.* You have a right to feel and express pain.

- *When someone takes the time to give you advice, you should take it very seriously. They are often right.* You have a right to ignore the advice of others.

- *Knowing that you did something well is its own reward. People don't like show-offs. Successful people are secretly disliked and envied. Be modest when complimented.* You have a right to receive formal recognition for your work and achievements.

- *You should always try to accommodate others. If you don't, they won't be there when you need them.* You have a right to say "No."

- *Don't be antisocial. People are going to think you don't like them if you say you'd rather be alone instead of with them.* You have a right to be alone.

- *You should always have a good reason for what you feel and do.* You have a right not to have to justify yourself to others.

- *When someone is in trouble, you should help them.* You have a right not to take responsibility for someone else's problem.

- *You should be sensitive to the needs and wishes of others, even when they are unable to tell you what they want.* You have a right not to have to anticipate others' needs and wishes.

- *It's always a good policy to stay on people's good side.* You have a right not to worry about the goodwill of others.

- *It's not nice to put people off. If questioned, give an answer.* You have the right to choose not to respond to a question or situation.

This list makes a good topic for a journal discussion with yourself. These issues also would make good support group discussion material.

The Fatigue Issue

The fatigue of FMS/MPS Complex is often overwhelming, and it may be the main symptom interfering with your ability to function in your family role. As an example, a woman once said to me, "I have a choice today—I can either wash my hair or unload the dishwasher." Everything takes more time for fibromites. Some days, even the effort of breathing can cause you to be short of breath!

It's also important that you allow time to clean up messes when you spill things, cut yourself, or otherwise fibrofumble.

Some of your awkwardness may be due to sleep deprivation (see Chapter 10, Sleep). Do everything you can to improve the quality and quantity of your sleep. Have a family meeting to discuss this issue. It is in your family's interest that they help you with this.

> I was horrified when I counted the number of times I have to clean up messes in the course of preparing a meal. I try to do a lot of preparing before my partner reaches home. That way, only the cats hear me complain.
>
> D.J.S.

Often authorities advise people who can't sleep to avoid naps during the day. You may find, however, that a short nap during the day is essential to your functioning. Go with what works for you. If you're not sleeping at night, avoiding rest during the day may squelch the only sleep you can get.

One fibromite stated that the only decent sleep she got was on the sofa in the afternoon. She tossed and turned all night long in her bed. Her mattress was a superfirm type, touted as healthy. Her sofa was very soft. She used a sofa cushion as a pillow when she napped, and it was one of the kinds with a button in the middle. She put her head in the depression the button made, and she had neck support. Without her "cervical pillow" and soft sofa, she couldn't sleep.

She had to try several cervical pillows before one would fit. Because of neck muscle tightness and range of motion restriction, many people with FMS/MPS Complex find it very difficult to find a cervical pillow to properly support their necks. Cervical pillows are a real challenge. When they fit, they can be lifesavers. If they don't fit, your misery will be compounded. Check with your chiropractor, physical therapist, or hospital supply shop. They will often let you buy one on a trial basis, if you don't remove the plastic. At least, that way you can see if it fits.

The woman who slept on the sofa finally had the superfirm "posture" mattress exiled to the spare room. She bought a SOMMA—a compartmented bed that many FMily members have found works very well. JC Penney carries them. These are waveless flotation waterbeds with foam-filled seamless cylinders. The next time you need a bed, consider checking out a SOMMA.

> I need a soft waterbed. I need to use an egg-crate pad with it, and it still feels hard to me. I can tolerate an air mattress. When my FMS/MPS Complex was developing, we went to many furniture supply shops, and all the beds were too hard. The first time I plunked my weary body down on a waterbed, I didn't want to get up. It was such a relief to lie down without feeling extra pain!
>
> D.J.S.

Some people with FMS or FMS/MPS Complex need hard mattresses, and some don't. There is no set rule. A lot depends on what TrPs you have, and what kind of muscle involvement is implicated. Try out different kinds of mattresses. Stay overnight in a place that has a waterbed. Find out what is available to try. Ask your doctor for suggestions. The right bed is as important as the right medication for your health.

FMS/MPS fatigue may last a long time or a short time, and you never know when it may strike. Be prepared. Have extra meals in the freezer or on the shelf. Fatigue makes you irritable, so warn your family. Don't overdo, or try to hide your fatigue.

At times, you may become so sensitive that loud noises, droning noises, changes in temperature (sometimes it isn't the air-conditioning, per se, but the temperature change that activates pain), uncomfortable furniture, stairs, and long waits all add to your fatigue. Become aware of what is affecting you. Make a list in your journal of these stressors and try to find ways to minimize them.

Fatigue can affect your ability to function in a big way. It paves the road for the fibrofog to roll in. It's a sign you need to stop the world and get off for a while. "Veg out," take a walk, laugh, play. Make sure to schedule time for enjoying these things in your life.

Save your energy. Listen to your body. Avoid tasks that stress your body. Make your work easier. Plan ahead, simplify, use short cuts, labor-saving devices, self-help devices, organize, ask for help. And don't forget to save some of your precious energy for fun.

The Chair

One of the most common perpetuating factors of TrPs can probably be found right in your own home. It is the poorly designed chair. Janet Travell offers some suggestions.

Check your chairs. When you are seated comfortably, the backrest should overlap the bottom of your shoulder blades by several inches. When you sit back, your elbows should comfortably rest on the arms of the chair, and your feet should touch the ground with a space under your knees large enough to fit your hand. If you have short lower legs, you can avoid cutting off your circulation from your hamstrings by using a footrest.

Coping with Visitors

Many people with FMS or FMS/MPS Complex can experience a flare even if they stay up one hour later than usual, undergo any disruption in their routine, or suffer increased stress. The best tactic in this case may be to "give in" and take it easy. Respect the pain. It is your body's way of telling you to slow down, stop, or even back up. This is particularly important when you have house guests. There are ways to forestall a flare at times like this.

Be Assertive

One of the best things you can do is to be assertive. Prepare statements like the following:

- "Because of my illness, I can only do so many things per day."

- "I can't do what you asked me to do because that would push me beyond my physical limits right now. Is there an alternative you can suggest?"

Sometimes you have to just say *"No."*

Post a "House Rules" List

Try leaving a list like the one below to keep your house guests (and family!) from making extra work for you:

- If you sleep on it, make it up.

- If you wear it, hang it up.

- If you drop it, pick it up.

- If you lay it down, put it away.

- If you eat out of it, wash it, or put it in the dishwasher.

- If you make a mess, clean it up.

- If you open it, close it.

- If you use the last of it, replace it.

- If you borrow it, put it back where it belongs.

- If it rings, answer it.

- If it cries, love it.

The Management

You can also post individual signs around your house. For example, if your home has only one bathroom, you might want to add something like "If you close it, open it" to your bathroom door. That way you won't have to wait in pain, only to find that there is no one inside. Of course, signs are helpful only when your visitors read them.

Educate Your Guests

Teach your visitors about FMS and FMS/MPS Complex. Send them some handouts ahead of the time you expect them to arrive for their visit. If *you* are going for a visit, you can do the same. Let your guests know what you need—pure water, time for rest, walks, meals at certain hours with certain types of foods, what you can and cannot do. Don't sacrifice your exercise, medications, therapy, or other healing routines. You may have to pay for the extra trauma of a visit or trip anyway, but buy it as cheaply as you can.

If you're expecting guests, tell them, "Please don't come if you have a cold." You don't want anyone who is sick to visit you, especially if you can't take antibiotics without suffering dire consequences. In this case, communication is a survival skill.

One man we spoke with told a story about visiting his brother, a New York executive, who would spend lavishly at Christmas time. The whole family would go to his house for the holidays, drink a lot, eat a lot of rich foods and sweets, and stay up late at night. It put a burden on both his health and his finances, trying to "keep up." The following year he stayed home in Vermont and had the happiest holiday he could remember.

Always remember that life is not a competition. Competition takes energy you may not have to spare. And the key to surviving family holiday "one-upmanship" is simple: *let them win*. That's the only way *you'll* win.

> In our house we post strategic signs, such as the one in our bathroom: "We have many cat water bowls but only one toilet. Please close the lid." I have found out that I can get away with nearly anything if I do it with a sense of humor.
>
> D.J.S.

Home Sweet Home?

Everyone needs a place to go to escape the hassles of daily life. In ideal situations, this place should be your home. For people with FMS and/or MPS, that often isn't the case.

At home, you're surrounded by things you "should" do. There are constant reminders of your limits. There may be steps to climb that loom like the Matterhorn. There may be enough "dust kitties" to open your own SPCA. Your spirit may be willing, but your body says "It's not my job." You may feel like a child, nose pressed against the window of today, wanting to join the action, but knowing that for anything you do, you will have to pay.

You can take steps to work within your limits. For example, rather than doing all the housecleaning, yard work, or similar types of physical activity in one long day, break up your tasks and do what needs to be done over several days. Hold onto mindful awareness of your body, and listen to it speak. In addition, meet with your family once a week to divide household chores.

Use no more than 70 percent of your energy at one time. This gives you a reserve. Don't wait until you have reached your limit and then collapse; you must learn to say "No." Also, avoid taking on any extra stressful activities. Whatever you do, find the easiest way to do it.

Rules for Surviving the FMS/MPS Game of Life

Following the rules described in this section can keep you on the right track, so you can accomplish what you need to and let go of the rest.

Rule 1: Simplify

Bed-making, as an example, is an frustrating task. Tucking in the sheets under the mattress can be enough to cut the skin around your cuticles. If you have certain TrPs, folding sheets can be agonizing. But if you strip a bed, wash the sheets, and put them back on, you don't need to fold at all.

Janet Travell suggests trying to make your bed on your knees. That will help the folks who have only back and arm TrPs, but if you have bodywide TrPs, it's murder. Instead, get a nice comforter. It works very well for hiding the evidence of a messy bed.

Rule 2: Delegate

Is there something that you must do that you no longer enjoy, because it has become so painful? You may be able to delegate it. It may take time to teach someone else to do a task that you now do. But once you do delegate the task, you may wonder why you struggled with it for so long.

Little children love to help, and they need to learn responsibility. If you have no children of your own, borrow some. If you can't afford to pay for help from older children, perhaps you can trade with them by supplying tutoring. There is always a way to work it out.

> Working on this book has been a challenge. I've pushed my limits and have been enlightened as to how ill I am. I have had to institute the "Law of Rectangles": While I'm focused on the book, parts of the house will be a wreck, and other parts will be tangles.
>
> D.J.S.

Here's another technique that may help with your family communications. Ask your Significant Other to do a task for you, just once. It may save you from being taken for granted so much. And your Significant Other will better understand just how much work there is in planning meals, shopping, canning salsa, and so on. It is surprising how fast the word gets around not to buy gifts of clothing that must be ironed, if someone else has to do the ironing.

Rule 3: Educate

When a relative or friend places unreasonable demands on your time and energy, use the experience as a chance to educate. Give that person options. For example, you might say, "You know, Aunt Tillie, I have fibromyalgia and myofascial pain syndrome. I am quite limited in what I can do. I can either take you food shopping or out to dinner. Which would you prefer?"

Rule 4: Set Limits

Learn the difference between complaining and clarifying the issues. Don't take the blame for your condition. Do take responsibility for optimizing it. Use "either/or" choices when confronted with too much to do. Learn the true meaning of "the spirit is willing, but the flesh is weak." Once you understand that, you must learn to say "No," gently, and perhaps with regrets, but firmly, nevertheless.

Rule 5: Pace Yourself

Organize your day so you have time to rest. Try not to do more than one activity in a small time period using a particular set of movements or muscle group. For example, if you must climb steps, allow yourself some time after climbing them to recover. Give yourself permission to admit that you have a medical condition.

Rule 6: Modify

You can modify areas of your home to be as fibrofriendly as possible. For example, you can organize your closet so that coordinated tops and bottoms of outfits are on the same hanger. You can button your shirts except for the top two buttons when you hang them up. That way, you can pull them over your head, if that is easier for you.

You can also modify your kitchen. For instance, consider having no upper cabinets you have to climb up to or reach for—just lots of windows. This provides an open feeling. Keep your kitchen stocked with paper plates and plastic utensils for the times when your grip strength isn't great. It's also a good idea to use a microwave oven often, which helps to minimize cleanup.

Rule 7: Find Alternatives

One woman in our support group was upset at the holidays. Each of her children wanted her to slow down and take it easy, but each one also said, "The holidays wouldn't be the holidays without your_____. One child wanted chocolate chip cookies, and another wanted peanut butter. There were the brownies, and the daughter who waited all year for the special "old country" recipes. This grandmother had no energy left to enjoy the special time.

But last year she did enjoy the holidays. As gifts, she had made booklets of her favorite recipes and had given them to her children, along with little stories of her childhood and theirs, complete with pictures. It was now time, she explained, to learn how to make those wonderful treats, and she would help with the tasting. Now she can enjoy herself during the holidays, and her children have priceless heirlooms.

Rule 8: Adjust Your Point of View

Think of your work list as a tool that helps you achieve your goals, not as a chore. Let the "relentless grind" of FMS, MPS, or FMS/MPS Complex become the "never-ending challenge." One person said she often feels as if she is in a maze. Well, mazes have been used both as endurance tests and as amusing puzzles and pastimes. It's all in how you look at it.

Rule 9: Delete

Whenever you are faced with a routine task you have to do every so often, and yet you loathe it, try re-evaluating the task. Sometimes it isn't necessary. If ironing is incredibly painful for you and washing things out by hand is no fun, you can simply decide not to do those things anymore!

Another rule might be added to this list: Inasmuch as it is in your power to do so, never allow yourself to pay for the mistakes of others, for in doing so, you will help them not to make so many mistakes in the future.

> When I first started my support group, I invited people to my home for free counseling sessions, to help them cope. I thought there would be a limited number of people. Before long, I found that this activity was not only perpetuating my TrPs and FMS, it was making things dramatically worse. Now I know that there is no way I can see everybody who wants to come. That is part of what this book is about. I found that I must schedule time for my first patient, me, or I will have nothing left for others.
>
> D.J.S.

Helpful Tricks to Make Your Life Easier

In addition to the other suggestions in this chapter, there are some simple tricks you can use to improve the quality of your home life. These ideas came from the local and Internet FMily. If you have any to add, please feel free to write c/o the publisher with your suggestions.

For Greater Physical Comfort

- Use grain-filled small pillows covered with flannel. Heat one in the microwave, it will stay warm for hours, providing relaxing warmth to painful areas. Chill it in the freezer, and it makes a good "ice pack." You can also fill a "solo" knee sock with grain and do the same: knot the toe end, fill, and knot the other end. Just don't get it wet.

- Get up slowly and deliberately after lying down or sitting, especially if you are having dizzy spells.

- If you get the chills, put on a warm hat—even in the house.

- Keep your personal telephone book on a hook next to the phone.

- Use the automatic redial on your phone. Think of using a phone with "memory" numbers for people you call frequently, as well as for emergency calls.

- The next time you buy a car, look for comfort. Choose power steering, automatic cruise control, adjustable seats, air-conditioning—look for as much help as you can get. Avoid deep bucket seats.

- Use felt tip pens. They are easier on the hands.

- Look for special garden tools at your garden store or in catalogs. They have bent handles for easier use. Find ways you can cultivate your health by cultivating a few plants. Don't be too ambitious. Start small.

- Ask your optician to help you find frames for your glasses that aren't too tight but that won't slide down your nose. Consider using a tube or chain "holder" to keep glasses around your neck when you aren't wearing them.

- Put your keys on a large key chain—one that is easy to find. The kinds that can be hooked onto a belt or belt loop are especially handy.

- Keep several sets of ear plugs by the bed. If you can't sleep at night because of noise interruption, or if you haven't slept well and don't have to get up at a certain time, use them to cut down on sensory overload. Keep at least three—you are sure to drop one or more when fumbling for them at night.

Clothing Issues

- Sit when you are dressing, especially when putting on socks, stockings, and shoes.

- Avoid buying garments that need hand-washing as much as possible.

- Check your closets. Rid yourself of tight, constricting clothes—they may be just the thing to put in a tag sale.

- Look for loose, well-made clothes with pockets for handkerchiefs and medications at tag sales. Pay special attention to elasticized waists, which can be very comfortable.

- Dress for comfort.

- Ensure that your shoes are wide enough, fit properly, and have flexible soles.

- Whenever you're faced with a choice, don't compromise function for packaging. For example, always choose the comfortable shoes rather than the stylish high heels.

- You may need to cut out the labels from your clothes before they cut you.

- A fanny pack may be more useful than a pocketbook, and will hurt your body less. Just keep weeding through the contents to keep it light. You need only a small assortment of change.

For Easier Housework

Housecleaning is all in the way you look at it. Once you've attained your FMS/MPS degree, you are intelligent enough not to be a slave to old habits. A little disorder in the house is good for the soul. It says that you have more important things to do—like taking care of yourself.

- When your daily chore list looks too formidable, see what can wait until next week, or next month, or can be deleted all together. Don't overload tomorrow.

- Get a soft, new paintbrush to clean pleated shades, knickknacks (or better yet, give the knickknack "heirlooms" away as presents).

- When making a bed, put some large tucks in the bottom to leave room for your feet. That will help to alleviate foot cramping.

- Organize your work areas with lightweight items placed higher than heavy items.

- Close all doors and drawers when they aren't in active use.

- Make sure rugs are anchored on pads that prevent slipping.

- If you need to do a task that might involve climbing or reaching, wait until a friend is there with you, in case you fall. Better yet, ask the friend to help.

- Use thinner, cheaper washcloths—they are easier to wring out.

Keep pathways and stairways free of clutter. You can save trips up and down the stairs by piling things at the top and bottom and moving them when you absolutely have to make the climb.

- Hire household help if possible, especially for large tasks like window cleaning. Investigate local schools. You may find a junior high school student willing to clean or do lawn care for the summer who won't charge a great deal.

- Do necessary chores while listening to positive thinking tapes or books on tape. Dust off your mind while you dust your shelves. Check your library for tape selections.

- Jar openers, sharp knives, scissors, loop handles and other self-help aids are available. Check your library, medical supply store, or with an occupational therapist for information.

- Return everything to its place after you use it.

For an Easier Time in the Kitchen

- When you need to replace kitchen equipment, purchase easy-to-grasp utensils and bowls with nonskid bases. These are also good choices to ask for as presents.

- At the grocery, buy smaller, easier to handle sizes of the products you use.

- Consider using a grocery scooter on bad days.

- Even if you are only picking up a few things at the grocery, use a cart. It is great to lean on.

- Open plastic bags with scissors. Keep several pairs of scissors—each in a handy location.

- Whenever you are making one dinner, make more of the same and freeze the extra in usable portions for a quick easy meal when you're having a bad day.

- Carry a container of "good" water around with you. A small plastic soda container partially filled with water is good to keep in the freezer for this. Then you can just fill it with water and you'll have a cool drink when you need it. The new straw-like tops make for easy drinking and avoiding spills.

- Consider buying a commercial-type ingredient mixer that you don't have to hold.

- Keep insulated rubber gloves handy for when you must handle cold things. Use insulated oven mitts when carrying freezer items.

- To deal with plastic produce bags at the grocery, wet your fingers. That makes it easier to separate the two sides.

- Rather than grating cheddar cheese for cooking, freeze it in portion size. After it is defrosted, the cheese will crumble readily.

- Paper plates are light, and they don't break. The Dixie plates are relatively sturdy and environmentally friendly.

- Some salad forks and some pickle or junior forks are much lighter than regular forks and therefore easier to lift and use.

- Finger foods and sandwiches are easy to eat—just don't fill the sandwiches too full. Pre-cut food dinners, such as stir-fry (in a microwave or frying pan with little oil or butter), casseroles, pot pies, and salads are good. Many things can be made ahead and heated later in the microwave, so you can clean up preparation dishes and lessen dinnertime stress.

- Boil water in the microwave, and leave the door closed for a few minutes. You can then clean the microwave with a paper towel.

- Put your toaster on a metal tray. The crumbs will be easier to clean.

- Spray furniture wax on your stainless steel sinks and appliances. Things won't stick to them as easily.

In Conclusion

One goal of this chapter has been to show you how to keep your home comfortable, attractive, and a haven that you want to return to in spite or having FMS or FMS/MPS Complex. The other goal has been to present some advice and tips to help you get along better with your family and friends. As with almost everything else in life, the key to successful relationships is good, open, honest communication.

CHAPTER 31

Building Your Support Structure

A structured support system with which you have ongoing contact is essential for optimizing the quality of your life. Healthy people can afford to take more casual approaches to arranging support, but for those with chronic pain, a casual approach is a recipe for trouble.

You need to develop a support plan and stick to it, to ensure that you always have support ready for you when you are in flare, when you need encouragement, or when you just need companionship.

Consider this statement:

"A human being is an entity having an emotional structure, as well as a physical and mental structure."

John W. Campbell, Jr.

The personal stories of people with fibromyalgia (FMS) or FMS/MPS Complex who moved from having no support at all to structured group support are vivid testimony to the power of support groups. One man revealed, "I now realize that my attempts at suicide were the result of poor coping behavior, failure on my part to take responsibility for improving my quality of life, and failure to educate my support team. Now I know what to do, and my support network is in place."

A woman said, "The daily grind of FMS/MPS was wearing me down. I met someone at a support group meeting. Then I met one of her friends. Before we knew it, we had a support network. I feel so much better knowing that I can give help as well as get help. It feels so good to be able to be useful again."

A good rule of thumb is to have at least five reliable friends or family members (or FMily members from support groups) whom you can call upon when you need support. These should be people who can count on you when they need a friend, as well. When you begin your journey on the road to healing, you may not have five supporters. But, gradually, as you put time and energy into developing a strong support system, you can increase the number of your supporters and strengthen and deepen their roles in enhancing your wellness.

What You Need/What Your Supporters Need

Perhaps the most valuable trait of a good supporter is the ability to listen *without judging, criticizing, or giving advice*. A good supporter lets you freely express all of your feelings and emotions.

At the beginning of the time you plan to spend with a supporter, let the supporter know what you want. For instance, you might say, "Today, I just need you to listen to me while I vent and express my angry feelings. Then I want to figure out this situation for myself." Another time you might say, "Today, I'd like some feedback and advice. I need a reality check." Being clear in stating your needs is the best way to get what you need for yourself.

Don't give up on supporters immediately because they criticized, judged, and advised you without having been asked. First, explain to them what it is you want and need and also what you don't want. Then, see if they can support you in the way that you described your needs to them. Many people are not accustomed to listening to someone talk without making some comment about what they hear. They feel that if you are saying something, it's their job to respond to you by telling you whether you are right or wrong and what you should do about it. But, if you state your wishes clearly, eventually most people can learn how to listen without feeling the need to respond.

In return, spend as much time listening to your supporters as they spend listening to you. Using the peer counseling structure is a good way to ensure that you both get equal time to be heard. (See the "Peer Counseling" section at the end of this chapter.) Do for them what they do for you: Allow them to express their feelings and emotions freely without being judged or criticized, and provide advice and feedback only when requested.

Good supporters allow you the space to change, grow, make decisions, and even make your own mistakes. They allow you your feelings and emotions, your needs and wants. You don't want them to have all the answers, and they feel the same way about you.

Your supporters need to be educated about FMS, myofascial pain syndrome (MPS), and FMS/MPS Complex issues, and people with these conditions need to know about those issues that are important to their supporters. For instance, if a supporter is diabetic, make it a point to learn about how that illness impacts that person's life.

You may want, and ask for, your supporters to work with you in deciding the next best step to take in a difficult situation. Then, when you have figured out what to do, your supporters can assist you in taking that step. Your supporters provide sympathy and encouragement when you need it. You, in turn, offer sympathy and encouragement to them when they need it.

Finding Personal Supporters

Your supporters will be people you like, respect, and trust, with whom you share common interests and rapport, and with whom you can share anything. They also need to understand thoroughly the concept of confidentiality—as do you.

You must choose your supporters yourself. No one else can determine who should be your supporter. You may want to ask someone who already is a supporter to help you find others—but the choice is always yours. It has to be someone with whom you feel absolutely comfortable. These are some good places to look:

- **Support Groups:** Support groups are excellent places to find supporters. These are people who can really understand what you are going through because they have already experienced or are going through very similar life experiences themselves.

When you've talked with the same person several times at a support group, you may decide to exchange phone numbers. After several conversations, you may decide to share an activity, like going out to lunch or a movie. The relationship may become more and more supportive as you get to know each other, or it may not. The choice is always yours to make about how much you want to be supported by and give support to someone from a support group.

- **Coworkers:** If you are working, some of your workmates may be appropriate supporters. (You will also get a chance to educate them.) If you cannot work, check out volunteer activities, where you can meet other people with similar interests, but be careful not to overwork. Most communities have a clearinghouse for potential volunteers. Check it out. Just make sure they understand your limitations. Too many people choose to overwork as volunteers.

- **Community activities:** Many communities offer a broad range of activities and special interest and action groups where you can meet people and develop supportive relationships. Use your local newspaper as a guide for finding these groups. Attend those activities and events that interest you. Perhaps you've often looked through the newspaper and said to yourself, "That looks like it would be fun," or "That would be interesting," but you've never followed up on it. Now is the time to make it a practice to attend those events that interest you. When you see the same people several times, initiate conversations. Give friendships and supportive relationships the opportunity to develop in this way.

Working with Your Supporters

When you feel you have identified or made a connection with people who meet all your criteria for supporters, there are several things you need to do:

- Ask them if they are willing to be one of your supporters. (Don't do this until you know the person very well. Explain in detail what you want and need from your supporters.)

- Tell them that, in return, you will be their supporter, providing for them all that you expect of them. (It needs to be very clear that this will be a two-way relationship that you are requesting.)

- Help them understand that you have several supporters and that it is not necessary for one individual supporter to be available to you at all times. At any given time, supporters will have reasons why they are unavailable, including work responsibilities, family responsibilities, other plans, illness, or vacations. Make it clear that you expect your supporter to have similar limitations on availability.

It is very important that if you ask a supporter for company or assistance and that supporter says he or she is unavailable, you respect that response and find another person to meet your needs. Contact another person on your list. This keeps supporters from becoming "burned out," and keeps you from interfering with their lives.

- Spend time listening to and supporting each other. Many people find it useful to make a contract to do this on a regular basis. For instance, every Friday afternoon from 1 p.m. to 2 p.m., you can contract to meet with a supporter for a shared listening session. Have an appointment book and keep it up-to-date.

- If you note early warning signs of flare, contact supporters and schedule time with them. Also schedule time for additional support when you have a crisis, such as the loss of a job or a disagreement with a family member. Then you will have someone to listen, help you make decisions and take necessary action.

Keeping Your Support System Strong

You don't want to wear out the people you've chosen to support you. In addition to making the support relationship one of give-and-take, as described, this section lists some steps you can take to keep things in balance.

- **Support your own good health:** Others will enjoy being supportive of you if you do everything you can to keep yourself as healthy as possible, using the strategies you have learned from this book, other resource books, your health care professionals, and others who have FMS, MPS, or FMS/MPS.

- **Find out about yourself:** If you have a hard time making and keeping friends, ask your health care professionals or others you respect and trust if you have social habits or behaviors that others find offensive—are you too loud, too "pushy," too negative? Listen to what they say without getting angry or being defensive. Ask others to verify these opinions. If you do have such habits, work with your health care professionals and friends to rid yourself of them. Admitting to others that you are working on eliminating these behaviors may be difficult. It will take work. You will need support while you do it.

- **Delegate responsibility:** If you are having a really hard time with fibrofog, flare, or depression and are unable to make decisions for yourself, you may need members of your support team to make decisions for you. For this reason, it's important for at least two supporters to know what treatments are all right with you and work well for you, and what treatments are either unacceptable or have not worked for you in the past. They need to know what procedures are necessary to get you help, if and when you are unable to seek help for yourself.

- **Arrange meetings:** You may want to arrange meetings between your key supporters and health care professionals when you are well. Then, if they need to contact each other when you are having a hard time, they will already be acquainted. Let supporters know who your health care professionals are, what roles they play in your life, and how they can be contacted. This facilitates the process of getting you help fast—when you need it.

At these meetings you can explain what you want from your supporters, describe and explain the symptoms that indicate you are having a hard time, and let supporters know what your health care professionals would like them to do about it.

This is also a good time for members of the support system to get each other's phone numbers and the phone numbers of your health care providers so they can coordinate efforts if necessary. It is a good idea to invite your support team members to a local support group meeting.

- **Plan on enjoyment:** Most of the time you spend with your supporters should be focused on enjoying each other's company and having a good time—in other words, being friends. It is just as important to be there for each other in the good times as it is in the more difficult times.

- **Plan ahead for phone calls:** Ask supporters the time of day they prefer to take phone calls. Avoid late night or early morning calls unless you have a true emergency. (Remember, irritability is one of the FMS symptoms.) The person you call at 8 a.m. may have fallen asleep only a few minutes ago.

- **Keep a list:** Make a list of your support team members with their phone numbers. As you implement the strategies described in this chapter and gain new supporters, update your list. The time when it is hardest to remember who your supporters are is also the time when you most need to reach out to them. Have copies of the list by your phones, on your bedside table, in your journal, and in your pocket or purse.

- **Assess the appropriateness of the support you are asking for:** Have you been using your professional health care team as moral support? If you have a mental health counselor, psychologist, or psychiatrist, this kind of support is appropriate. Frequent calling of other members of your health care team when you need attention or reassurance is not.

Frequent calling for moral support is a good way to trigger "burnout" in the health care professional; it leaves your doctor, physical therapist, or other professional very frustrated. If you have a psychologist, social worker, or other counselor, you may want to talk to that person about this problem. He or she can help you set up a healthy support system.

Support Groups

Support groups are wonderful places to make new, understanding friends. It is a place where you can form long-lasting friendships, or perhaps even find a life partner. Your support group can help to counteract the social isolation that many people with FMS, MPS, or FMS/MPS Complex experience.

The most common emotion new members of our local support group feel is profound relief. At last, someone believes them. They belong. Instead of being met with skepticism, they are met with compassion and understanding. There is an incredible feeling of compassionate sharing when a roomful of people express their understanding of what you have been going through.

Often, many people find that they have more in common with people in their support group than they do with their own relatives. Unless, of course, someone in their family is also afflicted—it isn't unusual to have more than one family member with FMS and/or MPS.

Support groups provide an opportunity to be with people who have similar problems and issues; people who understand and can be supportive. They remind you that you are not alone. Communication is easy in the group, because you all share so much. People there help you to appreciate your own circumstances and you begin to understand that things aren't as bleak as they might otherwise seem. You learn that others with similar problems are managing very well, and you find hope there.

There may be FMS/MPS or chronic pain support groups in your area. They are generally listed in the community calendar section of the newspaper. Your local hospital, health agency, or health care professionals can also refer you to local support groups.

Attend a support group several times before making a decision about whether it is the right one for you. Every group can have an off night where things just don't "gel." Include your support group as an essential part of your support system. You may even find that members of the support group will become members of your personal support network.

Starting Your Own Support Group

There may not be a specific FMS/MPS support group in your area. In that case you may need to start your own. This is easier than it sounds. The Fibromyalgia Network has an information packet that can help you get one going. Contact them for "How to Run a Support Group: A Guide for Leaders" (see Appendix A, Resources). The National Foundation for Fibromyalgia also has a packet that can guide you in starting a local support group.

When starting a support group, here are some things to keep in mind:

- It helps to have a physician, nurse practitioner, or physician's assistant associated with your group. Someone like this may be able to speak only once a year but can be an ongoing resource for information, nevertheless.

- The first time you hold a support group meeting can be scary. Janet Travell said something about emergency situations that applies here. "The secret is always to do something, no matter how trivial, and no matter how helpless you feel at first. That gives you time to think."

- It is a good idea to spend the first part of the meeting having all the people present give their names and say a little about themselves. That helps to get things going. To break the ice, you can start with yourself.

- Make it plain that everyone can come or go as they choose, as long as they are not disruptive. People need to feel free to get up and stretch. Everyone can share information, and can also choose not to share. Sharing, not comparing, is the best focus for the group.

- Do your best to ensure confidentiality. Remember, the main element of a support group is sharing. *Group members should agree at the onset that anything personal that is shared at the group is confidential.* In addition, group members should agree not to share with people outside the group information about who is attending the group.

- Support groups are about acceptance and empowerment. No criticizing or judging is allowed. Expression of emotion is encouraged.

- Allow some social time, time to discuss what has helped others and what has not helped, and time to discuss individual problems and possible solutions.

- If someone comes to the group who is depressed and possibly suicidal, be prepared. It happens. Don't leave people alone in that situation. Invite them to tell their story if they wish. You may want to set up a smaller group to discuss possible solutions to an individual group member's problems. Let the person know that you will be glad to stay after the meeting to talk with him or her. Be sure that person has a safe way to get home and people to be with who are protective and supportive.

> When I started our local group, I first met with the hospital community liaison person, a representative of the state Arthritis Foundation, and my friend Pat Remick. Pat was a person whom I had met at an FMS/MPS support group in another town. The idea of forming a local support group was Pat's. At that meeting, we were given a conference room in the hospital and were assigned a specific time that we could have that room. The community liaison person set up radio interviews for me, as well as getting a story about FMS/MPS into the newspaper to let the community know the group was available.
>
> D.J.S.

Warning: Know the signs that indicate someone may commit suicide. If you don't know these signs, contact a local agency health care professional to find out about them. If a group member exhibits clear signs of feeling suicidal, contact your local suicide prevention agency to find out what to do.

- Spread out the group's workload as much as possible. Find an assistant leader to chair some of the meetings, and to be there when you can't. You don't want to wind up totally drained after every meeting.

- Your group may decide to have to guest speakers or educational programs. Possible topics include: hypnosis, massage, acupuncture, chiropractic, medications, well-spouse support, easy cooking, FMS/MPS and the family, how to deal with insurance companies, and exercises.

- If new people show up, you may find it wise to have a newcomer's packet, with basic handouts and information. You might also want to have a special session with them, turning over the main group to an assistant until you can explain the basics to the new people and help them to feel welcome. On the other hand, you may have a knowledgeable assistant take over the welcoming. It helps to have a side room where they can talk confidentially.

Peer Counseling

Many people with FMS or FMS/MPS Complex have found peer counseling, a structured form of mutual attention and support, to be a valuable technique that gives them an opportunity to express themselves anyway they choose, while supported by a trusted ally. It's an excellent way to deal with the pain and frustration of FMS/MPS. Peer counseling, when used consistently, is a free, safe, and effective self-help tool that encourages full expression of feelings and emotions.

Peer Counseling Sessions

In a peer counseling session, two people who are mutually supportive spend a previously agreed upon amount of time together, dividing the time equally, paying attention to each other's issues, needs, triumphs, and distresses. Sessions usually last one hour but can be shorter or longer. Half of the time is spent addressing one person's issues while the other person listens, pays attention, asks appropriate questions, and gives appropriate feedback. Then, they switch roles for the other half of the time.

In peer counseling, there is an ongoing agreement of complete confidentiality. Judging, criticizing, and giving advice are not allowed.

Although most people prefer sessions where they meet in person, peer counseling can be conducted over the phone when necessary. Sessions should take place in a comfortable, quiet atmosphere where there will be no interruptions or distractions, and where the session cannot be heard by others. Disconnect the phone, turn off the radio and television, and do whatever is necessary to eliminate other distractions.

The content of the session is determined by the person who is receiving attention—the talker. This person can use the time however he or she wants. The session may include eager talk, tears, crying, trembling, perspiration, indignant storming, laughter, reluctant talk, yawning, singing, or punching a pillow. The person may want to spend some time planning his or her life and goals. The only thing that is not OK is hurting the listener.

Most people find that peer counseling sessions are most effective if they focus on one issue. But that is not always the case. At the beginning of a session, the talker may want to focus on one particular issue, but as the session proceeds, he or she may find other issues coming up that take precedence.

The person who is listening and paying attention needs to do only that—be an attentive listener and supportive. If it enhances the process and is acceptable to the talker, the listener can ask questions or encourage the expression of emotion. The listener must never demand anything of the talker. Full control must remain at all times with the talker.

Many people feel that supporters view the expression of emotion as symptoms of illness rather than as a vital part of feeling well. Perhaps you have been treated inappropriately for expressing emotion or have learned not to express emotion because it has not been safe. In peer counseling, the expression of emotion is *never* seen as a symptom.

Some people feel that because they are having a difficult time in their own lives, they can only listen or share for a short time. They need to honor those feelings, increasing or decreasing the length of sessions as it feels right.

Many people who try peer counseling have never received anyone's full attention to their issues, concerns, and feelings. They often find that sharing with a person committed to paying close attention yields amazing results.

Steps for Peer Counseling

The steps listed in this section provide a way for you set up effective peer counseling for yourself:

1. Find someone you feel comfortable with who you think will be able to listen and pay attention to you, as well.

2. Agree to exchange time listening to each other on a regular basis (weekly, daily, biweekly).

3. Agree on the amount of time to exchange. The time may vary from week to week—it may be five minutes for each over the phone, one hour each way in person, or anything in between.

4. Find an environment where you will not be disturbed; take the phone off the hook or have calls held; find a childcare person or a baby-sitting cooperative to watch your child.

5. As a listener, listen intently with your focus entirely off your own problems.

6. As the talker, trust the listener by sharing all that you can about yourself. Say what you *really* think as much as you can.

7. Take charge of your own time as talker. Bring up and work on what you think will help you most.

8. It is a good idea to start sessions by recounting something good that happened in the past week. End sessions by sharing something you are looking forward to. This technique imbues your sessions with positive feelings for both the past and the future.

In Conclusion

Your supporters are all around you. If you take the time to figure out the best way you and your supporters—whether they be family, friends, support group members, or peer counselors—can help each other, you're well on your way to a having a healthy support system.

CHAPTER 32

Past Issues

It appears that many people with FMS or FMS/MPS Complex have a history of having been abused or traumatized. Sometimes, FMS, MPS, or FMS/MPS Complex may be one result of the *physiological* effects of tension, anger, determination, fear, or other intense emotions. If you hold your body very tensely all the time, as many people do who have been abused, even long after the abuse has ended, it can start a cascade of symptoms. Therefore, abuse may, at times, be implicated in triggering FMS/MPS Complex.

Many people with FMS/MPS remember a precipitating event or series of events, a set of life circumstances, or ongoing misperceptions and guilt about the past that created intense stress, which seemed to start the cascade of FMS/MPS symptoms. A close look at some of these circumstances and issues may provide important clues about factors that may worsen FMS or FMS/MPS Complex.

Although you cannot keep traumatic events from happening or life issues from influencing your thoughts and feelings, you can learn to respond to them, deal with them, and work through them in ways that allow you to relieve tension and to feel much better.

In addition, there may be various circumstances in your life *now* that need to be addressed. In some cases, major changes are necessary to allow you to take charge of your own journey to healing. The past is a shadow that follows us, mostly unnoticed, throughout our lives. We become aware of it only when certain conditions occur. It is then, only then, that the past emerges as a recognizable companion and undeniable part of our reality/existence.

Examining Your Issues

As you are considering your particular issues, decide whether they are major or minor influences in your life. Do you think about them daily? Have they had a major effect on how you feel, on your thought patterns and your lifestyle? Or are they are only minor issues that have minimal effect on your moods and your life, and that you think about only occasionally? At some time in your life, some of them may have been major issues, but with the passage of time, everything in life changes. If you enjoy satisfying relationships and hard work today, these past issues may now be only minor influences. Decide which issues are the ones that need immediate attention and action and which are important for you to work on for the long term.

If this process is hard for you, if it brings up frightening images (called flashbacks) or it makes you feel uncomfortable in any way, don't try to think it all through now. You may want to think about this slowly, over a long period of time, when you will be supported by a counselor or by some other person with whom you feel safe.

The following is a list of issues that may be affecting your condition:

- **Abuse:** Many people with FMS or FMS/MPS Complex report a history of abuse—sexual, physical, or emotional—that they believe either caused or worsened their symptoms. In fact, some people are still being abused, even as adults. Although it is well-known that abuse has been going on for a long time, its disastrous effects on the psyche have not been completely understood or validated until recently.

In the past, those who reported such abuse often were not believed. Upon reporting the abuse, they were told to "forgive and forget" or, worse, that they had just imagined it. One predictable result for abuse victims who experienced such responses has been poor self-esteem, as well as a wide variety of ongoing physiological symptoms, including FMS/MPS.

Those of us who have worked at overcoming the effects of such abuse—and have succeeded—have regained our feeling of self-worth, some measure of control over our lives, a greater sense of security, and a strong sense of well-being.

Warning: If you are currently being abused by anyone—a spouse, family member, coworker, or acquaintance—you must take steps immediately to end this abuse. Reach out to organizations in your area that deal with abuse for immediate help.

- **Neglect:** People whose parents were absent or whose needs for affection, protection, food, clothing, and warmth were never or seldom met must work hard to overcome the long-term effects of such neglect. Long-term, ongoing childhood neglect is devastating.

- **Crime Victim:** The traumatic effect of crime on its victims cannot be overstated. A world once considered comfortable and safe suddenly becomes a terrifying, hostile place. If you have been the victim of criminal activity (i.e., robbery, mugging, rape, assault, attempted murder, etc.), you may have observed that the incident (or incidents) coincided with the onset of your FMS/MPS symptoms.

- **Witness to Violence or Crime:** If you have witnessed violence, particularly violence against a loved one, such as the beating of a parent, you may experience intense, long-lasting effects.

- **Natural Disasters:** Hurricanes, floods, earthquakes, fires, mud slides and other disasters disrupt daily life, damage social support systems and increase feelings of insecurity.

- **War:** The Vietnam War brought American society to a new level of awareness regarding the damaging effects of wartime activity on the well-being of involved individuals. We are now beginning to see FMS-type symptoms in veterans of the Persian Gulf War.

- **Poverty:** At any given time, many people in the world are living in dire poverty without adequate housing, food, clothing, health care, and other necessities. Those of us who deal with such survival issues on an ongoing daily basis have few resources left to deal with the other problems that may be determining factors in our illness.

Claiming Control and Taking Action

If you can relate to any of the issues described above or you know there are other issues in your life that are getting in the way of your wellness, you can do something about them.

Making Changes

If you have been exposed to circumstances in your life that were largely out of your control, you may feel that your life continues to be out of your control. However, your life *is* under your control now, and you can choose to make some changes to your life or lifestyle. These changes may include:

- Ending a long-term abusive relationship

- Finding a new, safe place to live that is appropriate to someone with your symptoms

- Applying for disability benefits so you can more appropriately meet your needs

- Changing or leaving a work situation

Some of these changes may be difficult and may take a long time to accomplish, but you can do it.

Reconnecting

When people have been traumatized in some way, they often report that they feel disconnected from everyone else. Reconnecting with others who are understanding and supportive will increase your level of wellness.

The first person you reconnect with may be a counselor. Counseling is often the best place to start dealing with abuse issues. Be sure the counselor avoids criticism and judgments, and is supportive and validating. As your relationship with your counselor becomes stronger, start reconnecting with others who have had similar experiences and who can validate your feelings. Support groups are a great way to do this.

Gradually, reconnect with others in the community who share your interests and help you to feel good about yourself. (See Chapter 31, Building Your Support Structure.)

Validation

Validation is an important part of letting go of the effects of trauma, even the trauma of an ongoing chronic illness like FMS/MPS Complex. Focus on spending time with those people who understand and validate what you are going through. Avoid those people, even health care professionals and family members, who criticize you and blame you.

Reclaim Yourself

Through trauma and chronic illness, people lose their self-esteem. They forget that, in spite of their experiences and limitations, they are wonderful, valuable, unique human beings who deserve to be alive and who deserve all the best that life has to offer. (If you think the preceding statement doesn't apply to you, *it does*.) Jot down that statement on a piece of paper, or write your own statement of your personal worth, and carry it around with you. Every time you have a free minute, pull it out and read it to yourself or to some other understanding person. Keep doing that until you really believe it.

Reach Out

Reach out to agencies and organizations that deal with issues of trauma for advice and support (see Appendix A, Resources).

Educate Yourself

Read articles and books on how to heal from traumatic experiences and how to achieve personal growth that validates your experience. There is a ever-growing body of literature in these areas that will give you ideas on how to proceed with your healing (see Appendix B, Additional Readings).

Avoidance

"Avoidance" is a loaded term—it can mean you're side-stepping your own issues. But to help yourself resolve past issues, there are certain people you should avoid:

- Any family member, counselor, doctor, psychiatrist, so-called friend, or spouse who tries to tell you what to do and insists that you must do it. *You* must be totally in charge of every aspect of your healing process. Others can give advice and support, but you have to do what feels right to you. It's your life, not anyone else's.

- Anyone who tells you that your current symptoms or your past trauma are your fault.

- Anyone who judges you or criticizes you. Tell these people they can do that when they have walked a mile in your shoes.

In Conclusion

The process of healing from trauma and rebuilding lost self-esteem can take a long time. Go slowly—one small step at a time. Good luck! Remember, we are all there, walking this difficult path with you.

CHAPTER 33

The Workplace

People with FMS, MPS, or FMS/MPS Complex who are not fully disabled are frequently a costly burden to their employers because of their increased work-loss time. But even if you are a fibromite who can still work, having FMS, MPS, or FMS/MPS Complex often forces you to make major changes in your job or career.

Perhaps you have had to cut back hours, shift responsibilities, or change jobs entirely. Such changes can be especially tough if, as many people do, you tie your self-respect and self-esteem to your job description or to your paycheck. And, of course, FMS, MPS, or FMS/MPS Complex also puts a lot of pressure on those who are the sole money-earners for themselves or their families.

Maybe you lost your job because of pain, depression, or mood instability—in other words, because your job was not appropriate to your special needs. However, as a person with FMS/MPS, having a job may be part of your solution. A job keeps your mind off your problems and gives you healthy ways to interact with other people and be accepted as you are.

On the other hand, your job may be a basic part of your problem. It can increase stress, both physical and mental. It may be time for you to take a good look at your job and examine how it affects your entire life.

Risks in the Workplace

Certain physical activities associated with the workplace often aggravate FMS. These include typing, prolonged sitting, prolonged standing and walking, heavy lifting and bending, repeated lifting and moving, climbing stairs, any prolonged repetitive activities, working with conveyor belts, and/or maintaining one position for sustained periods. It almost goes without saying that high-stress jobs also aggravate FMS, and that these aggravations are greatly increased if myo-fascial pain syndrome (MPS) is also present.

As you know, chronic strain and repetitious motions reactivate and perpetuate trigger points (TrPs). This effect is worsened if you have developed poor work habits; if you have workstation problems, such as a too high keyboard, a sticking doorknob, or a stuck drawer; if you have posture problems, such as slouched shoulders; or if you experience a great amount of stress as a normal everyday part of the job.

If the source of physical strain is not obvious, it is important that you help to identify it. Ask your physical therapist which kinds of movements are likely to overload your muscles with TrPs. Note these in your journal. Record any movement at work that increases your pain. The two of you, working together, can usually figure out what is causing your problem. Your physical therapist may be able to teach you how to avoid or modify that movement—that is, how to perform that task without aggravating your muscles.

You may be able to come up with a list of activities that are less aggravating to FMS; for example, walking on a level surface, some types of teaching, light desk work, and light sedentary occupations that allow varied tasks and changing positions—unless FMS is also accompanied by chronic severe MPS.

Note: Another subject for you to research is your company disability plan. *Some companies refuse to underwrite anyone with FMS.*

Making Things Easier

You can take a number of steps to make your job easier. Some may not apply. Try the ones that do.

Some General Rules

- Read through the survival skills discussed in Chapter 30, The Home Front. Some of them may apply.

- Break huge, seemingly overwhelming tasks into smaller pieces.

- Whenever you begin to do a task, ask yourself if there is an easier way to do it before starting.

- Find a freezer at work that you can use to store gel packs (or bring your own cooler); find an outlet for a heating pad.

- Accept that you can't change your boss or coworkers. Any adaptation has to come from within yourself.

- Focus on how much you've accomplished. The power of positive thinking—"I'm really doing well"—often helps to delay fatigue.

- Laugh whenever you can. It boosts your immune system and lowers your blood pressure. Don't compare yourself with others or focus on your failures. Frustration and lack of control are destructive to your sense of well-being.

- Consider alerting your supervisors to your medical condition(s) formally and in writing, especially if you are taking medication or have symptoms that can have an impact on your job. Some symptoms of FMS/MPS Complex can be mistaken for drug or alcohol abuse symptoms, so it may be important that you educate your supervisors.

- Streamline what you need to do to prepare yourself for work. Do whatever it takes to allow yourself to move through life as effortlessly as possible. You may find it necessary to take shortcuts—sometimes literally, where your hair is concerned. If you are unable to fuss with long hair, crop it. You'll gain time, extra freedom, and the knowledge that you look fine without a lot of effort.

- Check out your closet at home. Not only do some people with FMS/MPS need to keep three sizes of clothing to accommodate body swelling and shrinking, but their feet often swell to the point where none of their shoes fit. Soft slippers and adjustable (Velcro), flexible sandals are helpful for those days. Avoid constricting clothing. If your wardrobe money is limited, check out tag sales. It hurts less when you spill indelible ink on a pair of pants that cost only a dollar.

- Find out what time of the day is your best, most energetic and clear-headed time. If possible, tackle more difficult jobs during those hours.

- Don't work through your lunch period. You need the break. And don't take work home.

- Set priorities. Focus your energy where it can be used most effectively.

- Keep a pencil and paper by the phone to keep track of messages.

- Keep lists of what you need to do, and keep them where you will find them when you need them.

- Ask your physical therapist for some exercises you can do at work that will help you to avoid muscle strain.

- If you can, wrap up each day by writing out a list of the tasks that you want to tackle the next day. That will give you a head start on tomorrow. Then, leave your list, and your worries, on your desk for the day and go home.

Optimizing Your Workstation

If you have FMS/MPS Complex, working at a desk, especially with a computer, can be a real challenge. This section describes some techniques for working at your workstation that might mean the difference between success at your job and hopeless frustration.

- When you talk to someone, turn your chair to face that person so you don't have to twist your body.

- Keep work close to your body, with your upper arms held vertically. This is especially difficult for people with short upper arms. If you do have short upper arms, find a comfortable chair, or adjust your chair to work for you. You may need to bring in sponges to tape to the chair arms to elevate them to a height more suitable for your needs. Discuss this problem with your supervisor. She or he may have some other suggestions.

- If you have TrPs, it is important to get up to stand and stretch every 20 minutes. Set a timer. Flex your fingers. Check to see that your shoulders aren't hunching. Move your neck around and do circular eye exercises, taking care to look up to the ceiling without moving your head upwards. This helps to avoid eye strain.

- Use what ever health aids you can to help you do your work comfortably, such as back supports, elastic supports, armrests, and wrist rests.

- If you don't already have them, request soft pads to place under your keyboard, fax, and other electronic devices to absorb the noise they produce. You don't need the added stress.

- If you spend a lot of time on the phone, get a speaker phone to avoid neck and arm strain.

- Arrange your workstation so that the things you use most are the things most convenient to reach.

- Avoid hunching your shoulder to cradle the phone receiver to your ear.

- Make sure your computer screen is 18 to 30 inches from your eyes—about an arm's length.

- Make sure your chair does not compress circulation. The chair seat must not compress your hamstring muscles. Fit your hand under your hamstrings when you sit. If your hand doesn't fit, you need a footrest.

- If you get shin-splint pain, try a triangular- or wedge-shaped footrest. Place the footrest with the point toward you. A large ring binder can serve this function.

- If your throat becomes dry and you must make a presentation, keep a supply of pure, room temperature water close by. Adding a lemon or lime twist will give it a touch of refreshment, and make it "special."

Keyboard/Mouse Issues

People with FMS/MPS Complex often struggle with their inability to type/keyboard as efficiently as they feel they "should." One hand doesn't work as fast as the other, and each finger may work at a different speed. One day it takes "x" amount of effort to reach "y" number of keys. The next day it takes the same amount of effort to reach only "y minus 2," so every letter you type is actually two letters off. If this was consistent, it could make you a fine career in cryptography, but it's frowned upon when you are trying to be understood.

One woman claimed to be able to type 150 words per minute on the computer, even with FMS. She said you'd have to count all the forward spaces and all the backward spaces she did correcting the errors, though, and not just the one sentence she managed to complete.

Fortunately, there are ways to make your life easier—and your typing better—whether you use a keyboard or a mouse. The first thing you can do is to make sure your fingernails are short. The tips of your fingers should touch the keys on the keyboard.

A product called "Hand-eze" is available from a company called Dome (see Appendix C, Suppliers of Health Care Items). These are fingerless gloves, made of a special type of Lycra that supports and massages your hands. These gloves must fit your hands very well. The company will send you a form to size your hands properly, before you order a pair.

Wrist rests are also important—not for use when typing, but to rest your hands when you are not typing. Develop the habit of keeping your hands *off* the wrist rest when you aren't resting them.

Rodent-based computer work can be aggravating. Mouse alternatives, such as Trackball, Glidepoint, or a graphic tablet may be the answer, but try before you buy. Each person works differently. Some accessories are made to order for the "rodentially challenged" who "don't do mousework."

> I have FMS/MPS-acquired dyslexia of the fingers. My right and left hand work at different rates of speed. It was an exciting challenge to write this book. In many cases, I have written these words twice, and sometimes even three times.
>
> Typing Chapter 8 took three tries, and I twice deleted two hours' worth of work instead of saving it. The logic behind having "F2" as a "find" function and "2" as a delete function is beyond my grasp.
>
> D.J.S.

Scanners are a wonderful way to avoid typing in new data, but they are expensive and therefore not widely available. Investigate copyholders, pen expanders, and other health aids (see Appendix C, Suppliers of Health Care Items).

Here are some rules to follow to maximize your keyboard and mouse achievements:

- Keep your wrists straight and held in neutral position, not bent up, down, or to either side.

- Don't stretch your fingers to reach for far-away keys—use your arm to put your fingers within reach.

- Keep your fingers curved as you type, with your thumb relaxed.

- Occasionally drop your arms and shake your fingers.

- Hold your rodent (mouse) loosely, and don't rest your arm on the surface while you work the mouse.

- Use your entire arm to move the mouse, not just your hand.

Environmental Issues

You may find that a working environment that is quiet, uninterrupted, smoke-free, with clean air and adequate, well-positioned lighting, is essential to your well-being. (You may also find it difficult to find such an enviroment.)

When your neurotransmitters are "jangly," normal office noises can drive you up the wall. You may find the droning hum of fluorescent lights unbearable. An air compressor can give you such a headache you may have to go home. What is annoying or even unnoticeable to others may be intolerable for you. These conditions in the workplace can also interfere with your ability to hear. If you don't want your boss to have to call the fire department to retrieve you from the ceiling light fixture, see what you can do about these situations. Ask if the annoyance can be moved, eliminated, or modified.

Check out the lighting at your workstation. Be sure to keep glare away from your screen. You also may need to adjust your screen's brightness or contrast for better viewing.

People at Your Workplace

As a person with FMS, MPS, or FMS/MPS Complex, you have special issues when dealing with your employer and your coworkers.

Your Employer

The Americans with Disabilities Act of 1992 (ADA) states that employers need to make "reasonable accommodations" for both apparent and nonapparent disabilities. If you are in a situation in which your health will affect your ability to do your job, or changes to your job will be necessary to protect your health, notify your employer.

If you are changing jobs, consider telling your prospective employers what you will need (although you're not obliged to—you can put off giving that information until after you're hired). By making a careful job choice, you may find that special accommodations are not necessary.

The ADA guarantees equal opportunity to people with disabilities in the areas of employment, state and local government services, public accommodations, and telecommunications. If you feel that FMS, MPS, or FMS/MPS Complex is in any way affecting your work situation or your ability to be employed, contact the National Rehabilitation Information Center (see appendix A, Resources). They provide a resource guide that contains information on a variety of ADA materials, including guides, manuals, publications, training programs, and technical assistance programs. For a free booklet on ADA, contact the Office of Equal Employment Opportunity. (See Appendix A, Resources.)

Your Coworkers

With a chronic "invisible" illness, you may find that other employees become jealous of any special accommodations your employer may make for you. Educate your coworkers when you can. And remember, you're not in a competition. Try to avoid whatever work stress you can. Learn to recognize exploitive behaviors. Set limits. Don't become a martyr to the "good sport syndrome."

If you keep cold gel packs around, they provide a visible reminder of the extra effort required of you just to do your job. The slight smell of a mentholated rub may also help to remind your workmates that you aren't a superhero. You're just doing the best you can.

Time for a Change?

Due to the nature of your job, you may not be able to modify it to suit your physical needs. You may require an occupational therapist to help you in making this decision. If so, ask your doctor for a referral.

Evaluating Your Job

1. What do you value about your job? _____

_____

2. What would you like to change? _____

_____

3. What jobs have you enjoyed in the past? _____

_____

4. What are your favorite hobbies and activities? _____

_____

5. Could you turn these into a job? _____

_____

6. What skills do you have? (You may have skills that you don't even know are valuable. Take an inventory of them all.) _____

_____

7. Are you satisfied with your current work or career? _____

_____

8. Does your work enhance your health? _____

_____

9. Would you like to pursue a different career, one that matches your special needs, interests, and abilities? _____

_____

> It has taken a long time to get to this place—where I really feel as if the work I am doing is the work I am supposed to be doing. It required great changes, both in me and in my career.
>
> My first vocational goal was to be a researcher and technical writer. I planned to develop the skills necessary for such a career. I met these goals with ongoing support and assistance from vocational rehabilitation and the financial assistance of a Social Security Plan to Achieve Self Sufficiency (PASS). The PASS gave me the funds needed to purchase a computer, develop research materials, and gather data.
>
> As a result of interest in my research, I gave several presentations that were very successful. I also found interest in

Creative Job Development

When making decisions about work and career, consider the fact that many people with disabilities are able to use the skills they acquired in dealing with their disorders to develop careers in special education, support, counseling, advocacy, and administration. Their life experiences make them especially effective in these roles.

Many people have found that creative job development (which in many cases means self-employment) is the best way to meet their needs for flexible scheduling, low stress, private space, and creativity in their careers.

When you have created your own job, you can take a break when you need it. If you feel like working late into the night, that's all right, too. You can schedule your work to meet your personal needs. Your new career, directed only by you, will make good use of your abilities and creativity.

You Aren't Alone

Take advantage of the available resources to find a job that is right for you or to assist and support you in creating a career for yourself. For contact information, see Appendix A, Resources.

Vocational Rehabilitation

The federal government, in cooperation with state governments, has set up a nationwide system of vocational rehabilitation services. Vocational rehabilitation services provide various kinds of vocational assistance and support to people with disabilities.

Don't wait until you know exactly what you want to do. If jobs or careers are an issue for you, establish your connection with your local or state vocational rehabilitation services right away. They have a wide variety of resources available to guide and assist you in all phases of career development, and they can help you develop a step-by-step approach to achieving your goals.

Contact your local or state Office of Vocational Rehabilitation. Note that to receive services, you may need to present medical documents or a statement from your physician to verify your condition.

Employment and Training Services

States are federally mandated to provide individuals with free employment and training services, such as aptitude testing, job screening, job referrals, placements, and vocational counseling. These offices have comprehensive listings of local area employment opportunities.

SCORE

SCORE is an acronym for Service Corps of Retired Executives. This is a program of volunteer retired executives who give free assistance to people who are starting up new businesses. Depending on their experience, they may help to develop business plans, set up bookkeeping systems, fill out loan applications, or develop marketing plans and strategies. SCORE is listed in the white pages of your telephone book, usually under U.S. Government, sometimes under the subheading Small Business Administration.

a workbook based on my findings for use by people suffering from depression or manic depression. I set up a new goal for myself— to become a public speaker and author. I got another PASS to help me meet these new goals. My new career has taken me to new levels of personal and financial achievement, satisfaction, and independence. At the time that I was accomplishing all of these goals I was unaware that I had FMS/MPS Complex.

M.E.C.

Small Business Administration

The Small Business Administration guarantees business loans to people in the labor force. Check the phone book for a branch office near you. You can find it under U.S. Government in the white pages.

Small Business Development Centers

Each state has federal and state funded Small Business Centers that provide in-depth counseling assistance at no cost to people starting new businesses or to existing firms. Their services include a comprehensive resource referral library. They sponsor workshops on a variety of business-related topics. Phone 1-800-SBDC for more information.

Office of Economic Development

Many larger towns and regions have offices of economic development that provide a range of services to businesses. Check the phone book to find such offices in your area. You can try looking under your state listing in the white pages. For example, Vermont lists this as the "Office of Economic Opportunity." Sometimes it is listed under county or region. If you have trouble locating an office, ask your librarian to help you find them.

Women's Support Networks

Gender-related issues often are obstacles to women who want to start their own business or develop a career. Through women's support networks, women can receive information on business assistance programs for women. Your state governor's hotline should have information on these networks and programs. If your state does not have a governor's hotline, contact the Project on Women and Disability, One Ashburton Place, Room 1305, Boston, MA 02108, 617-727-7440, and ask your librarian to help you find a local resource.

Libraries

Libraries are an excellent source of information to use in your job development plan. They are great for finding educational facilities and programs, career ideas, organizations, corporations, and how-to references. Your librarian can guide you to the proper resources.

Note: Check with your local Office of Vocational Rehabilitation and Employment and Training Services for information on other programs with services that may be useful to you.

Education and Training

If you're planning on changing jobs, this may entail returning to school. Returning to post-secondary education can be exciting and challenging. To make it work for you, here are some things you can do:

- Take responsibility for your own wellness and develop a program for managing your symptoms. A good support network, both personal and professional, will increase your chances of a successful educational experience.

- Many schools have an Office of Disability Support Services (ODSS). Let that office know you have a disability. You may need documentation (such as a medical report) of your disability to present to the ODSS.

- It is often helpful to take a reduced number of classes the first several semesters until you become acclimated to the new environment and lifestyle.

- Become familiar with the resources on your campus. There may be a learning center or its equivalent that will assist you in sharpening your study skills and also may provide tutoring services. Some counseling centers provide support groups for students returning to campus after a long absence.

- Before you return to school, contact the college's financial aid officer for information on the financial awards available, such as Pell Grants. When all other resources have been used, you may be eligible for financial assistance from the Department of Vocational Rehabilitation. This assistance could help you to finance your education.

- If your disability prevents repayment of student loans, contact the lender immediately and request a medical deferment. Note that granting deferment of your payments is not automatic. You must continue to make payments until you are notified that the deferment has been processed and approved. If you do not continue payments, you may be in default. Once your loan is in default, it can be very difficult to change that status.

- If you have to leave school, be sure to withdraw officially so that you do not fail your classes by default. In some cases you may be able to have the designation "Incomplete" recorded, thereby earning the right to complete the requirements later.

In Conclusion

Work can be wonderful therapy if it's something you love doing and you aren't in pain. It is important, however, no matter how much you love your work, to leave your workday when you leave your work and not to overwork. Remember, you now have tools to help you control how stress affects you. Use them.

CHAPTER 34

Disability: There Oughtta Be a Law

In 1989, Dr. Frederick Wolfe found that 30 percent of all fibromyalgia (FMS) patients surveyed had changed jobs because of FMS, 17 percent could not work at all, and 54 percent had problems performing daily functions (Wolfe 1989). If you are among those with FMS, MPS, or FMS/MPS Complex who cannot work, you will need to investigate the possibility of receiving disability benefits.

There are many kinds of disability benefits. Supplemental Security Income (SSI) is a federal needs-based disability program for people with very low incomes. You may also qualify for Medicare and food stamps, although eligibility requirements for these are being changed. Social Security Disability (SSD) is not needs-based, but is part of what you pay for with the Social Security (FICA) taxes that are taken out of your earnings. SSI and SSD are both Social Security benefits. Medical requirements for both of these programs are the same, and personal disability is determined by the same process. For information packets about these programs, call your local Social Security office or 800-772-1213.

Social Security Administration (SSA) disability benefits range from $350 to $1000 a month. The laws governing Social Security are being changed as this chapter is being written, but for now, Supplemental Security Income is payable from the date the application is filed.

You may qualify for short-term disability. Call your local Social Security office to find out. Another possibility of receiving some kind of financial help might be Personal Injury Protection—the PIP portion of your auto insurance—if you can prove that an automobile accident has contributed to your condition.

If you experience a precipitating event on the job, such as a fall or some other type of accident, you may qualify for workers' compensation. This may include payment for medical bills and, in some cases, payments toward job retraining.

And remember this:

"Governments exist to protect the rights of minorities. The loved and the rich need no protection—they have many friends and few enemies."

Wendell Phillips

People who work for the Social Security Administration are trying to do their best to protect the system. Unfortunately, the system is not set up for the person with FMS/MPS disabilities. There are ways to help the system work for people with FMS, MPS, or FMS/MPS, however, and you will find them in this chapter.

Do You Qualify?

To determine whether you can qualify for any of these programs, you first must establish whether you meet the particular agency's definition of "disabled."

In most cases, you must be incapable of performing *any* work, although this rule has some flexibility if you are over the age of 50. Most jobs require regular attendance, the ability to concentrate and to follow instructions, and so on.

"A claimant's case is greatly furthered by a report that reads: 'Patient's past work required sitting all day, analysis of complex data, and lifting to 10 lb. Now the patient can sit a maximum of 20 minutes, cannot concentrate because of medications and pain, and is always exhausted because of lack of sleep. Patient is irritable, argumentative, and misses appointments. Measured lifting is now to 3 lb. Cannot and should not work. . . .'" (Potter 1992).

Often you may have to see several physicians before you obtain a diagnosis of FMS, MPS, or FMS/MPS Complex. (One man we know was sent from specialist to specialist and then was accused of *"doctor shopping."*) You tell the doctors that you are in pain, but where's the proof? Your tests results are normal. Research now indicates that patients are predisposed to get FMS (Pellegrino 1989 (a) and *Fibromyalgia Network Newsletter* January 1996), but some doctors don't even believe in the reality of FMS, MPS, or FMS/MPS Complex. Clearly, more education is needed.

When you speak to your doctor or attorney, be sure to describe the ratio of your good days to bad days. Mention level fluctuations. Explain everything. Write your explanation in this form: "This is how I used to do _____ and now I can't do it or I must modify _____." Use simple language and assume that wherever it is possible to misunderstand, everything will be misunderstood. Social Security Administration officials find it very difficult to grasp the concept of variable symptoms.

If the medical notes on your chart are vague, you can forget about receiving any disability benefits. When you are choosing your medical team, make sure your key player, your primary physician, is caring, careful, and articulate. Your doctor should *specify* your pain symptoms and list the *specific* factors that make it worse.

Note: A complete report, if supported by a good medical record, need be only two to three pages long.

The fact that FMS or MPS isn't on the SCI's "List of Impairments" (contained in "Disability Evaluation Under Social Security," available from the Office of Medical Evaluation of the Office of Disability, SST, 6401 Security Blvd., Baltimore, MD 21235) is a real impediment. This is another reason why it is imperative that those with FMS or FMS/MPS Complex must educate others as well as themselves.The Social Security Administration defines disability as:

> "An inability to perform any substantial gainful activity because of a medi-
> cally determinable physical or mental impairment . . . for a continuous period
> of not less than 12 months." (Potter 1992)

Many of the frequently asked questions about qualifying for benefits are covered in articles by Joshua W. Potter, Esq. (see Bibliography). This attorney has written some fine articles, and he tells it like it is. Receiving disability benefits depends on how well your doctors document your case and how much they know about how they have to document it for you to become eligible for benefits.

The cards are stacked against you even more in terms of getting a positive settlement in an insurance case. The Fibromyalgia Network had a good article on this subject in the July 1990 edition of the *Newsletter.* Alan T. Radnor, an attorney, pointed out that because many doctors don't believe there is such a disease as FMS, they think that the symptoms are all psychosomatic.

When trying to qualify for benefits, always be prepared for a Catch-22 situation to present itself. For example, one man in Maine was receiving disability payments, but he was filmed working in his garden, and his benefits were canceled. His doctors are still writing letters to the state office explaining that they prescribed yard work as exercise. His ability to do a few hours of garden work a week doesn't translate to being able to work nine-hour shifts in a hospital (his previous job) and now this man can't afford his medication because his income has been cut off. It's time for a reality check here. Two essential components in the system are missing: compassion and understanding.

One person on the Internet commented that, like the rest of society, most people with FMS/MPS Complex are hard workers. They enjoy doing a good job and they don't seek help until there is no other recourse. They are then treated like people who are trying to take advantage of the system.

Here's an interesting sidelight: at least two people from our Internet group had applied for disability benefits only to find that they were listed as dead. One of these people said that someone had already applied for her death benefits. It may be easier for the living to prove that they are dead than it is for them to get disability benefits!

Dr. Mark Pelligrino (1993) says that FMS is recognized by the courts, Workers' Compensation, and Social Security as a bonafide medical condition. So why do they play these games?

One long-term (eight years) follow-up study reported that with fibromyalgia, the symptoms remained stable over the years. The muscle function was markedly reduced. *And the condition had and continues to have a marked impact on work capacity* (Bengtsson et al. article to be published in 1996).

Another study (Burkhardt et al. 1993) administered a "Quality of Life" test scale to women with fibromyalgia, insulin-dependent diabetes, chronic obstructive pulmonary disease, osteoarthritis, rheumatoid arthritis, and permanent ostomies, as well as to a control group. The fibromyalgia patients consistently scored *among the lowest in all measurements.*

This isn't much comfort, but based on Internet communications, it appears that in other nations, the requirements for disability eligibility for FMS and FMS/MPS Complex are just as biased and illogical as they are in the United States. Most hadn't heard of MPS.

Starting the Claim Filing Process

You start the process of applying for disability insurance by making your claim at the local SSA District Office, in person or by telephone. This agency will need to know the nature of your medical condition; your physician's (or physicians') name(s), address, and telephone; and your job background and education. When you call, the agency will set up an appointment for an interview. They will also send you a packet with information and forms.

You must make the SSA understand what kind of problems you have. Describe your problems with fingering, dexterity, depth perception, changing vision, sensitivity to fumes and dust, and so forth—things that they have some familiarity with. See the Fibromyalgia Residual Functional Questionnaire at the end of this chapter.

The Forms

The SSA likes forms. They want you to fill out lots of them. It doesn't matter if writing is excruciatingly painful for you. It doesn't matter if the forms are biased against chronic pain patients and completely irrelevant for FMS, MPS, or FMS/MPS Complex patients. That is why the Fibromyalgia Residual Functional Questionnaire form at the end of this chapter, which is based on the Fibromyalgia Impact Assessment form, is so important to you. Its questions are meaningful to the person with FMS, MPS, or FMS/MPS Complex. You are allowed to add many pages of comments, but the people at SSA go by the forms.

> I couldn't fill out the forms by hand, so I typed the requested information on the computer. Then I got a call telling me I still had to fill out the forms. One person has suggested gluing typed responses onto the SSD forms.
>
> D.J.S.

The Interview

There is one rule you should always follow, whether you are having an initial interview, a follow-up interview, or appealing your claim: *Take a tape recorder with you.* Your interviewers will probably tell you that you can have a copy of *their* tape, but that may take quite a while to get to you.

The Review Process

The request you make triggers an in-depth investigation of your problem and disabilities. The SSA also investigates your medical history: the initial description of your condition, including your capacity for lifting, walking, standing, and sitting; your job history—the date you last worked and a description of past work; and proof of citizenship and insurance status.

You must be examined by a physician working for the Disability Determination Service. "Frequently, waits are long, examinations are brief, and medical records are not available for review by the SSA physician, who is paid approximately $88 for the examination and report" (Potter 1992). A number of insurance doctors have licenses to practice in ten or more states, just so they can work for insurance companies. No bias at all there. Right?

In addition, be aware that the physician-reviewer who is part of the reviewing team is usually not a practicing physician and probably knows little or nothing about FMS or MPS.

To receive a response after this review may take six to eight months. (How the people filing for SSI are supposed to eat during these months is a mystery.)

If Your Claim Is Denied

Be prepared: *Initial applications for disability are routinely denied.* Apply again and again until you are accepted. Hire a disability lawyer through your local legal aid organization, if there is one available.

If you receive a denial, it usually will offer suggestions for alternative work—suggestions that usually have no relation whatsoever to your work history or ability to work. You don't have to act on these alternatives.

You must make an appeal to the SSA within 60 days of the denial mailing. *The SSA will not hear your appeal if it is filed late.* Get it in there. This appeal is called a "Request for Reconsideration." You can file it at the SSA District Office or through an attorney who deals with these cases. The attorney will usually charge 25 percent of back benefits from six months after the first date that you reported yourself as unable to work. (You aren't entitled to SSD benefits for the first six months.)

At the time of a second denial, you must file another "Request for Hearing" within 60 days. This will result in a trial by a judge, usually within four months. At this time, "experts in forensic medicine and trial advocacy are needed" (Potter 1992). You must be sure that the lawyer you pick is a specialist with SSD and/or SSI and knows something about FMS, MPS, or FMS/MPS Complex, or is willing to learn.

The information sheet both offices sent to me had no local numbers, only state capital lawyers, lawyers on the coast at the other side of the state, and an 800 number that didn't work and had been obsolete for some time! Your tax money at work.

My hearing was near by. I was lucky. I had a judge who knew about David Simons and MPS. I brought a tape recorder with me but didn't use it, since the judge said I wouldn't need it. He said they would send me a tape if I requested it. By then I was so sick I couldn't remember how to use it. It took all my focus and energy to answer his questions about my condition. I slept all that afternoon.

Before my hearing, I had gone to my doctors with the Fibromyalgia Impact Assessment Form. (See the end of this chapter.) I had each doctor and the hospital physical therapist document every step and some of the disability. Many months later I was informed by mail that I had qualified for Social Security Disability payments.

D.J.S.

You will testify, as well as your physician. Maybe. Some people on the Internet have indicated that their references were not even contacted. The key to the hearing is a comprehensive medical chart and report. Your physician must be familiar with the SSA "Listing of Impairments."

As mentioned earlier, there is no specific listing for FMS or MPS. Sometimes, you have to utilize other headings, since you have many of the criteria for a psychiatric or some other disability evaluation. In your detailed medical record, your doctor must have recorded your *adaptive reactions*, *physical limits*, and *dysfunctions*, in addition to your medical signs and symptoms.

"Every patient visit should result in entries concerning physical capacities (verified with measured weights); time durations for sitting, standing, and walking (by history); the nature, location, and intensity of pain (by history); psychosocial and adaptive behavior, including the ability to interact appropriately with others, follow instructions, and adhere to a regular schedule; and the complex of depressive symptoms" (Potter 1992).

If the judge rules that you are not disabled, you may appeal to the Appeals Council within 60 days after the judge's ruling. Their decision, usually reached within seven months, almost always agrees with the judge. You can appeal this decision by filing suit in the U.S. District Court. (Note that an attorney handling this type of case must be licensed to appear before a U.S. District Court.) Usually, the District Court will return the matter for a new hearing (this hearing is called a "remand"). This is based on the initial application. Now you understand why they call you "patient."

Worksheet for Explaining FMS, MPS, and FMS/MPS Complex to People Who Don't Want to Know

Use the following worksheet to help you describe the information you must give to the agency to which you are applying for disability benefits:

1. Are any of these functions disrupted by your condition? If so, how?

a. Breathing: _____

b. Eating: _____

c. Dressing: _____

d. Walking: _____

e. Hygiene: _____

f. Bathing: _____

g. Continence: _____

h. Grooming: _____

i. Communication: _____

j. Standing: _____

k. Sitting: _____

l. Sleeping: _____

m. Lifting: _____

2. Do you use assistive devices? If so, which ones?

_____

3. Which of the following activities are influenced by your illness? How?

a. Writing: _____

b. Reading: _____

c. Meal preparation: _____

d. Shopping: _____

e. Doing laundry: _____

f. Climbing stairs: _____

g. Telephoning: _____

h. Taking medicine: _____

i. Managing money: _____

j. Working: _____

k. Travel: _____

l. Dealing with people: _____

m. Hearing: _____

n. Seeing : _____

o. Speaking: _____

p. Using hands: _____

In Conclusion

The process of applying for, qualifying, and finally receiving financial aid is a long, hard road. Sometimes the good guys win. Sometimes the dragon wins. The system makes it very tough on you, and you have to grit your teeth and endure. Even if you win, you usually will have been thoroughly battered by an unfeeling system. Make sure you have a good support system—physical and emotional—in place before you start you start applying. You will need it.

Fibromyalgia Residual Functional Questionnaire

Fibromyalgia Residual Functional Questionnaire (modified from the *Fibromyalgia Impact Assessment Form* developed by J. Mason, et al. (*Arthritis Care Resident* 4:523, 1991))

This questionnaire has been modified from the Fibromyalgia Impact Assessment Form developed by John Mason and others (1991 (b)). It was created especially to fill the need for a meaningful form to show specific disabilities common to people with FMS and FMS/MPS Complex. Filling out copies of this form with your doctors may make the difference between receiving or being denied disability benefits.

To: _____

Re: _____ (name of patient)

_____ (Social Security number)

Please answer the following questions concerning your patient's impairments:

1. Nature, frequency, and length of contact: _____

2. Does your patient meet the American Rheumatological criteria for Fibromyalgia?
   _____Yes _____No

3. List any other diagnosed impairments: _____

_____

4. Prognosis: _____

5. Have your patient's impairments lasted or can they be expected to last at least 12 months?
   _____Yes _____No

6. Identify the clinical findings, laboratory and test results which show your patient's medical impairments: _____

7. Identify all of your patient's symptoms:

_____Multiple tender points   _____Numbness and tingling

_____Nonrestorative sleep   _____Sicca symptoms

_____Chronic fatigue   _____Raynaud's phenomenon

_____Morning stiffness   _____Dysmenorrhea

_____Subjective swelling   _____Anxiety

_____Irritable Bowel Syndrome   _____Panic attacks

_____Depression   _____Frequent severe headaches

_____Mitral valve prolapse   _____Female Urethral Syndrome

_____Hypothyroidism   _____Premenstrual Syndrome

_____Vestibular dysfunction   _____Carpal Tunnel Syndrome

_____Incoordination   _____Chronic Fatigue Syndrome

_____Cognitive impairment   _____TMJ Dysfunction

_____Multiple trigger points   _____Myofascial Pain Syndrome

8. If your patient has pain:

a. identify the location of pain, including, where appropriate, an indication of right or left side or bilateral areas affected:

_____Lumbosacral spine   _____Cervical spine   _____Thoracic spine   _____Chest

	Right	Left	Bilateral
_____Shoulders	_____	_____	_____
_____Arms	_____	_____	_____
_____Hands/fingers	_____	_____	_____
_____Hips	_____	_____	_____
_____Legs	_____	_____	_____
_____Knees/ankles/feet	_____	_____	_____

b. Describe the nature, frequency, and severity of your patient's pain: _____

_____

c. Identify any factors that precipitate pain:

_____Changing weather   _____Fatigue   _____Movement/overuse

_____Stress   _____Hormonal changes   _____Cold   _____Heat

_____Humidity   _____Static position   _____Allergy   _____Other

9. Is your patient a malingerer? _____Yes _____No

10. Do emotional factors contribute to the severity of your patient's symptoms and functional limitations?

_____Yes _____No

11. Are your patient's physical impairments plus any emotional impairments reasonably consistent with symptoms and functional limitations described in this evaluation?

_____Yes _____No

12. How often is your patient's experience of pain sufficiently severe to interfere with attention and concentration?

_____Never _____Seldom _____Often _____Frequently _____Constantly

13. To what degree is your patient limited in the ability to deal with work stress?

_____No limitation _____Slight limitation _____Moderate limitation

_____Marked limitation _____Severe limitation

14. Identify the side effects of any medication which may have implications for working, e.g., dizziness, drowsiness, stomach upset, etc: _____

_____

15. As a result of your patient's impairments, estimate your patients's functional limitations if your patient were placed in a competitive work situation: _____

a. How many city blocks can your patient walk without rest or severe pain?_____
   Comment_____

b. Please circle the hours and/or minutes that your patient can continually sit and stand at one time:

Sit   Stand/walk

_____   _____   Less than 2 hours

_____   _____   About 2 hours

_____   _____   About 4 hours

_____   _____   At least 6 hours

c. Does your patient need to include periods of walking during an 8-hour day?

_____Yes _____No _____Cannot work 8-hour day

d. Does your patient need a job which permits shifting positions at will from sitting, standing, or walking?

_____Yes _____No

e. Will your patient sometimes need to lie down at unpredictable intervals during a work shift?

_____Yes _____No

f. With prolonged sitting, should your patient's legs be elevated?

_____Yes _____No _____Cannot tolerate prolonged sitting

g. While engaged in occasional standing/walking, must your patient use a cane or other assistive device?

_____Yes _____No _____Sometimes

h. How many pounds can your patient carry in a competitive work situation? In an average workday, "occasionally" means less than one-third of a workday, "frequently" means between one-third to two-thirds of the workday.

	Never	Occasionally	Frequently
_____Less than 10 lbs	_____	_____	_____
_____10 lbs	_____	_____	_____
_____20 lbs	_____	_____	_____
_____50 lbs	_____	_____	_____

i. Does your patient have any significant limitations in reaching, handling, or fingering?

_____Yes _____No _____Sometimes

If yes, please indicate the percentage of time during a workday on a competitive job that your patient can use hands/fingers/arms for the following repetitive activities:

HANDS (grasp, turn, twist objects)   FINGERS (fine manipulation)

Right _____%   _____%

Left _____%   _____%

ARMS (reaching—incl. overhead)

Right _____%

Left _____%

j. Does your patient have the ability to bend and twist at the waist?

_____Not at all _____Occasionally _____Frequently

k. On the average, how often do you anticipate that your patient's impairments and treatments or treatment would cause the patient to be absent from work?

_____Never _____Less than once a month

_____About twice a month _____About three times a month

_____About once a month _____More than three times a month

16. Please describe any other limitations that would affect this patient's ability to work at a regular job on a sustained basis: _____

_____

_____

17. Does your patient have:

_____headaches, _____migraines, _____sleep deprivation, _____morning stiffness,

_____weakness, _____fatigue, _____shortness of breath, _____dizziness,

_____reflux esophagitis, _____pelvic pain, _____speech difficulties,

_____visual perception problems, _____memory impairment,

_____motor coordination problems, _____nausea, _____cramps,

_____sensitivity to cold/heat/light/humidity, _____panic attacks, _____buckling ankles,

_____buckling knees, _____leg cramps, _____sciatica, _____confusional states,

_____muscle twitching, _____numbness/tingling, _____problems climbing stairs,

_____anxiety, _____lack of endurance, _____mood swings, _____irritability,

_____handwriting difficulties, other _____

Date: _____ Signed: _____

Print/type name: _____

Address: _____

CHAPTER 35

Travel

Everyone with FMS, MPS, or FMS/MPS Complex has a different degree of disability. There are several downhill skiers with FMS, and even a few marathon racers. Most fibromites find it a real challenge to go on vacation, however. The extra work needed to get ready, the trip itself, and the recovery period sometimes seem more trouble than the trip is worth.

Perhaps you've been on "vacations" that turned out to be endurance sessions. You may have appreciated the beauty around you, but not nearly as much as you would have if you hadn't been severely handicapped by pain and other disruptive symptoms. Fortunately, there are steps you can take to enjoy your travels, as described in this chapter.

Visiting Relatives

At times your vacation will simply be a visit to your relatives (see Chapter 30, The Home Front, for more information on dealing with relatives). Family members may try to understand your situation, but if you look fine, it's hard for them to know how bad you feel.

The secret may be to involve them in your preparations for travel. Let them know what you need. For example, you may need time to "decompress" when you arrive—time for a bath and/or a nap. You will probably also want to schedule time to relax. Be especially clear about dietary needs, including time restrictions.

If you are traveling all or part of the way by car, get out and stretch at least every hour. Walk around the car. You needn't take a lot of time, but use the time you have wisely. If you are driving, and sometimes it is more comfortable if you do some of the driving, use cruise control and automatic everything if possible. (The next time you buy a car, it should be as comfortable as possible.) Adjust your seat to your maximum benefit. If you have bucket seats, try a pad in back to "delete" the bucket effect.

No matter how carefully you plan, there can be disasters. We were careful to book waterbed rooms for a long trip to the Canadian Rockies. Every step was carefully planned. The one night we couldn't get a waterbed (there were none in Banff) was the most expensive night of the trip, both in money and in pain. I didn't sleep at all. Fortunately, the hotel we stayed at in Jasper not only had a waterbed, it had a hot tub at the right temperature. I did a lot of physical therapy on the way, and was in reasonable shape when we returned to Calgary. The hotel where we had a room with a "guaranteed waterbed" informed us that the person who had been staying there had decided to stay another day, and there was nothing they could do about it. (I suppose saying

New Experiences

If you are able to travel somewhere you have never traveled before and will be staying at hotel-type accommodations, you need to think about your travel plans carefully. Decide what you want to see beforehand. Check out books and videos from your library. Talk to friends. Ask people in your support group what they know.

Send away for information packets whenever you see something that looks interesting. Read the "Travel" section of your Sunday paper.

There are tours for people with limited mobility. Ask your travel agent about them.

Some hotel chains have rooms designed for people with disabilities. Find out exactly what each hotel means by this. Get written confirmation.

When you check out hotel accommodations, be sure to ask about:

- Walking distance and number of stairs to the room, eating facilities, pool, and shops

- Tours available from the hotel, transportation to and from the airport, train, and so on

- Temperature of the pool and hot tub

- Availability of room service and laundry service (you can carry less luggage if you can wash your clothes)

- Types of beds available

Travel Tips

Here are some things to keep in mind when planning a trip:

- Begin a trip in the best shape you can be. You may want to schedule physical therapy before and after the trip.

- Always try to find the easiest air routes with the fewest plane changes, and allow enough time to change planes when you must.

- Find out about trip cancellation insurance.

- Dress for success. Research the conditions of the area where you are traveling. Travel as light as possible, but pack what you need. Remember that altitude changes bring weather and temperature changes. A day or so before your trip, give your hotel a call and ask whether you should expect rain, cold, or heat.

- Consider taking trips midweek and at nonholiday times when fewer people are traveling.

- If you're taking your vacation on a cruise ship, make sure there are ramps for boarding and exiting. Contact the cruise line to ensure accessibility on the ship itself. Some areas may be off-limits to you because of stairs.

- Find out whether you will be able to purchase items you might need at reasonable prices.

- When you arrange for a rental car, ask for power everything, with cruise control.

- Avoid alcohol, sugar, and salty foods. Learn when to say "No."

- Be aware that sometimes the medications you take are available in other countries, even over-the-counter medicines, but the names will be different. For instance, trazodone is called Molipaxin in England. Call and find out what you need to know before you go, or ask your travel agent to take care of that for you.

- It may pay you to arrive early at your destination to do a little food shopping. Ask if there is a nearby grocery or health food store. Also, you may be able to rent accommodations where you will have a food preparation area.

- Use hotel hot tubs unless they are too hot. Don't stay in too long.

- Put your feet up whenever possible when traveling. Change position frequently. Tense and relax your muscles. Remove your shoes, if possible.

- Allow time for resting and organizing once you reach your destination.

- Take a shower or brief walk on flat ground after you arrive.

- Keep up your normal exercise regimen while on vacation.

> "No" was beyond their understanding.) Their guarantee meant nothing.
>
> I spent about 20 minutes on the phone, and was able to find a waterbed hotel. I will never forget the "Royal Wayne." I am very grateful to them and their pleasant accommodations. I was actually in fairly decent shape when we returned home, and it was a long flight.
>
> D.J.S.

Travel Resources

There are agencies and other resources you can contact to help you have the vacation you want.

Greyhound and Trailways buses have special accommodations for people of limited mobility. Check with your travel agent.

Some hotels in the states and elsewhere are offering "Evergreen" rooms. These offer purified air, bottle-quality water, and chlorine-free showers. Call 1-800-929-2626, or write Evergreen Rooms by Hartford, 432 Landmark Drive, Wilmington, NC 28412. There are 100 hotels with Evergreen Rooms, and the number is growing. Their lists are updated twice a year. If you want to be put into their database, let them know, and they will send you a new list when it is updated.

For more organizations that can help you to plan your traveling, see Appendix A, Resources.

Jet Lag

There are biological rhythms to everything, including respiration, heart action, and immune response. Travel upsets these rhythms. Your body is already in a susceptible state, because of FMS, MPS, or FMS/MPS Complex. Travel makes it more so. Take it easy, and baby yourself.

With time-zone changes, regularity is disrupted. Eating times are changed. People with chronic illnesses who must take medications at certain times of the day, such as diabetics needing insulin, should consult their doctor or pharmacist if they are planning a trip that will cross time zones.

Some medications known to be affected by changes in biochemical rhythm are antihistamines, sedatives, anti-anxiety medications, and some pain relievers.

You can prepare your body to adapt to the changes you will encounter by beginning your day earlier or ending it later *before* you go on a trip. Keep the lights on later at night, or turn them off earlier, depending on which way you are traveling. Your biological clock responds to light, so you can use the light to "reset" it before the trip.

If you fly east to west, stay outside for several hours the afternoon of your arrival. Light suppresses melatonin release from your pineal gland (see Chapter 22, Enhancing Your Medications). When traveling west to east, it's important to get out in the sun early in the morning to reset your clock.

Checklist for Traveling

Use the following list to help you organize your trip with as few stressors as possible.

- Keep a tennis ball in your carry-on luggage, and place it under your hamstrings or between your back and the seat, to compress different TrPs while you are traveling.

- On airlines, use small pillows to support your lower back and neck.

- You may want to wear an upside-down and backward soft collar to "splint" your neck. This will help to avoid compression on your neck TrPs if you go over bumpy roads or hit air turbulence. (Airline personnel will also be more helpful.)

- Carry healthy foods, and eat lightly.

- Bring a medical history, including medications. If you are going overseas, you may want to write for the names of the local equivalents. Ask your travel agency for the address of the United States Embassy in the country you wish to visit. They will give you the name of a local contact.

- Carry more than enough medications for the trip, and pack them in your carry-on bag—not in a checked-in bag that might wind up in another state or country.

- Keep liquid medications in their original bottles, sealed in plastic bags.

- Wear a Medic-Alert bracelet, if needed.

- Carry the names and phone numbers of your doctors. You may also want to carry a note from your doctor listing the medications you need.

- Remember to bring any special aids, such as light eating utensils, a folding cane, gel cold packs, a small collapsible cooler, an egg-crate mattress, an inflatable air mattress, an air pump, a cervical pillow, a footrest, and loose clothing. (Don't wear tight clothes on any trip.)

- Keep your master list with you, as well a copy of this list in your luggage.

- Drink plenty of water. Most airline air is very dry. If you wish, keep several bottles of "good" water for taking pills. Consider taking a portable filter.

- You may need to wear thin socks or support hose under regular socks. Try them at home at first with the shoes you plan to wear traveling, and see what combination of shoes and socks or stockings are the most comfortable and functional.

In Conclusion

You may feel that planning for a trip is more trouble than the trip is worth. The benefits and pleasures of travel are numerous, however, and taking the proper steps both before and during your trip can make your time away from home a refreshing and enriching experience.

CHAPTER 36

Children with FMS or FMS/MPS Complex

Most adults with fibromyalgia (FMS) and/or myofascial pain syndrome (MPS) may believe that their problems started fairly recently. When questioned closely, however, they often remember experiencing "growing pains," especially in their hips. Quite often this was the first warning sign of a genetic predisposition towards FMS/MPS Complex. There is a trigger point (TrP) in the gluteus maximus that often causes considerable pain in a rapidly growing child.

If you suspect that your symptoms began in childhood, you'll find this chapter interesting. If you are caring for a child with FMS, MPS, or FMS/MPS Complex, the information in this chapter is crucial.

The Child's Point of View

If you are an adult, FMS/MPS can confront you with a seemingly unending obstacle course. This perception is intensified and amplified if you are a child. Adults have a little more leeway in charting their course in life. Adults get a little more respect. This should not be so, but it is so. Too many adults don't treat children as if they were people at all. At no other time in life do people change so rapidly and yet have so little authority in planning their day-to-day lives.

Go back to Chapter 8, Common Symptoms and Why They Occur. Think about these symptoms and the impact they might have on a child. The exhaustion, the lack of sleep, the inability to

> I can remember experiencing excruciating leg pain when I was a child.
>
> M.E.C.

concentrate, the detrimental impact on memory. . . . Kids are creatures in rapid flux. They are growing, and rapid body changes can cause even the healthy child a respectable amount of grief.

An undiagnosed child developing FMS, MPS, or FMS/MPS Complex may stumble over his or her feet, trying to coordinate muscles in a world of jump ropes, gymnastics, fast food, and shaky self-esteem. Think of them carrying heavy school books to and from school. Imagine them attending classes, perhaps with fluctuating vision and hearing, and symptoms that change from day to day and hour to hour, including dizziness and balance difficulties. In school, an invisible, variable illness can lead to the label "problem child." The FMS/MPS child sometimes becomes the class clown, or withdraws, just to cope.

School Issues

In youth, FMS/MPS Complex often starts with a flu-like illness and then manifests as "growing pains." With FMS/MPS Complex, the cognitive problems can be intense. Often, their teachers consider these kids lazy or discipline problems. Some of these kids are very smart and ask questions their teachers don't expect and can't answer—a situation some teachers are unable to handle well.

There are some adult artists with FMS/MPS Complex who can do calligraphy and elaborate drawings yet they can't handle cursive writing. This can be an added problem for school kids. They may bring home notes like "How come your child can't write legibly, and yet he doodles all the time? Why can't he spend that energy on something constructive!" In a situation like this, the teacher has no idea that the writing assignment can mean severe pain for someone coping with trigger points (TrPs) in the upper body.

The Pain Issue

Children vary tremendously in their pain perceptions and pain management. There is no cookbook dosage for medications. FMS children, like adults, respond in individual ways to different medications.

Some children, especially very young children, may have difficulty communicating the nature or intensity of their pain. It is vitally important that parents become active advocates for their children and represent them in the matter of symptom relief. Be honest with your child about treatments that may hurt. Ensure that communications are two-way. You can learn a lot from your kids.

> I remember having horrible pain in my hips and legs when I was a child. There was a doctor who made a house call when I was about eight, who said he wanted to "try something." He pressed an area in my hip, and suddenly the pain vanished.
>
> This experience made me want to become a doctor and to learn how that doctor could relieve pain so fast and with so little effort. Unfortunately, I found out that they weren't teaching that brand of magic in medical school. It was only later, when I saw the Trigger Point Manuals, that I understood what had been missing in my education.
>
> D.J.S.

There is a helpful booklet, *Fibromyalgia Syndrome and Chronic Fatigue Syndrome in Young People* (see Appendix B, Additional Readings). Unfortunately, it does not deal with myofascial trigger points, which are frequently involved and can be remedied (often quickly) to lighten the child's pain load. The booklet also blurs the distinction between FMS and MPS and says that many physicians consider them the same. Remember the old joke, "How many legs does a dog have if you call its tail a leg?" The correct answer is four, because calling a tail a leg doesn't make it one.

One difficulty for children with chronic pain conditions, especially very young children, is they often have no self-references to health issues. They don't know that their classmates get refreshing sleep while they themselves wake up exhausted. Their mental confusion, memory problems, frequent illnesses, and pains (often met with disbelief by classmates and teachers) are often *all* that they know, and they have no reason to believe that other children aren't dealing with the same obstacles. When even raising an arm in class can quickly become extremely painful, school days can be extremely difficult. Guilt is piled on top of sometimes insurmountable pain and dysfunction. They can't cope and don't know why, so they think that somehow all of their difficulties are their own fault.

Symptoms Later in Childhood

When a child grows older, the symptoms of FMS, MPS, or FMS/MPS Complex often increase. Depression can set in because of the child's inability to keep up with the other children and take part in extracurricular activities.

Puberty magnifies all of the problems. Young girls are often stricken with severe cramps and premenstrual syndrome (PMS). Often they are effectively disabled by their menstrual periods.

Communications

Talk to your children. If you have FMS/MPS Complex, there is a good chance your children may also have it. Don't withhold the diagnosis from them. Explain simply. Tell them there are a lot of things that can be done to improve the quality of their life, especially since they are starting when they are young.

Your children may already feel miserable. They may recognize the symptoms when they are described to them, and it will be liberating for them to know that it isn't their fault. Give

By the time I was 16, severe cramps (I know now they were more like labor pains than menstrual cramps, as I passed blood clots, etc.), disabled me for an entire week of agony. By age 20, I was having severe symptoms for the week before my period and the week after, with "mittelschmerz" ovulation pains in between, radiating down my legs. By age 30, I was in constant pain, but I "looked just fine."

I got lost in the school building a lot. The administration mandated rotating the class periods. That meant that we didn't have the same classes at the same time every week. For six years, I was unable able to figure out where I was supposed to be. One day I became so confused I walked home instead of going to class.

D.J.S.

the problem a name, and help your children to cope. On the other hand, there may be a stage of denial at first, but let your child know that the sooner she or he starts treatment, the sooner she or he will feel better.

Teach your children to stretch. Help them to find alternatives. Be pro-active, and ensure that their teachers know, for example, that when tiny hands just let go, it is due to grip failure, and not to naughtiness. Meet with your child's teacher(s). Make sure they understand that your child's pain and limitations are real.

It is never too early to start a parent/child dialogue. There are wonderful stories of coping behavior on the Internet. One mother on the Internet group has invented a product she calls "Monsters Be Gone." When her kids are troubled by bizarre FMS dreams and fears, she sprays this under their beds to help her allay her kids' fears and to help them feel safe at night.

> I didn't have parents, just guardians. I had to learn how to be independent, and how to cope, at an early age. I made friends with the snakes under my bed, and they kept the monsters away. Try it, kids. It worked for me.
>
> D.J.S.

In Conclusion

If you are caring for a child with FMS, MPS, or FMS/MPS Complex, it's important to see things from the child's point of view. From that vantage point, you can make sure your child has the tools to deal with the symptoms of FMS or FMS/MPS Complex, and you can ensure that teachers and others who spend time with your child learn how to accommodate their requirements to your child's needs.

CHAPTER 37

Finding Your Primary Care Physician

If you have FMS, MPS, or FMS/MPS Complex, finding a primary care physician (PCP) may be difficult. If you already have an excellent physician, and she or he knows little or nothing about FMS, MPS, or FMS/MPS Complex but is willing to learn, stay with that doctor and provide her or him with as much information as you can find. Your doctor can always become educated. But learning to be compassionate is something else.

A good doctor works for *you*, not the insurance company or your employer. Your doctor's most important task is to help you find the direction and tools to manage your condition. Of course, to do that effectively, the doctor must know the direction in which to go. Recently, someone on the Internet posted this message: "I'm teaching a course in FMS. Translation: I have a new doctor."

What to Look for in a Primary Care Physician

When choosing your primary care physician, whether that person is a Medical Doctor (M.D.), a Doctor of Osteopathy (D.O.), a Doctor of Chiropractic (D.C.), or a Doctor of Naturopathy (N.D.), you'll want someone who is willing to work with a patient who has a chronic pain condition. Perhaps the most important criterion, though, is finding someone you can trust and who trusts you.

You'll want someone who believes that FMS, MPS, and FMS/MPS Complex exist, who is willing to keep current on therapies and research, and who will treat you in accordance with the most up-to-date information.

One woman said she always asked new members of her health care team this question: "Do you respect my knowledge of my body, and are you willing to work as my partner in meeting my health care needs?" These are vitally important issues because your body is often the best "doctor" available.

Medicine is a service occupation. You hire a doctor and his or her staff to help in your care. *You* are the employer in this unwritten contract. If there is a problem, speak up. You need a PCP who knows how to listen and how to communicate—and will take the time to do both. Your PCP should be your consultant and your partner.

Because FMS/MPS Complex does not respond to "cookbook medicine" (there is no one cause, and there is no one treatment), there is no "quick fix" for either FMS or chronic MPS. Dealing with FMS/MPS is even more challenging. It's a real bonus to find a doctor who actually enjoys dealing with complex issues.

You need a doctor who knows how to work with a health care team. Your PCP also needs to understand the basic concepts of FMS, MPS, and chronic pain states. A doctor who understands the nature of these conditions, and who is aware of the complex issues that arise in their treatment, usually enjoys treating FMS/MPS Complex patients because so much can be done to improve their quality of life.

Finding a good doctor is more difficult than just finding someone you like. You may want to ask your friends for recommendations. You may also want to talk with the people in your support group about potential doctors. It is important to interview a potential doctor *before* making a decision to work together.

One way to ensure that you make the right decision is to schedule a "compatibility interview" with any potential doctor, during which you describe your previous bad (or good) experiences with health care providers; find out whether the doctor is comfortable dealing with lesser-known conditions such as FMS/MPS Complex; and discuss important lifestyle choices.

Worksheet for Interviewing Doctors

1. When are the best times to reach you? _____

_____

2. What are the best ways to get in touch with you? _____

_____

_____

3. Are you willing to talk with and work with other family members or supporters? _____

_____

4. Who will be available to answer questions and provide support when you are not available? _____

_____

_____

5. What kind of health care program do you recommend? _____

_____

_____

6. What is your opinion about alternative, noninvasive treatments? _____

_____

_____

7. Are you willing to work with other health care professionals in determining the most appropriate treatment for me? _____

   If not, why not? _____

8. Are you comfortable dealing with chronic pain conditions? _____

_____

9. Are you comfortable dealing with patients who are educated about their conditions and manage their own health care? _____

10. Will you be comfortable if I want a second opinion? _____

_____

Note: When evaluating a new doctor, make sure you're being honest with yourself. You may get less than you deserve if you are using denial as a coping mechanism.

The "Good Doctor" Checklist

How does your doctor rate on the following "good doctor" checklist? If he or she does not rate high, perhaps it's time to discuss these issues with your doctor and/or to seek out a new one.

The following characteristics are typical of good medical practitioners. A good doctor:

- Believes that steps can be taken to relieve your symptoms.

- Accepts FMS, MPS, and FMS/MPS Complex as legitimate medical conditions.

- Enforces your self-esteem rather than diminishing it.

- Listens well.

- Believes you.

- Is knowledgeable and sympathetic to those with FMS, MPS, and FMS/MPS Complex.

- Is willing to advocate for you.

- Is trustworthy.

- Permits you to bring a family member or friend along on visits.

- Encourages you during a visit to ask the questions that might be bothering you.

- Encourages you to ask for explanations if you don't understand what you're being told.

- Allows you to disagree.

- Is honest with you about your diagnosis.

- Willingly supplies copies of your test results.

- Is understanding about your bringing lists of questions, a tape recorder, and so on, to your office visits.

- Shows an interest in and reads any material you bring in concerning FMS, MPS, or FMS/MPS Complex.

The Initial Visit

A thorough medical evaluation begins with a careful medical history. This includes a completely honest and frank discussion of all symptoms, even those that seem irrelevant or unimportant, such as tingling sensations and digestive disturbances.

The physician you choose for this examination needs to be sensitive, compassionate, and willing to listen to and address your concerns. You need to feel comfortable, safe, and validated during the examination.

Gather the information specified below and take it with you when you go for your initial evaluation. It will be of great benefit both to you and the physician in adequately addressing your symptoms and deciding on a treatment protocol.

Checklist for Initial Visit

- A list all medications, vitamins, and health care preparations you are using for any reason, and their dosages.

- A medical history of yourself and your family. Make it thorough. You may remember your mother talking about her thyroid disorder or your growing pains, or Uncle Jake describing his diabetes or lapses of memory. For help in compiling this information, talk with one or several family members who might have some valuable input for you.

- A list describing any changes in your appetite, diet, weight, sleep patterns, sexual interest, ability to concentrate, memory, and bowel and/or urinary habits.

- A detailed list of the following symptoms if you have recently had any of them: headaches; numbness or tingling anywhere (indicate where); loss of balance; double vision or vision problems; periods of amnesia; mood swings; coordination changes; weakness in arms or legs; fever; nausea or diarrhea; fainting or dizziness; seizures.

- A detailed list of any recent stressful life events, such as the loss of a loved one, job changes or problems, family problems, or moving.

- A detailed account of your diet, use of caffeine-containing substances (coffee, tea, chocolate, soft drinks), use of alcohol, and any smoking habits.

A complete physical and neurological examination should be part of your initial visit. Depending on the findings, an EEG and/or CAT scan may be required. Testing for tender points and trigger points (TrPs) should also be part of this physical, although many of your TrPs may be evident from your history.

Ask your doctor to explain your test results and what they indicate relative to your overall wellness. This is an important part of assuming responsibility for your own health. The more you know, the better the decisions will be that you make in your own behalf.

Be sure to ask your physician for copies of all of your test results. You may not understand what they mean (most of us don't), but these copies should be in your possession. You then can make your records available to other health care providers, eliminating the need for expensive duplication of tests, or lengthy time delays while new testing is completed.

These records also provide an accurate history of the changes you undergo through the years. Again, obtaining and retaining these records is an important part of assuming responsibility for your own health.

If the doctor advises particular medications, diet, exercise programs, or other courses of treatment, you have a responsibility to investigate every aspect of this recommendation thoroughly. Only then will you be able to determine whether it is something you are willing and able to do, what might stand in the way of your ability to implement this treatment plan, whether there are possible side effects, and so on. Such an investigation will facilitate every aspect of your treatment and give you more information on which to base questions to ask your doctor.

One physician said that some of his patients apologize when they come to see him armed with extensive information and related questions. He says no apology is necessary; he appreciates the information. It makes his job easier and ensures greater success in getting to the root of his patients' problems. Some patients fax their doctor with questions.

Repeat Visits

When a new symptom occurs, don't automatically assume that FMS, MPS, or FMS/MPS has caused it. Discuss it with your doctor. The symptom may be caused by another illness. It is wise to have a complete physical examination *periodically* so that your PCP can monitor your progress and keep communication lines open between the members of your medical health care team.

Specify your problems. Tell your doctor whether you are having difficulty brushing your teeth, taking a bath/shower, grocery shopping, handling change, writing, brushing your hair, walking, lifting, climbing stairs, getting dressed, picking up children, driving, exercising, eating, making love, and so on. Be specific in describing your symptoms and in how they disrupt your life.

Many people find it helpful to make lists of questions before going to see their doctors. Here are some questions you may want to ask:

- What do my symptoms mean?

- Could my symptoms be side effects of my medications?

- What is the purpose of the test you're recommending, and why is it necessary?

- What are the risks involved in the treatment you're prescribing?

- Do I have any other options?

- Do I have to limit my activities during this treatment?

Then, during your office visit, take notes. Get clarification. Make sure you understand what is said to you. You may have memory and cognitive deficits, so take a tape recorder or ask for detailed instructions in writing. (Most FMS/MPS patients have even worse penmanship than most doctors.)

Problems: What You Don't Need

In many cases of long-undiagnosed chronic pain syndromes, the doctor shoulders the burden of convincing the patient that the condition is treatable. In cases of FMS, MPS, or FMS/MPS Complex, it is often the other way around. And, unfortunately, in some cases, the doctor doesn't know that either of these conditions exists or she or he thinks that "it's all in your head."

You don't need doctors who don't listen and/or don't believe you. And you certainly don't need doctors who blame you for your symptoms. If your self-esteem is low, this kind of ignorant blaming can destroy what little self-esteem you have left.

Does your doctor seem cold, abrupt, and too busy to talk? Are you afraid of or intimidated by your doctor? If you are assertive, does your doctor become impatient with you? Has your doctor ever said, "I don't want to hear that," when you say you aren't doing well? If you answered "Yes" to any of these questions, you're having problems.

If you have had many misunderstandings with your doctor or bad experiences with other doctors, you may want to visit your present doctor or a new doctor with a "handler"—someone who can run interference for you, as they say in football. Your "handler" should be able to supply details when you forget, be

> I find it very important to keep a pad of paper handy for several days prior to my doctor's appointment so I can write down questions as I think of them. I have so much on my mind when I go in that, without my list, I would forget to ask for important information until long after I left the doctor's office.
>
> M.E.C.

knowledgeable about FMS, MPS, and/or FMS/MPS Complex, know what questions you want to ask, and be willing to ask them if you become too stressed or forget to ask them.

Diagnostic Issues

In 1990, Frederick Wolfe, M.D., Director of the Arthritis Center in Wichita, Kansas, reported in the *Fibromyalgia Network Newsletter* (October 1990) that only 6 percent of the patients with FMS who came to his clinic came in with the correct diagnosis. FMS is often coupled with another condition and tends to intensify the symptoms of that other condition. Dr. Wolfe says, "FMS lowers the pain threshold and makes other subclinical conditions clinically important."

One local doctor suggested that patients should be warned not to mention FMS at the beginning of a visit, or they will be automatically tuned out. Do you really need a doctor like that?

> When I first set up a session to teach physicians about FMS and MPS at the hospital where we hold our local support group, I was warned, "Some of them won't want to know." I found this to be true. Fortunately, the number of such physicians is growing smaller.
>
> D.J.S.

The Medication Issue

Chronic pain patients are often treated like drug addicts when they ask for pain medications. However, if you have FMS/MPS Complex, before you begin to understand what is going on in your body and mind—and sometimes even after—you have no way of knowing when you're going to hurt a lot. If you have to beg for pain medication, this situation is compounded by guilt. Sometimes you're placed in this uncomfortable position by a "gatekeeper"—a doctor's receptionist or nurse who keeps asking, "What, you need *more* pills? Why, we gave you ten only a few weeks ago!"

Certainly, your doctor should check you carefully if you suddenly need a great deal more medication. There may be another reason for your pain. However, doctors often have been on the receiving end of education about narcotics that is just plain wrong. Most have no idea that there is a one-percent chance, or less, of addiction occurring when narcotics are used for chronic severe pain (McCaffery 1989).

One person said, "I wish a doctor would view me as part of the solution rather than as a big part of the problem. Sometimes I feel the doctor is blaming me for my illness, that I must not be following each and every instruction as stated. I can't help it if his suggestions don't work. I know FMS is not easy to treat. I don't want to get high. I just want to feel as normal as possible."

The Wrong Words

One woman from the Internet support group developed a new symptom—a troubling rash. Because of the FMS amplification effect, this rash began to irritate her to the point of interfering with already troubled sleep. It was not a minor matter. Yet all her doctor could offer in the way of help was, "Do you always wear those cheap dangling earrings?"

This woman asked for a snappy comeback to use the next time she felt insulted and "put down" by her doctor. Often, when if you're faced with such abrupt rudeness from a professional

I once spoke to a group of health care workers in Vermont. My topic was the difference between FMS and MPS. Some of the doctors there thought I should have brought slides to convince them that there were such conditions. Some stayed and asked questions. One told me frankly that I was actually making people sick and that neither myofascial pain syndrome nor fibromyalgia existed. I was amazed.

If ignorance is bliss, that was one happy man. I wish I could say the same for his patients. Your doctor cannot begin to treat a condition successfully until he or she admits that it exists.

D.J.S.

in addition to the burden of FMS, MPS, or FMS / MPS Complex, you tend to go into a mute state of shock. Sometimes, you may cry or express rage, but usually not until the initial hurt has passed and you are in the privacy of your own home, or at least the car.

Snappy comebacks have their place. But yielding to the temptation to say, "With your fees, that's all I can afford, " won't score any points with your doctor. Physicians have bad days, too. Earrings *can* sometimes cause a rash, even if the manner this doctor chose to convey this information was not appropriate.

If you find yourself in a situation like this, try to take a deep breath and repeat to the doctor what she or he said. Ask for an apology, and ask to be taken seriously in the future. If you are in the numb, mute state such remarks often cause, you might want to wait until the shock wears off and then send a note to the doctor. This avoids a confrontation and allows both of you some time to think it over. Something like this might be in order:

> Dear Doctor,
> I am very unhappy about your attitude during my last visit. I feel your remark about my earrings was thoughtless and unkind. I come to you for advice on my medical symptoms, not for a fashion opinion. I chose to wear those earrings to brighten my day, since I knew it would be stressful. It isn't easy for me to get out to your office. Those earrings have no causal relation to my problem. Right now, your words do. You are supposed to be part of my team. Instead, you chose to dampen my hard-won enthusiasm for life by disparaging my taste and my economic station.
>
> I would appreciate an apology and more considerate treatment in the future. Please don't write off my complaints. Give me a thoughtful and professional evaluation of my symptoms, to lighten my pain and stress load. It is important for my well-being that we maintain a good relationship. A prerequisite of that is mutual respect.
>
> I don't expect you to have all the answers. If you don't know what is causing a symptom, let me know that. I accept the fact that you are doing your best to help me. I understand that fibromyalgia and myofascial pain syndrome are confusing and often frustrating for both of us. Let me know what I can do to help avoid this kind of misunderstanding in the future.
>
> (Signature)

What Your Doctor Needs from You

Here are some guidelines for developing a good relationship with your doctor:

- Be reasonable. Your doctor has many patients.

- Don't expect a cure.

- Don't expect hand-holding. (That's what support groups, friends, and family are for.)

- Don't waste your doctor's time on irrelevant talk.

- Have specific questions in writing ready for the doctor.

- Be honest with your doctor. If you aren't going to comply with a treatment or medication regimen, say so. Perhaps there are alternatives.

- Repeat back what you hear, in case of misunderstanding. For example: "Did you mean for me to take this three times a day while I'm awake, or three times in 24 hours?"

- Remember that listening should go both ways. You are paying for your doctor's advice, so listen well.

- If your doctor recommends a treatment program, share your concerns, but remember that *you* decide. However, don't change a treatment plan on your own; communicate with your doctor.

The cost of medical care is an issue for many of us. Discuss these concerns openly with your health care providers. They may be able to steer you to programs that assume some or all of the costs of your treatment or medications. (And remember to advocate for health care that is equally accessible to people with all kinds of symptoms and from all socioeconomic levels.) Most doctors are becoming more aware of the rising cost of health care and may be able to suggest ways to help you minimize the financial impact of your treatment.

In Conclusion

The quality of your rapport with your primary physician will have a direct impact on your quality of life. It is worth your time and effort to do whatever you can to find the best primary care physician you can, and to do your part to help the relationship work as smoothly as possible. Both your state of health and your peace of mind will benefit.

Appendix A: Resources

This appendix lists a number of agencies and organizations, audio aids, and video aids that both you and your health care team will find helpful.

Agencies and Organizations

Acupressure Institute, 1533 Shattuck Ave., Berkeley, CA 94709

Alexander Technique, NASTAT (North American Society of the Teachers of Alexander Technique) POB 517, Urbana, IL 61801 (217-367-6956)

Allergy and Asthma Information Center and Hotline, POB 1766, Rochester, NY 14603 (800-727-5400)

American Academy of Environmental Medicine, POB 16106, Denver, CO 80216 (303-622-9756)

American Association of Naturopathic Physicians, POB 20386, Seattle, WA 98102

American Association of Professional Hypnotherapists, POB 29, Boones Mill, VA 24065

American Center for the Alexander Technique, 129 West 67th St., New York, NY 10023

American CFIDS Association, 4500 Summer Ave., Suite 149, Memphis, TN 38122 (901-680-0466)

American Chiropractic Association, 1701 Clarendon Blvd., Arlington, VA 22209

American Chronic Pain Association, POB 850, Rocklin, CA 95677 (916-632-0922)

American Coalition of Citizens with Disabilities, 1200 15th St. N.W., Suite 201, Washington, DC 20005

American FMS Association, Inc., POB 9699, Bakersfield, CA 93389 (805-633-3777)

American Foundation for Alternative Health Care, 25 Landfield Ave., Monticello, NY 12701

American Foundation of Traditional Chinese Medicine, 1280 Columbus Ave., Suite 302, San Francisco, CA 94133

American Guild of Hypnotherapists, 2200 Veterans Blvd., New Orleans, LA 70062 (504-468-3213)

American Massage Therapy Association, 1130 West North Shore Ave., Chicago, IL 60626-4670

American Occupational Therapy Association, 1383 Piccard Dr., Rockville, MD 20850 (301-948-9626)

American Osteopathic Association, 142 E. Ontario St., Chicago, IL 60611

American Physical Therapy Association, 1111 North Fairfax St., Alexandria, VA 22314 (703-684-2782)

American Sleep Disorders Association, 604 Second St. S.W., Rochester, MN 55902

Amtrak, Office of Customer Relations, POB 2709, Washington, DC 20013. Booklet, "Access Amtrak."

ASSIST, 3080 Yonge Street, Suite 4020, Toronto, Ontario M4N 3N1 Canada. Travel assistance.

Biofeedback Certification Institute of America, 10200 West 44th Ave., Suite 304, Wheat Ridge, CO 80033

Bonnie Prudden Institute for Physical Fitness and Myotherapy, 3661 N. Campbell Ave., POB 102, Tucson, AZ 85719

Brazilian Medical Society of Acupuncture, Campus Universitaio, Tridad, CP 476 LIS 88000, Florianopolis, Santa Caterina, Brazil

Bruce Kumar Frantzis, POB 99, Fairfax, CA 94978-0099. He has written several books and has several tapes available on alternate Asian therapies.

Callanetics book and tapes can be ordered through Avon Books (800-238-0658). Tapes can be ordered through MCA Home Video, Inc., 70 Universal City Plaza, Universal City, CA 91608

Candida Research Foundation, 1638 B St., Hayward, CA 94541 (501-582-2179)

Choice Travel International, Inc., 7101 N. Green Bay Ave., Milwaukee, WI 53209

Chronic Pain Outreach Association, Inc., 7979 Old Georgetown Rd., Suite 100, Bethesda, MD 20814 (301-652-4948)

Clearinghouse on Disability Information, Office of Special Education and Rehabilitation Services, U.S. Department of Education, Room 3132, Switzer Building, 330 C St. S.W., Washington, D.C. 20202

Disability Rights, Technical Information Office, 145 Newberry St., Portland, ME 04101 (805-446-4ADA or 800-949-4232)

Environmental Health Network, POB 1155, Larkspur, CA 94977 (415-541-5075)

Evergreen Travel Service, 19505L 44th Avenue West, Lynnwood, WA 98036

Eye-Robics Vision Training Institute, 11303 Meadow View Rd., El Cajon, CA 92020

Feldenkrais Guild, POB 489, Albany, OR 97321-0143

Fibromyalgia Association of Central Ohio, POB 21988, Columbus, OH 43221-0988

Fibromyalgia Network, POB 31750, Tucson, AZ 85752-1750 (520-290-5508/800-853-2929) Owner/publisher: Kristin Thorson. (They publish the *Fibromyalgia Network Newsletter*.)

Fibromyalgia Network Newsletter, POB 31750, Tucson, AZ 85752-1750 (520-290-5508/800-853-2929)

Focusing Institute of Chicago, 401 S. Michigan, #710, Chicago, IL 60605

Healing Alternatives Foundation, 1748 Market St., Suite 205, San Francisco, CA 94114 (415-626-4053)

Health Equations, Lynne August, M.D., POB 323, Newfane, VT 05345 (802-365-9213)

Herb Research Foundation (800-748-2617)

HOW (Handicapped Organized Women) national organization, POB 35481, Charlotte, NC 28235

Hypoglycemia Association, Inc., POB 165, Ashton, MD 20861-0165 (202-544-4044)

Internet listserv support group: The address you use is as follows:
listserv@vmd.cso.uiuc.edu
Contact this e-mail address with the following command which you place *alone* in the space allowed for the body of the letter.
subscribe Jane Doe (substituting your name) fibrom-l
You will receive an automated response. The people in this group will direct you to the many World Wide Web sites and other groups on the Internet.

National Center for Homeopathy, 801 N. Fairfax St., Suite 306, Alexandria, VA 22314 (703-548-7790)

National Center for Post-Traumatic Stress Disorder, V.A. Medical Center, 116D, White River Junction, VT 05001 (802-296-5132)

National Chronic Pain Outreach Association, Inc., 7979 Old Georgetown Rd., Suite 100, Bethesda, MD 20814 (301-652-4948)

National Digestive Diseases Information Clearinghouse, POB NDDIC, 9000 Rockville Pike, Bethesda, MD 20892

National Family Caregivers Association, 9223 Longbranch Parkway, Silver Springs, MD 20901

National Foundation for Fibromyalgia, POB 3429, San Diego, CA 92163-1429 (800-251-9528)

National Organization for Rare Disorders, POB 8923, New Farifield, CT 06812-8923 (800-999-6673)

National Organization for Seasonal Affective Disorders, POB 40133, Washington, DC 20016

National Organization of Social Security Claims Representatives (800-431-2804)

National Rehabilitation Center. ABLEDATA Database of Assistive Technology, 8455 Colesville Road, Suite 935, Silver Spring, MD 20910-3319 (V/TT: 800-227-0216 or 301-589-3563). Resource guide on ADA materials.

National Self-Help Clearinghouse, 25 West 43rd St., New York, NY 10036

National Society of Hypnotherapists, 2175 N.W. 86th St., Suite 6A, Des Moines, IA 50325 (313-270-2280)

Office of Equal Employment Opportunity (800-669-3362). Free booklet on ADA.

Pharmaceutical Research and Manufacturers of America, 1100 15th Street N.W., Washington, D.C. 20005 (202-835-3400).(They publish the *Directory of Pharmaceutical Indigent Assistance.*)

Project on Women and Disability, One Ashburton Pl., Room 1305, Boston, MA 02108 (617-727-7440)

Social Security Administration (800-772-1213)

Social Security Claims Representatives (800-431-2804)

Society for Light Treatment and Biological Rhythms, POB 478, Wilsonville, OR 79070 (503-694-2404)

Special Needs Project. To order book list (800-333-6867)

United States Travel Service, United States Dept. of Commerce, Washington, DC 20230. "Travel Tips for the Handicapped."

Well Spouse Foundation, POB 28876, San Diego, CA 92198 (619-673-9043) Executive director: Peggy Meisel; support groups, newsletter.

Audio Aids

"Living with Depression and Manic Depression," Mary Ellen Copeland. Oakland, CA: New Harbinger Publications.

I.M.P.A.C.T. Publishing, Inc. (800-426-3963). Subliminal tapes: "Be Positive," "Codependency to Self-Discovery," "Freedom from Guilt," "Freedom from Worry," "I Want to Be Happy," "Insomnia," "Pain Relief," "Peace of Mind," "Relaxation," "Relieve Stress and Anxiety," "Self-Confidence," "Self-Healing," "Stop Being Angry," "Up From Depression."

"How to Handle Conflict and Manage Anger," Denis Waitley. Simon and Schuster Audio, 1994 (800-223-2348)

Video Aids

Anderson, Bob and Jean, "Stretching, The Video," Stretching, Inc., POB 767, Palmer Lake, CO 80133 (800-333-1307)

Bourne, Patty, Kinesiologist, "Fibromyalgia Exercise Video." OTM Hospital, Psychotherapy Dept., 327 Reynolds St., Oakville, Ontario L5J3L7 Canada

Copeland, Mary Ellen, "Coping with Depression." Oakland, CA: New Harbinger Publications.

Daitz, Ben, M.D., with Janet Travell, M.D., "Myofascial Pain Syndromes: The Travell Trigger Point Tapes." William's and Wilkins, 800-527-5597.(No physical therapy department should be without this six-tape series.)

Gallagher, Paul, Deer Mountain Taoist Academy RD3 #109A Guilford, UT 05301 Chi kung/tai chi tapes deermt@sover.net

Maoshing Ni, PhD "Self-Healing Chi Gong for the Five Organ System," 2-hour videotape. Seven Star Communications, 1315 Second St., Santa Monica, CA 90401

St. Amand, R. Paul and Nancy Medeiros, "Fibromyalgia: A New Approach to Treatment (guaifenesin)," $20, Nancy Medeiros, P.O. Box 461377, Escondido, CA 92046-1377.

Appendix B: Additional Reading List

Advances in Research. No date. Fibromyalgia Network, POB 31750, Tucson, AZ 85751-1750 (520-290-5508).

A Guide to Legal Rights and Options for People with Disabilities. No date. Order from The Special Needs Project (1-800-333-6867).

Budget Health and Fitness Travel Tips Brochure. No date. POB 23375, Milwaukee, WI 53223. (Send self-addressed envelope with two stamps.)

Careers and the Disabled. No date. EOP, Inc., 150 Motor Parkway, Suite 420, Hauppauge, NY 11788-5145.

Depression Is a Treatable Illness: A Patient's Guide. April 1993. Pamphlet available from the Department of Health and Human Services, Agency for Health Care and Policy Research, 2101 East Jefferson St., Suite 501, Rockville, MD 20852, Publication Number AHCPR 93-0553.

Directory of Pharmaceutical Indigent Assistance. No date. Pharmaceutical Research and Manufacturers of America, 1100 15th St. N.W., Washington, DC 20005 (202-835-3400).

Fibromyalgia Network Newsletter. Fibromyalgia Network, POB 31750, Tucson, AZ 85751-1750 (520-290-5508).

Fibromyalgia Syndrome/Chronic Fatigue Syndrome in Young People. 1994. Fibromyalgia Network, POB 31750, Tucson, AZ 85751-1750 (520-290-5508).

Getting the Most Out of Your Medicines. No date. Fibromyalgia Network, POB 31750, Tucson, AZ 85751-1750 (520-290-5508).

How to Get Services by Being Assertive. 1993. The Family Resource Center on Disabilities in Chicago. Special Needs Project, 3463 State St. #282, Santa Barbara, CA 93105 (800-333-6867), snpbooks@eworld.com.

Personal Counselors, Inc.: Fundamentals of Co-Counseling Manual. 1982. Seattle, WA: Rational Island Publishers.

United States Pharmacopeia Drug Index. Volume II. No date. This is the *Advice for the Patient, Drug Information in Lay Language* volume. It is comprehensive and very clear. It also lists Canadian equivalents. For information on this book, contact USP Customer Service Dept. POB 560, Williston, VT 05495-0560. (800-877-6209).

Adair, Margo. 1984. *Working Inside Out.* Oakland, CA: Wingbow Press.

Adams, K. 1990. *Journal to the Self.* NY: Warner Books.

Anderson, Rob. *Stretching.* 1980. NY: Random House.

—— and Sally Carlson. 1988. *Stretching for Working America.* Stretching Inc., POB 767 Palmer Lake, CO 80133 (800-333-1307).

Appleton, Nancy. 1985. *Lick the Sugar Habit.* Garden City Park, NJ: Avery Publishing Co.

Backstrom, Gayle, *The Resource Guide for the Disabled.* No date. Order from G. Backstrom, 2212 Ft. Worth Dr. #94, Denton, TX. 76205.

—— and Dr. Bernard R. Rubin. 1995. *When Muscle Pain Won't Go Away.* Order from G. Backstrom, 2212 Ft. Worth Dr. #94, Denton, TX 76205.

Baldwin, Christina. 1991. *Life's Companion: Journal Writing as a Spiritual Quest.* NY: Bantam Books.

Bek, Lorna, R.N. and Eudora Seyfer. 1982. *Gentle Yoga.* Berkeley, CA: Celestial Arts.

Bergman, Thomas. 1994. *Determined to Win: Children Living with Allergies and Asthma.* Special Needs Project, 3463 State St. #282, Santa Barbara, CA 93105 (800-333-6867), snpbooks@eworld.com.

Bolles, Richard. 1994. *Job Hunting Tips for the So-Called Handicapped.* Special Needs Project, 3463 State St. #282, Santa Barbara, CA 93105 (800-333-6867), snpbooks@eworld.com.

Borysenko, Joan. 1990. *Guilt is the Teacher, Love Is the Lesson.* NY: Warner Books.

Brown, Beverly. 1989. *I Choose to Live: How to Cope with Chronic Illness.* Special Needs Project, 3463 State St. #282, Santa Barbara, CA 93105 (800-333-6867), snpbooks@eworld.com.

Burns, David. 1980. *Feeling Good: The New Mood Therapy*. NY: William Morrow.

Carter, Jay. 1989. *Nasty People: How to Stop Being Hurt by Them without Becoming One of Them*. Chicago: Contemporary Books.

Catherall, D. *Back From the Brink*. 1992. NY: Bantam Books.

Cohen, Kenneth S. No date. *Qi gong: The Chinese Way of Health*, POB Box 234, Nederland, CO 80466.

Cousins, Norman. 1989. *Head First: The Biology of Hope*. NY: E.P Dutton.

Davis, Stephen H. 1994. *Accessible Gardening for People with Physical Disabilities*. Special Needs Project, 3463 State St. #282, Santa Barbara, CA 93105 (800-333-6867), snpbooks@e-world.com.

de Langre, Jacques. 1994. *Sea Salt's Hidden Powers*. Magalia, CA: Happiness Press.

Dunkell, Samuel. 1994. *Goodbye Insomnia, Hello Sleep*. NY: Birch Lane Press.

Ediger, Beth. No date. *Coping with Fibromyalgia*. LRH Publications, Box 8, Station Q, Toronto, Ontario M4W 3P2 Canada.

Freedman and Gersten. 1987. *Travelling Like Anybody Else*. Special Needs Project, 3463 State St. #282, Santa Barbara, CA 93105 (800-333-6867), snpbooks@eworld.com.

Goldfarb, Brotherson, Summers, and Turnbull. 1986. *Meeting the Challenge of Disability*. Special Needs Project, 3463 State St. #282, Santa Barbara, CA 93105 (800-333-6867), snpbooks@eworld.com.

Greenspan, Miriam. 1983. *A New Approach to Women and Therapy*. NY: McGraw-Hill Book Co.

Hamachek, Alice. 1995. *Coping with College* (section on learning disabilities). Special Needs Project, 3463 State St. #282, Santa Barbara, CA 93105 (800-333-6867), snpbooks@eworld. com.

Hanh, Thich Nhat. 1987. *Being Peace*. Berkeley, CA: Parallax Press.

Hankins, Gary and Carol Hankins. 1993. *Prescription for Anger*. NY: Warner Books.

Johnson, Rebecca and Bill Tulin. 1995. *Travel Fitness: Feel Better, Perform Better on the Road*. Human Kinetics. POB 5076, Champaign, IL 61825-5076.

Kabat-Zinn, John. 1990. *Full Catastrophe Living*. NY: Delacorte Press.

Keleman, Stanley. 1981. *Your Body Speaks Its Mind*. Berkeley, CA: Center Press.

Kelin, Stanley D. and Macwell Schliefer. 1993. *It Isn't Fair: Siblings of Children with Disabilities*. Special Needs Project, 3463 State St. #282, Santa Barbara, CA 93105 (800-333-6867), snpbooks@eworld.com.

Larson, Georgiana. 1988. *Managing the School-Age Child with a Chronic Health Condition.* Special Needs Project, 3463 State St. #282, Santa Barbara, CA 93105 (800-333-6867), snpbooks@ eworld.com.

Le Maistre, JoAnn. 1993. *Beyond Rage: Mastering Unavoidable Health Changes.* Special Needs Project, 3463 State St. #282, Santa Barbara, CA 93105 (800-333-6867), snpbooks@ eworld.com.

Magalaner, Jillian. 1994. *Great American Vacations for People with Disabilities.* Special Needs Project, 3463 State St. #282, Santa Barbara, CA 93105 (800-333-6867), snpbooks@eworld.com.

Matsakis, A. 1992. *I Can't Get Over It: A Handbook for Trauma Survivors.* Oakland, CA: New Harbinger Publications.

Maze, M. and D. Mayall. 1991. *The Enhanced Guide for Occupational Exploration.* Indianapolis: JIST Works, Inc.

McKay, M., M. Davis, and P. Fanning. 1981. *Thoughts and Feelings.* Oakland CA: New Harbinger Publications.

———— and P. Fanning. 1992. *Self-Esteem.* Oakland, CA: New Harbinger Publications.

Meyer D.J., P.F. Vadasy, and R.R. Fewell. 1985. *Living with a Brother or Sister with Special Needs.* Special Needs Project, 3463 State St. #282, Santa Barbara, CA 93105 (800-333-6867). snpbooks@eworld.com.

Moyers, Bill. 1993. *Healing and the Mind.* NY: Doubleday.

Pisani, Emilia D'Agostino. No date. *The Wellness Daybook.* Boston, MA: Data Design Publishing (800-947-6688).

Pitzele, Sefra Kobrin. 1985. *We Are Not Alone: Learning to Live With Chronic Illness.* Workman Publishing: NY. POB 21988, Columbus, OH 43221-0988.

Potter-Efron, Ron. 1994. *Angry All the Time: An Emergency Guide to Anger Control.* New Harbinger Publications: Oakland, CA.

Rogers, Sherry. 1990. *Tired or Toxic?* Syracuse, NY: Prestige.

Rosenbaum, M. and M. Susser. 1992. *Solving the Puzzle of Chronic Fatigue Syndrome.* Tacoma, WA: Life Sciences Press.

Rosenthal, N. *Winter Blues* (SAD). 1993. New York, NY: The Guilford Press.

Saathoff, Mary Anne. 1992. *The Fibromyalgia Syndrome.* Fibromyalgia Association of Central Ohio, POB 21988, Columbus, OH 43221-0988.

Sandbek, T. 1986. *The Deadly Diet: Recovering From Anorexia and Bulimia.* Oakland, CA: New Harbinger Publications.

Sears, Barry and Bill Lawren. 1995. *The Zone*. NY: Harper Collins.

Sheehy, G. 1992. *The Silent Passage*. NY: Random House.

Siegel, B. 1986. *Love, Medicine and Miracles*. NY: Harper & Row.

————. 1990. *Peace, Love and Healing*. NY: Harper & Row.

Silverman, Harold. 1986. *Travel Healthy*. NY: Avon.

Solomon, Muriel. 1990. *Working with Difficult People*. Engelwood Cliffs, NJ: Prentice Hall.

Spencer, Bev. *Fibromyalgia: Fighting Back*. No date. LRH Publications: Box 8, Station Q, Toronto, Ontario M4W 3P2 Canada.

————. No date. *How to Run a Support Group*. National Foundation for FM: POB 3429, San Diego, CA 91263-1429.

Spiegle, Jan and Richard A. van den Pol. 1993. *Making Changes: Family Voices on Living with Disabilities*. Special Needs Project, 3463 State Street #282 Santa Barbara, CA 93105 (800-333-6867), snpbooks@eworld.com.

Steketee, G and K. White. 1990. *When Once Is Not Enough: Help for Obsessive Compulsives*. Oakland, CA: New Harbinger Publications.

Stolman, Marc. 1994. *A Guide to Legal Rights and Options for People with Disabilities*. Special Needs Project, 3463 State St. #282, Santa Barbara, CA 93105 (800-333-6867), snpbooks@e-world.com.

Strong, Maggie. 1988. *Mainstay* (for the well spouse). Special Needs Project, 3463 State St. #282, Santa Barbara, CA 93105 (800-333-6867), snpbooks@eworld.com.

Tallard, J. *Hidden Victims*. 1988. NY: Doubleday.

Thompson, W.G. 1989. *Gut Reactions: Understanding Symptoms of the Digestive Tract*. NY: Plenum Publishing Corp.

Thorson, Kristin. 1992. *Getting the Most Out of Your Medicines*. Fibromyalgia Network, POB 31750, Tucson, AZ 85751-1750.

Upledger, John. No date. *Your Inner Physician and You*. North Atlantic Books. Also available from the Upledger Institute, 11211 Prosperity Farms Rd., Palm Beach Gardens, FL 33401-4449.

Walsh, Alison, Jodi Abbott, and Peg Smith. 1994. *Able to Travel: True Stories By and About Travellers with Disabilities*. Special Needs Project, 3463 State St. #282, Santa Barbara, CA 93105 (800-333-6867), snpbooks@eworld.com.

Weiss, Louis. No date. *Access to the World: A Travel Guide for the Handicapped*. NY: Facts on File, Inc., 460 Park Ave. S, New York, NY 10016.

Wheeler, Genie G. and J. Dace-Lombard. 1989. *Living Creatively with Chronic Illness: Developing Skills for Transcending the Loss, Pain, and Frustration*. Ventura, CA: Pathfinder Publications.

Williamson, Miryam Ehrlich. 1996. *Fibromyalgia: A Comprehensive Approach: What You Can Do about Chronic Pain and Fatigue*. NY: Walker and Co.

Willis, Jan. 1994. *Beautiful Again: Restoring Your Image and Enhancing Body Changes*. Special Needs Project, 3463 State St. #282, Santa Barbara, CA 93105 (800-333-6867), snpbooks@eworld.com.

Zhang, Mingwu and Sun Xingyuan. 1985. *Chinese Qi Gong Therapy*. Translated by Yang Entang and Yao Xiuqing. Jinan, China: Shadong Science and Technology Press.

Appendix C:
Suppliers of Health Care Items

Part 1. Suppliers of Health Care Items for the Consumer

Adaptability, POB 515, Colchester, CT 06415-0515 (800-288-9941). Products to help improve quality of life, such as ice grippers for shoes and canes, easy-use flexible utensils and plates (with high lips), door openers, grip-extenders, ice/heat packs, supports, braces and more.

Apollor Light Systems, Inc., 352 West 1060 S, Orem, UT 84058. Light boxes.

Bio-Brite, 7315 Wisconsin Ave., Suite 900E, Bethesda, MD 20814 (800-621-5483). Information on light visors.

Brainstorms Catalog, 800-621-7500. Health aids, anatomical charts, diagrams, and general catalog.

Decent Exposures, 2202 115th N.E., Seattle, WA 98125 (800-524-4949) U.S.; Canada 9-9 PST. Pull-on/step-in "sports" style bras, with no hardware, in cotton, cotton-Lycra, and firm support cotton velour. They aren't cheap, but they custom-make large sizes.

Dome, 800-432-4352. Hand-eze gloves. Note: Dome will supply a size chart to anyone who calls for it.

Dr. Leonard's Healthcare Catalog, POB 7821, Edison, NJ 08818-7821 (908-225-0880). Canes, hot/cold therapy aids, cordless lights, book holders, other patient aids.

The Grain and Salt Society. POB DD, Magalia, CA 95954 (916-872-5800). Celtic Salt, whole grains.

JC Penney Special Needs Home Health Care and Easy Dressing Fashions, POB 2021, Milwaukee, WI 53201-2021 (800-222-6161).

Medic-Light, Inc., Yacht Club Drive, Lake Hopatcong, NJ 07849 (800-544-4825). Light boxes.

Armand Nadeau, 27 Black Mountain Rd., Brattleboro, VT 05301 (802-254-2900). Handmade, folding, portable, wood footstools.

Pilgrim Designs, Inc, POB 35306, Canton, OH 44735. FMS T-shirts with "Fibromyalgia Survivor" and tender points marked with red dots. (Not exactly a health aid, but might be a morale booster.)

Shoe Express, POB 31537, Lafayette, LA 70593-1537 (800-874-0469). Ladies' large and wide shoes.

Shop at Home, POB 221050, Denver, CO 80222-9050, (800-315-1995). Catalog of catalogs. All sorts of shopping-by-mail catalogs including clothes for larger sizes and clothes for shorter men.

Stretching, Inc., POB 767, Palmer Lake, CO 80133. Stretching books, video, charts, and physical therapy aids.

SunBox Company, 1132 Taft St., Rockville, MD 20850 (310-762-1786). Light boxes.

Wissota Trader, 1313 First Ave., Chippewa Falls, WI 54729 (800-833-6421). Regular and hard-to-find shoe sizes.

Part 2. Suppliers of Health Care Items for the Health Care Team

I. Information Sources

Journal of Musculoskeletal Pain. I. Jon Russell, M.D., PhD., Ed., The Haworth Medical Press: 10 Alice St., Binghamton, NY 13904.

"Choosing Electrotherapeutic Devices" by Thomas P. Nolan Jr., M.S., P.T. *PT Magazine* (July 1993).

Reprints, Physicians: Available from Gebauer 1-800-321-9348

"The Myofascial Genesis of Pain" by Janet Travell and Seymour Rinzler.

"Myofascial Trigger Points: A Need for Understanding" by David G. Simons.

"Myofascial Trigger Points: Clinical View" by Janet Travell.

"Temporomandibular Joint Dysfunction" by Janet Travell.

"Myofascial Pain Syndrome Due to Trigger Points" by David Simons.

From Williams and Wilkins

"Myofascial Pain Syndrome: The Travell Trigger Point Tapes" with Janet Travell, M.D. Set of six videotapes. Ben Daitz, M.D. 800-527-5597.

Myofascial Pain and Dysfunction: The Trigger Point Manual Volume I: The Upper Body by Janet G. Travell, M.D. and David G. Simons, M.D. Williams and Wilkins 1983. (Revision coming January 1997) (800-638-0672).

Myofascial Pain and Dysfunction: The Trigger Point Manual Volume II: The Lower Body by Janet G. Travell, M.D. and David G. Simons, M.D. Williams and Wilkins 1992 (800-638-0672).

II. Products

Fluori-Ethyl Vapocoolant Spray for Spray and Stretch
Ethyl-Chloride Vapocoolant Spray for Spray and Stretch
Salivart Oral Moisturizer from Gebauer Company
9410 Catherine St.
Cleveland, Ohio 44104
1-800-321-9348
1-216-271-5252 in Ohio

Electronic Muscle Stim and Ultrasound
David De Natale (multiple source tech)
POB 578
Shaftsbury, VT 05262
1-800-923-0118

Galvanic Muscle Stimulators
Rich-Mar
POB 879
Inola, OK 74036-0879
1-800-762-4665

Continental S.E.L. Health Care Products Catalog
(ultrasound, electrostim, hot and cold therapy, supports, other physical therapy aids)
4440 Southeast 53rd Ave.
Ocala, Florida 34480
1-800-826-9946

NMES (EMS 300) Electrotherapy personal device for patients
Commumed
120 Kedron Ave.
Holmes, PA 19043
1-800-848-5397

Bibliography

AHCPR guidelines recommend NSAIDS and acetaminophen—but how safe are they? 1993. *MPI's Dynamic Chiropractic* 94(5) (February 15).

Alvarez, A. 1995. *Night: Night Life, Night Language, Sleep and Dreams.* NY: W.W. Norton.

Anderson, R.M., N. Polansky, S. Bryden, S. Bhathena and J. Canary. 1987. Effects of supplemental chromium on patients with symptoms of reactive hypoglycemia. *Metabolism* 36 (4).

August, Lynne. April 1995. Food and Hormones. *Townsend Letter for Doctors.* No. 140, 911 Tyler St., Port Townsend, WA 98368-6541.

Batten, Mary. 1995. Take charge of your pain. *Modern Maturity* (Jan./Feb.).

Becker, Robert O. and Gary Selden. 1985. *The Body Electric.* NY: William Morrow and Co.

Bengtsson, A., E. Bäckman, B. Lindblom, T. Skogh. 1994. Long-term follow-up of fibromyalgia patients: clinical symptoms, muscular function, laboratory tests—an eight-year comparison study. *Journal of Musculoskeletal Pain* (2) 2.

———, K.G. Henriksson, J. Larsson. 1986. Reduced high-energy phosphate levels in the painful muscles of patients with primary fibromyalgia. *Arthritis and Rheumatism* 29 (7).

Bennett, R.M. 1994. Exercise and exercise testing in fibromyalgia patients: Lessons learned and suggestions for further studies. *Journal of Musculoskeletal Pain* 2(3).

———. 1990. Myofascial pain syndromes and the fibromyalgia syndrome: a comparative analysis. *Advances in Research and Therapy,* 17, 45-65.

————, H. A. Smith and F. Wolf. March 15, 1992. Recognizing fibromyalgia. *Patient Care*, 211-218.

Best and Taylor's Physiological Basis of Medical Practice. 1991. Ed. John B. West. Baltimore, MD: Williams and Wilkins.

Bohr, T. 1987. Painful questions about fibromylagia. *JAMA* 258(11).

Bonica, John J., John D. Loeser, C. Richard Chapman and Wilbert E. Fordyce. 1990. *The Management of Pain*. Baltimore, MD: Williams and Wilkins. (Originally published by Lea and Febiger.)

Boston City Hospital Clinical AIDS Team. 1992. Fibromyalgia syndrome in patients infected with human immunodeficiency virus. *American Journal of Medicine* 92 (4).

Bourne, Edmund. 1995. *The Anxiety and Phobia Workbook*, 2d ed. Oakland, CA: New Harbinger Publications.

Bruce, D.G., J.F. Golding and N. Hockenhull. 1990. Acupressure and motion sickness. *Aviation, Space and Environmental Medicine* 61 (4).

Bruusgaard D., A.R. Evensen and T. Bjerkedal. 1993. Fibromyalgia—a new cause for disability pension. *Scandinavian Journal of Social Medicine* 21 (2).

Burk, O. 1989. Effect of homeopathic treatment of fibromyalgia. *British Medical Journal*, No. 299: 685.

Burkhardt, C.S., S.R. Clark and R.M. Bennett. 1991. The fibromyalgia impact questionnaire: development and validation. *Journal of Rheumatology* 18 (5).

————, S.R. Clark and R.M. Bennett. 1993. Fibromyalgia and quality of life: a comparative analysis. *Journal of Rheumatology* 20 (3).

Butler, Sharon. 1995. *Conquering Carpal Tunnel Syndrome and Other Repetitive Strain Injuries*. Berwyn, PA: Advanced Press. RSI Solutions, 1273 Lancaster Ave., Suite 1-B, Berwyn, PA 19312-1244.

Calabro, J.J. 1986. Fibromyalgia in children. *American Journal of Medicine* 81: 3A.

————. 1986. Juvenile primary fibromyalgia syndrome. *Arthritis and Rheumatism* 29(3).

Carette, S. and L. Lefrancois. 1988. Fibrositis and primary hypothyroidism. *Journal of Rheumatology* 15 (9).

Cassisi, J.E., G.W. Sypert, L. Lagana, E.M. Friedman and M.E. Robinson. 1993. Pain, disability, and psychological functioning in chronic low-back pain subgroups: Myofascial versus herniated disc syndrome. *Neurosurgery* 33:379-385.

Catalano, E. 1990. *Getting to Sleep*. Oakland, CA: New Harbinger Publications.

Caudahl, Lurie M. and K. Johansson. 1990. Respiratory function in chronic fibromyalgia. *Scandinavian Journal of Rehabilitation Medicine* 22 (3).

Charmes, William. 1976. *Some Must Watch While Some Must Sleep*. San Francisco Book Co. (distributed by Simon & Shuster, NY).

Christiansen, Erik, Bente Dannerskiold-Samsøe, Birger Lund and Rasmus Bach Andersen. 1982. Regional muscle tension and pain (fibrositis) effect of massage on myoglobin in plasma. *Scandinavian Journal of Rehabilitation Medicine* 15:17-20.

Clark, Wesley. Craig Brater and Alice R. Johnson. 1988. *Goth's Medical Pharmacology*. St. Louis, Baltimore, Philadelphia, Toronto: C.V. Mosby Co.

Cleveland C.H., R.H. Fisher and E.P. Brestel. 1992. The association between rhinitis and fibromyalgia. *Journal of Allergy and Clinical Immunology* 89 (1).

Consensus Document on Fibromyalgia: The Copenhagen Declaration. Issued by the Second World Congress on Myofascial Pain and Fibromyalgia meeting August 17-20, 1992. Published *Lancet*, vol. 340, Sept. 12, 1992, and incorporated into the World Health Organization's 10th revision of the International Statistical Classification of Diseases and Related Health Problems, ICD 10, Jan. 1, 1993. Available from Bente Danneskiold-Samsøe, Department of Rheumatology, Frederiksberg Hospital, Ndr Fasanvej 57, DK-2000 Frederiksberg, Denmark. Also in the *Journal of Musculoskeletal Pain,* vol. 1, No. 3/4, 1993.

Copeland, Mary Ellen. 1992. *The Depression Workbook: A Guide to Living with Depression and Manic Depression*. Oakland, CA: New Harbinger Publications.

―――. 1994. *Living Without Depression and Manic Depression* Oakland, CA: New Harbinger Publications.

Cowan, Penney. 1987. *American Chronic Pain Assn. Workbook Manual*. POB 850, Charlotte, NC 28222-4398 (916-632-0922).

Cracchiolo, Camilla, R.N. No date. *Frequently Asked Questions about Vaginal Yeast Infection*. fibrom-l Internet. camilla@primenet.com (see Appendix A, Resources, for information on accessing the Internet).

Crofford, Leslie J. 1994. Neuroendocrine aspects of fibromyalgia. *Journal of Musculoskeletal Pain* 2(3).

Culclasure, T.F., R.J. Enzenauer and S. G.West. 1993. Post-traumatic stress disorder presenting as fibromyalgia. *American Journal of Medicine* 94 (5):548-549.

Danneskiold-Samsøe B., E. Christiansen and R. Bach Anderson. 1986. Myofascial pain and the role of myoglobin. *Scandinavian Journal of Rheumatology* 5: 174-178.

―――, E. Christiansen, B. Lund and R. Bach Andersen. 1982. Regional muscle tension and pain (fibrositis). Effect of massage on myoplasma. *Scandinavian Journal of Rehabilitation Medicine* 15: 17-20.

Davis, Martha, Elizabeth Robins Eshelman and Matthew McKay. 1995. *The Relaxation & Stress Reduction Workbook,* 4th edition. Oakland, CA: New Harbinger Publications.

de Aloysio, D. and P.Penacchioni. 1992. Morning sickness control in early pregnancy by neuguan point acupressure. *Obstetrics and Gynecology* 80 (5).

Deng, D.H., Tan Qi and J.S. Han. 1986. Observations on combatting nausea by finger pressure on the hegu point. *Journal of Traditional Chinese Medicine* 6 (2).

Diagnostic and Statistical Manual of Mental Disorders. 1989. Editor Janet B.W. Williams. American Psychiatric Association: Washington, D.C.

Does fibromyalgia qualify as a work-related injury? 1992. *Journal of Occupational Medicine* 34(10):968.

Donoghue, Paul J. Sick and Mary E. Siegel. 1992. *Tired of Feeling Sick and Tired.* NY: Norton.

Edie, Barbara. 1993-4. Fibromyalgia: cruel and unusual. *Canadian J. Pharm.* 126 (Dec./Jan.).

Eisinger, J., A. Plantamura and T. Ayavou. 1994. Glycolosis abnormalities in fibromyalgia. Centre Hospitalier, Toulon, France. *Journal of the American College of Nutrition,* 1994 edition.

Ferraccioli, G.F. S. Fontanna and F. Scita. 1989. EMG-biofeedback training in fibromyalgia syndrome. *Journal of Rheumatology* 16 (7).

Fibromyalgia Network Newsletter. POB 31750, Tucson, AZ 85751-1750.

Finestone, D.H., B.A. Sawyer and S.K. Ober. 1991. Periodic leg movements during sleep in patients with fibromyalgia. *Annals of Clinical Psychiatry* 3 (3).

Fitzcharles, Mary-Ann, Stuart Greenfield and John M. Esdaile. 1992. Reactive fibromyalgia syndrome. *Arthritis and Rheumatism,* 35 (6).

Frantzis, B. K. 1993. *Opening the Energy Gates of the Body.* North Atlantic Books: Berkeley, CA.

Frenstrom, J.D. 1987. Food-induced changes in brain- serotonin synthesis: Is there a relationship to appetite for specific macro-nutrients? *Appetite* 8 (3).

Fry, E.N.S. 1988. Acupressure and morning sickness. *Journal of the Royal Society of Medicine* No. 81.

Galloway, J. 1990. Maintaining serenity in chronic illness. *New York State Journal of Medicine* 90 (7).

Gedalia, A., J. Press and M. Klein. 1993. Joint hypermobility and fibromyalgia in children. *Annals of Rheumatic Diseases* 52 (7).

Gerster, J.C. and A. Hadj-Djilani. 1984. Hearing and vestibular abnormalities in primary fibrositis syndrome. *Journal of Rheumatology* 11 (5).

Giannini, A.J., Donald A. Malone, A. Thaddeus and J. Piotroski. 1995. The serotonin irritation syndrome—A new clinical entity? *Journal of Clinical Psychiatry* 41 (1) (January).

Goldenberg, D.L. 1994. Fibromyalgia and chronic fatigue syndrome. *Journal of Musculoskeletal Pain* 2 (3).

Grad, Marcia. *A Taste for Life* with foreword by R. Paul St. Amand. 1975. (Out of print. This book contains *great* recipes for people with reactive hypoglycemia. It was published by Charles Scribner and Sons, NY ISBN 0-684-14381-X.)

Griep, E.N., J.W. Boersma and E.R. de Kloet. 1993. Altered reactivity of the hypothalmic-pituitary-adrenal axis in the primary fibromyalgia syndrome. *Journal of Rheumatology* 20 (3).

Halpern, Lawrence M. 1989. Analgesic and anti-inflammatory medications. In *Chronic Myofascial Pain Syndromes*. Edited by C.D. Tollison, J.R. Satterthwaite, J.W. Tollison and C.G. Trent. Baltimore, MD.: Williams and Wilkins

Hawley, D.J., F. Wolfe and M.A.Cathey. 1988. Pain, functional disability, and psychological status: a 12-month study of severity in fibromyalgia. *Journal of Rheumatology* 15 (10).

Heimeyer, K., R. Lutz and H. Menninger. 1990. Dependence of tender points upon posture: a key to understanding of fibromyalgia syndrome. *Journal of Manual Medicine* 5 (4).

Henriksson, K.G., I. Gundmark and A. Bengtsson. 1992. Living with fibromyalgia, consequences for everyday life. *Clinical Journal of Pain*, 8 (2).

Hong, C-Z, Hsueh T-C and Simons D.G. 1995. Difference in pain relief after trigger point injections in myofascial pain patients with and without fibromyalgia. *Journal of Musculoskeletal Pain* 3 (Suppl 1):60 (Abstract).

Hunter, J.O. 1991. Food allergy—or enterometabolic disorder? *Lancet* 338:495-496.

Internet address. *See* Appendix A, Resources.

Johannson, G., M.G. Elam and B.D. Wallin. 1992. Do patients with fibromyalgia have an altered sympathetic nerve activity? *Pain* 48 (3).

Johannson, Valur 1993. Does a fibromyalgia personality exist? *Journal of Musculoskeletal Pain*, vol. 1 (3/4).

Joos, Erika, D. Eljuga, P. Capel, V. Bujan-Boza, A. Essalhi and J. P. Famaey. 1994. Fibrinolytic activity in fibromyalgic patients—the role of latent tetany. *European Journal of Physical Medicine and Rehabilitation* 4 (2) (June).

Journal of Musculoskeletal Pain I. Edited by Jon Russell. The Haworth Medical Press: 10 Alice Street, Binghamton, NY 13904.

Juhan, Deane. 1987. *Job's Body*. Barrytown, NY: Station Hill Press.

Kastner, Mark and Hugh Burroughs. 1993. *Alternative Healing*. La Mesa, CA: Halcyon Publishing.

Kaufman, L. 1993. Tryptophan: Current status and future trends. *Drug Safety* 8 (2).

Kemple, Kip L. 1989. Fingernail pits: Clinical markers for fibromylagia? *Modern Medicine,* vol. 57 (May).

Klein, Linda. 1989. Fibromyalgia syndrome shedding light on the mystery disease. *Arthritis Today* (May/June).

Koenig Jr., W.C., J.J. Powers and E.W. Johnson. 1977. Does allergy play a role in fibrositis? *Archives of Physical Medicine and Rehabilitation* 58 (2).

Kuch, K., R.J. Evans and C.P. Watson. 1991. Accidents and chronic myofascial pain. *Pain Clinic* 4 (2).

The leaky gut syndrome and fibromyalgia—what is the connection? 1995. *Let's Live.* (April) POB 74908, Los Angeles, CA 90004. (Sidebar to the Leichtberg article referenced below.)

Lehmann, K A. 1994. Tramadol for the management of acute pain. Dept of Anaesthesiology, University of Cologne, Germany 71 REFS *Drugs* 47 Suppl 1:19-32. *MEDLINE 94298535.*

Leichtberg, Joshua J. Can diet and nutrition affect the mind? 1995. *Let's Live.* (April) POB 74908, Los Angeles, CA 90004.

Lewis, P. J. 1993. Electroacupuncture in fibromyalgia. *British Medical Journal* 306:393.

London, Wayne. 1994. *Principles of Health.* London Research, 139 Main Street, Brattleboro, VT 05301.

Lowe, John C. 1993. The master of myofascial therapy. ACA *Journal of Chiropractic.* (November)

Lue, F.A. 1994. Sleep and fibromyalgia. *Journal of Rheumatology* 2 (3).

Mann, John, 1994. *Murder, Magic and Medicine.* NY: Oxford University Press.

Marwick, Charles. 1995. Should physicians prescribe prayer for health? Spiritual aspects of well-being considered. *JAMA,* vol. 273 (20) (May 24-31).

Mason, J., S.L. Silverman and A. L. Weaver. 1991. Fibromyalgia Impact Assessment Form. *Arthritis Care Resident* 4:523.

McCaffery, Margo and Alexandra Beebe. 1989. *PAIN: Clinical Manual for Nursing Practice.* St. Louis, Baltimore, Philadelphia, Toronto: C.V. Mosby Co.

McCain, Glenn A. 1994. Treatment of the fibromyalgia syndrome. *Journal of Musculoskeletal Pain,* vol. 2(1).

———, David A. Bell, Brancois M. Mai and Paul D. Halladay. 1988. A controlled study of the effects of a supervised cardiovascular fitness training program on the manifestations of primary fibromyalgia. *Arthritis and Rheumatism,* vol. 31 (9) (September).

Mengshoel, A.M., O. Forre and H.B. Komnaesh. 1990. Muscle strength and aerobic capacity in primary fibromyalgia. *Clinical and Experimental Rheumatology* 8(5):475-479.

Moldofsky, H. 1989. Sleep and fibrositis syndrome. *Rheumatic Disease Clinics of North America* 15 (1).

———. 1989. Sleep-wake mechanisms in fibrositis. *Journal of Rheumatology* 16 (Supp 19).

Moore, Larry. 1993. Talking with your doctor. *Coping* (March/April).

Mufson, M. and Q.R. Regestein. 1993. The spectrum of fibromyalgia disorders. *Arthritis and Rheumatism* 36 (5).

Murray, Michael. 1994. *Natural Alternatives to Over-the-Counter and Prescription Drugs.* NY: William Morrow Co.

Myofacsial pain diagnosis and treatment. *Fibromyalgia Network Newsletter* (October 1995).

Neeck, G. and W. Riedel. 1992. Thyroid function in patients with fibromyalgia syndrome. *Journal of Rheumatology* 19 (7).

Nunnelley, Hamilton, Eva May, Eleanor Noss Whitney and Frances Sienkiewicz Sizer. 1988. *Nutrition: Concepts and Controversies.* St. Paul, MN: West Publishing Co.

Pascarelli, Emil and Deborah Quilter. 1994. *Repetitive Strain Injuries.* New York: John Wiley & Sons, Inc.

Pelligrino, Mark J. 1993. *Fibromyalgia: Managing the Pain.* Columbus, OH: Anadem Publishing. 3620 N. High St., Columbus, OH 43214 (800-633-0055).

———, G.W. Waylonis and A. Sommer. 1989(a). Familial occurrence of primary fibromyalgia. *Archives of Physical Medicine and Rehabilitation 1989* 70 (1).

———, D. Van Fossen and C. Gordon. 1989(b). Prevalence of mitral valve prolapse in primary fibromyalgia. *Archives of Physical Medicine* 70 (7).

Potter, J.W. 1995. Swimming upstream. *Fibromyalgia Network Newsletter* (April).

———. 1994. Filing for Social Security Disability. *Fibromyalgia Network Newsletter* (July).

Raloff, Janet. 1995. Drug of darkness. *Science News*, vol. 147 (May 13).

Reilly, Paul A. and Geoffrey O. Littlejohn. 1990. Fibrositis/Fibromyalgia syndrome: the key to the puzzle of chronic pain. *The Medical Journal of Australia,* vol. 152 (March 5).

Romano, T. J. 1993. Report. *Fibromyalgia Network Newsletter* (January).

———. 1991. Fibromyalgia in children: diagnosis and treatment. *West Virginia Medical Journal* 87 (3).

———. 1988. The fibromyalgia syndrome. It's the real thing. *Postgraduate Medicine* 83 (5).

————. 1988. Coexistence of irritable bowel syndrome and fibromyalgia. *West Virginia Medical Journal* 84 (2).

Rosenhall, U., G. Johansson, G. Omdahl. 1987. Eye motility dysfunction in chronic primary fibromyalgia with dysthesia. *Scandinavian Journal of Rehabilitation Medicine* 19 (4).

Russell, I.J. 1994. Biochemical abnormalities in fibromyalgia syndrome. *Journal of Musculoskeletal Pain* 2 (3).

————. 1990. Treatment of patients with fibromyalgia syndrome: considerations of the whys and wherefores. *Advances in Pain Research and Therapy* 17: 303-314.

————. 1989. Neurohormonal aspects of fibromyalgia syndrome. *Rheumatic Disease Clinics of North America* 15 (1).

Schafer, Karen Moore. 1995. Struggling to maintain balance: a study of women living with fibromyalgia. *Journal of Advanced Nursing* 21, 95-102.

Sedgewick, John. 1991. Pain. *SELF* (July).

Selye, Hans. 1975. *Hans Selye, The Stress of My Life*. NY: Van Nostrand-Reinhold.

Sietsema, K.E., D.M. Cooper and X. Caro. 1993. Oxygen uptake during exercise in patients with primary fibromyalgia syndrome. *Journal of Rheumatology* 20 (5).

Simms, R.W. and D.I. Goldenberg. 1988. Symptoms mimicking neurologic disorders in fibromyalgia syndrome. *Journal of Rheumatology* 15 (8).

Simons, David G. 1995. Myofascial pain syndrome: One term but two concepts; a new understanding. *Journal of Musculoskeletal Pain*, vol. 3 (1).

————. 1994. Understanding myofascial pain syndromes. *Journal of Musculoskeletal Pain* 2(1).

————. 1990. Familial fibromyalgia and/or myofascial pain syndrome? *Archives of Physical Medicine and Rehabilitation* 71 (3).

———— and Lois Statham Simons. 1989. Chronic myofascial pain syndromes. In *Handbook of Chronic Pain Management*. Edited by C.D. Tollison, J.R. Satterthwaite, J.W. Tollison and C.G. Trent. Baltimore, MD: Williams and Wilkins.

————. 1988(a). Myofascial pain syndromes: Where are we? Where are we going? *Archives of Physical Medicine and Rehabilitation* 69 (3).

————. 1988(b). Myofascial pain syndrome due to trigger points. In *Rehabilitation Medicine*. Edited by Joseph Goodgold. St. Louis, Baltimore, Philadelphia, Toronto: C.V. Mosby Co. (reprinted by Gebauer Company).

Smythe, H. 1992. Links between fibromyalgia and myofascial pain syndromes. *Journal of Rheumatology* 19 (6).

Sola, A.E. 1985. Trigger point therapy. In *Chemical Procedures in Emergency Medicine*. Edited by J. Roberts and J. Hedges. Philadelphia: W.B. Saunders.

Some jobs tend to exacerbate muscle problems in fibromyalgia. 1991. *Medical Post* (Canadian) 27 (43).

Stack, Michelle. 1994. Handling insurance claims. *Fibromyalgia Network Newsletter* (April).

St. Amand R. Paul. No date. *Hypoglycemia*. (Handout) 4560 Admiralty Way, Suite 355, Marina Del Rey, CA 90292.

———. March 1993. *The Use of Uricosuric Drugs in Fibromyalgia*. (Handout) 4560 Admiralty Way, Suite 355, Marina Del Rey, CA 90292.

Starlanyl, Devin J. 1995. Comment on Granges and Littlejohn's article "Prevalence of myofascial pain syndrome in fibromyalgia and regional pain syndrome: A comparative study." *Journal of Musculoskeletal Pain*, vol. 3 (1).

———. 1994. Comment on article by Hong, Chen, Pon and Yu, "Immediate effects of various physical medicine modalities on pain threshold of an active myofascial trigger point." *Journal of Musculoskeletal Pain* 2 (2).

Steinhart, Melvin. 1992. Irritable bowel syndrome: How to relieve symptoms enough to improve daily function. *Postgraduate Medicine* 91 (6).

Stormorken, H. and F. Brosstad. 1992. Fibromyalgia: family clustering and sensory urgency with early onset indicate genetic predisposition and thus a "true" disease. *Scandinavian Journal of Rheumatology* 21 (4).

Thorsen, Kristin. *Fibromyalgia Network Newsletter*. Fibromyalgia Network, POB 31750, Tucson, AZ 85751-1750.

Travell, Janet G. 1968. *Office Hours Day and Night*. NY: World Publishing Co.

Travell, Janet G. and David G. Simons. 1992. *Myofascial Pain and Dysfunction: The Trigger Point Manual Volume II: The Lower Body*. Baltimore, MD: Williams and Wilkins. (800-638-0672).

——— and David G. Simons. 1983. *Myofascial Pain and Dysfunction: The Trigger Point Manual Volume I: The Upper Body*. Baltimore, MD: Williams and Wilkins (revision in-process) (800-638-0672).

Travis, John. 1995. Probing the cause of after-baby blues. *Science News*. vol. 148 (July).

Triadfiloupolis, G., R.W. Simms and D.I. Goldenberg. 1991. Bowel dysfunction in fibromyalgia syndrome. *Digestive Diseases and Science* 36 (1).

Upledger, John E. *CranioSacral Therapy I*. 1983. Upledger Institute, 11211 Prosperity Farms Road, Palm Beach Gardens, FL 33401-4449.

van Why, Richard. 1994. *Fibromyalgia Syndrome and Massage Therapy: Issues and Opportunities.* Self-published: Richard P. van Why, 123 East 8th Street, Frederick, MD 21701.

———. 1992. Fibromyalgia and chronic fatigue: My experience and a proposal for research. *Massage Therapy Journal* (Summer).

Vecchiet, L., P. de Bigontina, M.A. Giamberardino and L. Dragani. (To be published in the *Journal of Muscloskeletal Pain.*). Fibromyalgia and myofascial pain syndrome: Comparative sensory evaluation of parietal tissues in painful and non-painful areas. Inst. of Medical Pathophysiol. Univ. of Chieti, Chieti, Italy, presented at 7th World Congress on Pain.

Wallace, D.J. 1990. Genitourinary manifestations of fibrositis: and increased association with female urethral syndrome. *Journal of Rheumatology* 17 (2).

Wilke, W. 1995. Treatment of "resistant" fibromyalgia. *Rheumatic Disease Clinic of North America* 21 (1).

Wolfe, Frederick. 1993. Disability and the dimensions of distress in fibromyalgia. *Journal of Musculoskeletal Pain* 1(2).

———, H.A. Smithe, et al. 1990. The American College of Rheumatology criteria for the classification of fibromyalgia. *Arthritis and Rheumatism* 33 (2); 160-72.

———. 1989. Fibromyalgia: the clinical syndrome. *Rheumatism Disease Clinics of North America* (February).

Wurtman, Richard J. and Judith J. Wurtman. 1989. Carbohydrates and depression. *Scientific American,* vol. 260 (January).

Xenakis, Alan. 1993. *Why Doesn't My Funny Bone Make Me Laugh?* NY: Random House.

Yunus, Muhammad B. 1992. Towards a Model of pathophysiology of fibromyalgia: Aberrant central pain mechanisms with peripheral modulation. *The Journal of Rheumatology* 19:6.

Zhang, Mingwu and Sun Xingyuan. 1985 *Chinese Qi Gong Therapy.* Translated by Yang Entang and Yao Xiuqing. Jinan, China: Shadong Science and Technology Press.

Zimmermann, Manfred. 1991. Pathophysiological mechanisms of fibromyalgia. *The Clinical Journal of Pain* 7 (Suppl. 1) S8-S15. NY: Raven Press, LTD.

Subject Index

A

abuse
avoidance issues, 318; counseling for, 317–318; making changes, 317; overcoming, 316, 317; as triggering event for FMS/MPS Complex, 315

Achilles tendon, 98

achiness, as symptom, 68

ACTH hormone, 108

acupressure
Jin Shin Do technique, 248; for morning sickness during pregnancy, 135

acupuncture
and dermographia, 72; and endorphins, 268; and shiatsu, 268; theory of, 268

adrenal glands, defined, 140

adrenaline, 70, 73, 140

affirmations
in cognitive therapy, 187, 188; to raise self-esteem, 150, 151

AIDS
and HIV as coexisting condition, 43; and T-cell production, 216; thymus extraction for, 216

Alexander Technique (massage therapy), 247, 260, 261

allergies
and flare, 127; and FMS/MPS Complex, 69; to food, 229, 230, 231; and post-nasal drip, 69; prescription drugs for, 203, 204

alpha-delta sleep anomaly. *See also* sleep disturbances
defined, 37, 114, 115; and FMS fatigue, 43; psychoactive drugs for, 203

American College of Rheumatology, 9, 14, 141

American Medical Association, 8, 14

Americans With Disabilities Act of 1992, 326

antidepressant. *See also* medications
exercise as, 182

antifungal. *See* medications (general)

antihistamine. *See* medications (general)

apnea. *See* obstructive sleep apnea

appendicitis-like pain, 92, 124

asymmetry as perpetuating factor, 23, 56, 260

B

balance problems
in cerebral palsy, 43; and fibrofog, 172; and perception problems, 27; due to SCM TrPs, 27; as symptom of MPS, 103

belch button. *See* trigger points (specific), external oblique

biofeedback, 269

blackfly bites, 68

blood/brain barrier, defined, 37

blood circulation. *See* circulation

blood pressure, fluctuating, 79

body mechanics, defined, 260

bodywork. *See also* bodyworkers; healing therapies; massage therapy; self-administered bodywork
> acupuncture, 268, 269; chiropractic methods, 245, 246; defined, 237; headaches caused by, 19; and heart health, 238; inappropriate therapies, 244; massage therapies, 246–250; nausea caused by, 19; oxygen need, 238, 239; and pain, 238; spray and stretch, 249; therapeutic value of pleasurable touch sensations, 238

bodyworkers. *See also* healing therapies; massage therapy
> chiropractors, 244, 245; defined, 243; massage therapists, 246–250; and microstim use, 252; and neuromuscular electronic stimulator use, 252; pulsed ultrasound with electrical stimulation therapy, treatment regimen for, 251

Bowen therapy, 247, 248

brain
> decreased blood flow to, 173; injury to sensory moderating system, 30

breathing. *See also* self-administered bodywork
> and "fight or flight" response, 259; mouth, 259, 260; paradoxical, 259

bruxism, 74, 80, 118

buckling knee
> defined, 100; in pregnancy, 134; walking exercise for, 257

C

calcification, defined, 17, 18

capillaries, compressed, 20, 72

carbohydrate craving
> and electrolytic balance, 233; as FMS symptom, 70; and hypoglycemia, 234, 235; prescription drug for, 204; and SAD, 181

carbohydrate metabolism
> and insulin production, 228, 233; and reactive hypoglycemia, 233–235

carpal-tunnel syndrome, as coexisting condition, 42, 43

cerebral cortex, number of nerve cells in, 113

cerebral palsy, as coexisting condition, 43

cervical pillows, 294

Chi gung. *See* Chi kung

Chi kung, 249, 263, 275

children
> communication with, 353, 354; condition from child's point of view, 351, 352; genetic predisposition, 351; and growing pains, 68, 352; need for diagnosis, 352; and pain issue, 352, 353; school issues, 352

chiropractors, 144, 244, 245, 246. *See also* spine manipulation

chronic dry cough, as symptom of FMS/MPs Complex, 78

chronic fatigue
> caused by chronic pain, 109; as coexisting condition, 43; and family issues, 293, 294; thymus extract for, 216; as sign of depression, 180

chronic fatigue syndrome, 43

chronic illness and family issues, 286, 287, 288

chronic MPS

as cause of FMS, 35; as cause of TrPs, 36; defined, 30; diagnosis of, 32, 33; and hypoglycemia, 233, 234

chronic pain. *See also* pain
> and children's issues, 353; and depression, 43, 108, 141, 149, 179; and dreams, 119; and drug dependency, 111; drugs to control, 144; and endorphins, 107–108; as fatigue cause, 109; and FMS/MPS Complex patients' attitudes, 109, 110, 111, 141, 142; and journal keeping, 167; and low self-esteem, 141, 143, 148; medication for, 361; mild narcotics for, 111, 202, 203; misconceptions about, 32; negative influences, minimizing, 155, 156, 158; psychoactive drugs for, 203; and sleep deprivation, 115, 116, 117; tricyclic antidepressants for, 108; undertreatment, results of, 203

circulation
> and bodywork, 239; and heat therapy, 261; impaired by prolonged sitting, 58; meditation effects on, 141; and myofascia, 20; and soleus muscle, 100

clinician bias. *See* doctors

clothing. *See also* shoes
> choosing colors of, 162; socks, elastic, as perpetuating factor, 58, 59; tricks to make life easier, 300, 301; for workplace, 323

coexisting conditions. *See also* specific name of condition
> carpal-tunnel syndrome, 42; cerebral palsy 43; chronic fatigue syndrome, 43; depression, 43; HIV, 43; hypoglycemia, 44; hypermobility syndrome, 44; lupus, 44; mitral valve prolapse, 44, 45; multiple chemical sensitivity, 45; multiple sclerosis, 45; osteoarthritis, 24, 45; Parkinson's Disease, 45; post- polio syndrome, 45, 46; Raynaud's Phenomenon, 46; rheumatoid arthritis, 46; temporomandibular joint syndrome, 46; yeast infections, 46, 47

cognitive therapy
> affirmations for, 187, 188; and depression, 184, 185, 186; identifying destructive patterns, 184, 185, 186; and irrational beliefs, 186, 187

collagen fibers, 19, 37. *See also* muscle fibers

color, 161, 162

computer use, as perpetuating factor, 57

connective tissue
> composition of, 19; mitral valve as, 91; overgrown as symptom of FMS/MPS Complex, 71

constipation, 54, 55, 121, 124, 125

contractures
> defined, 21; and immobility, 141

Copenhagen Declaration, 9, 10

coping behavior
> color therapy as, 161, 162; daily, 157; enjoyable activities, 159, 160; for fibrofog, 173–175; for handling negative events, 155, 156, 157; journal keeping as, 162; laughter as, 160; lifestyle changes, 158, 159; for mornings, 156, 157; music for, 162; prayer as, 198; proactive, 158; water therapy as, 161; for yeast infections, 176, 177

craniosacral release, massage therapy, 248

cutaneous TrPs

and ear problems, 81; and eye problems, 81; and migraine, 83; prescription drugs for, 204

D

delta-level sleep, 37, 69

dependence on medication, 111

depression

and chronic pain states, 108, 109, 110; as coexisting condition with FMS/MPS Complex, 43; cognitive therapies for, 184, 185, 186; counseling for, 180; defined, 179; exercise for, 182; and flare, 128; and living quarters, 183; and low self-esteem, 149; and pain, 13; as perpetuating factor, 50, 51; and psychological aspects of chronic pain, 141; and SAD, 181; signs and symptoms of, 43, 180; and sleep, 183; support groups for, 311; tricyclic antidepressants for, 109

dermographia, 72

destructive thinking patterns, 184, 185

diagnosis

of FMS, 8–12; of FMS/MPS Complex, 35; of MPS, 32

Diagnostic and Statistical Manual of Mental Disorders, 180

diet. *See also* food allergies and sensitivities; nutrition

for Irritable Bowel Syndrome, 123, 124; for yeast infections, 177

disability

appeals process, 337, 338; claim filing process, 336; agency definition of, 334; Fibromyalgia Residual Functional Questionnaire for determining, 340–344; information worksheet for agency evaluation, 338–339; Medicare and food stamps, 333; percentage of unemployed FMS patients, 333; Personal Injury Protection, 333; "Quality of Life" test scale for, 335; records, need for accuracy, 334, 335, 337; short-term benefits, 333; Social Security Administration benefits, 333, 334; Social Security Administration investigation of claim, 337; Social Security Disability benefits, 333

dizziness

as symptom of flare, 128; as symptom of FMS, 75; as symptom of FMS/MPS Complex, 84

doctors. *See also* primary care physician

attitudes toward chronic pain, 109, 110, 111, 141; attitudes toward FMS, 8, 10, 14, 141, 179, 335, 360, 361, 362; checklist for initial visit, 358; and chiropractors, 244; and disability diagnoses, 334, 337; "Good Doctor checklist," 357; and insurance companies, 337; worksheet for interviewing, 356, 357

dopamine depletion

and Parkinson's Disease, 45; and SAD 181

double-jointed joints. *See* hypermobility

dreams

in pregnancy, 134; and REM sleep, 119

drug addiction

defined, 111; incidence of, 202, 361

drugs. *See* medications (general); medications (specific); nonprescription medications

E

ear problems

and cutaneous TrPs, 81; and masseter TrPs, 78; and SCM TrPs, 27, 77

education and training

Office of Disability Support Services, 330; Office of Vocational Rehabilitation and Employment and Training, 330; student loans, 330, 331

electrolytes

and dairy craving, 229; function of, 52, 228, 229, 238; and ionized salt, 228; and leg cramps, 98; and nerve function, 75; and reactive hypoglycemia, 234; and refined salt, 229

electromagnetic sensitivity

and craniosacral release therapy, 248; defined, 267; and serotonin deficiencies, 267, 268; as symptom of FMS/MPS Complex, 75

electronic devices, 250

endorphins

and acupuncture, 268; decrease over time, 202; defined, 107; and "fight or flight" response, 108; and nerve cell receptors, 108

esophageal reflux

and chronic dry cough, 78; defined, 86; and hiatal hernia, 86; and pregnancy, 135; prescription drug for, 206; process of, 86; treatments for, 86, 87

exercise for depression, 182, 183

extrinsic eye muscles and TrPs, 81

eye problems

asymmetry, 56; blurred vision, 8, 81; double vision, 81; floaters, 81, 82; internal eye muscle TrPs, 75; redness or tearing, 79; and SCM TrPs, 27, 76, 81; watering, 12

F

fallen arches, 60

family clusters, 104, 118, 220. *See also* genetic predisposition

family issues. *See also* home life

and chronic fatigue, 293, 294, 295, 296; courtesy, need for, 287; dynamics of, 285, 286, 287, 288; honesty, need for, 289; impotence, 292; journal keeping for, 288; list of rights, 292, 293; partner participation, 289, 290; and premenstrual syndrome, 291; receiving help, 287; relinquishment exercise, 290, 291; sexuality, 291, 292; verbalizing needs, 288

fasciculation

defined, 118, 128; and flare, 128

fatigue. *See also* chronic fatigue

and disrupted HPA axis, 69, 70; and disrupted neurotransmitters, 70; family issues with, 293, 294, 295, 296; as symptom of FMS, 69, 70

feet. *See also* foot slap

deformations of, 59; fallen arches, 60; intrinsic foot muscle TrPs, 102; Morton's foot, 60, 61; Morton's neuroma, 62; pain, 102; wedge-shaped FMS/MPS foot, 103

Feldenkreis therapy, 248

fibroblast, 36, 37
fibrofog
cognitive difficulties of, 172, 173; coping behaviors for, 173–175; defined, 171; and driving, 174; durable power of attorney, need for, 131; and flare, 129, 130, 131; and forgetfulness, 285, 286; and frustration, 172; and hospital facilities, 131; and journal keeping, 173; morning coping behaviors, 156; and sensory input, 175; symptoms of, 171, 172; and yeast problems, 47, 128, 173, 175, 176–177

fibromite
defined, 8; and insulin, 124

Fibromyalgia Syndrome. *See also* FMS/MPS Complex; FMS patients; symptoms of FMS
adrenal glands, role in, 73; and alpha-delta sleep anomaly, 13, 36, 43; as biochemical disorder, 31; blood test for, 9; defined, 9; diagnosis of, 8–9; differences with myofascial pain syndrome, 31–32; effect on grip, 13; Fibromyalgia Residual Functional Questionnaire for disability determination, 340–344; FMS Personality, myth of, 177, 178; genetic factor in, 12; and hypoglycemia, 44; inappropriate therapies for, 244; incidence in males, 14; laboratory tests for, lack of, 9; misdiagnosis of, 8; and mucus, 220; and multiple chemical sensitivities, 45; and multiple sclerosis, 45; myths about, 14; and neurotransmitter dysregulation, 13, 31; not inflammatory condition, 203; not progressive illness, 26, 30; official definition of, 9–10; physiological effects of trauma in, 315; and reactive hypoglycemia, 233–235; remission during pregnancy, 133; remission of, 12, 14, 133, 146, 147, 222, 223; sensitivity amplification aspect of, 13, 35, 37; social consequences of, 286, 287; temperature changes from exercise, 255; thermal fluctuation in, 12; traumatic, 12, 30, 32; triggering events of, 13-14; and uric acid, 220

"fight or flight" response
and breathing, 259; description of, 13; effect on musculature, 24; and endorphins, 108; and nervous system, 140; sensitivity amplification, 13; stress effect on, 17

fingernail ridges, 12, 71
flare
cognitive function changes, 129; defined, 127; and fibrofog, 171; getting through, 131, 132; medication use, 211; preparation for, 130, 131; supporters for, 308; symptoms of, 128–129; and yeasts, 128

FMily, defined, 8

FMS. *See* Fibromyalgia Syndrome

FMS/MPS Complex. *See also* symptoms of FMS/MPS Complex
abuse, as triggering event, 315; appropriate medications for, 201, 202, 203; as chronic pain condition, 35; coexisting conditions with, 42–47; and "deconditioning" myth of, 37; diagnosis of, 35; educational resources for, 145; fluid exchange disruption in, 36; and growth hormone, 37; and hypometabolic state, 191; as "invisible" illness, 156; medications during

pregnancy, 133; misdiagnosed as Reflex Sympathetic Dystrophy Condition, 46; myofascia function, disruptions in, 37; perpetuating factors in, 35; seratonin levels in, 37; skin tests not reliable for diagnosis, 69; trigger point injections for, 38, 39, 205; trigger points, role of, 23,35

FMS/MPS Complex patients. *See also* family issues
abuse, history of, 315, 316; attitudes toward chronic pain, 109, 110, 111; bending problems of, 260; brain tissue changes in, 139; coping behaviors of, 156–161; as crime victim, 316; electromagnetic sensitivity of, 267; and exercise, 182; Fibromyalgia Residual Functional Questionnaire for disability determination, 340–344; foot and callus pattern in, 60, 61; head roll exercises, danger of, 197; hoarding pain medication, 202; information worksheet for disability evaluation, 338–339; prayer for, 198; responses to drugs, 204; and restricted physical activity, 141; and short-term memory loss, 119; sleep patterns of, 116, 117; spine manipulation of, 245; stages of acceptance by, 140, 141; water therapy for, 161

FMS/MPS foot, 60, 61, 102. *See also* Morton's foot; shoes

FMS patients. *See also* family issues
abuse, history of, 315; attitudes of families and friends toward, 14, 15; bending problems of, 260; child's point of view, 351, 352; disability, determining, 340–344; electromagnetic sensitivity of, 75, 267; electronic stimulation for TrPs, 244; employment problems of, 12, 333; gender distribution of, 31; percent correctly diagnosed, 361; and puberty, 353; "quality of life" test scale, results of, 335; self-esteem of, 14, 15; seratonin, levels of, 37; support groups and networks for, 145, 146; and smoking, 146; treatment contra-indicated for MPS, 211

focusing exercise, 271, 272

food allergies and sensitivities, 229, 230. *See also* nutrition

foot slap, 98, 258

frozen shoulder, 42, 87

frustration, as symptom, 72

furniture
cervical pillows, 119, 294; chairs, 295; mattresses, 294; for offices, 324; as perpetuating factor, 57; rocking chair exercise, 256, 257; Somma bed, 119, 294; waterbeds, 119, 294

G

galvanic muscle stimulation, 224, 250, 251, 252

genetic predisposition, 12, 68, 104, 351

glial cell, 173, 174, 238

grip. *See* hand grip

ground substance
behavior of, 18, 37; and "fight or flight" response, 20; function of, 238, and glial cells, 238

growing pains. *See* genetic predisposition

growth hormone, 37

guaifenesin therapy

and blackfly toxin, 68; for cervical secretions, 224; and commercial expectorants, 219, 220; discovery of, 219, 220; dosages, 222; electrical bodywork devices, warning for, 250; and esophageal reflux, 86; guidelines for taking, 223, 224; and mucus secretions, 220, 222; remission of symptoms, 222–223; and reversal of FMS symptoms, 225 and salicyclates, 221, 224; side effects of, 224; treatment process, 220; treatment symptoms, 222; and uric acid, 220

guided imagery (A Walk in the Forest), 193–196

H

hair loss, 70, 71, 222

hamstring pain, 102, 103

hand grip
in children, 92, 354; and flare, 128; FMS effect on, 13; TrPs effect on, 25, 92, 84, 86, 87, 88, 89; weakness of, 13, 25

headache, 82, 83, 239. *See also* migraine

healing therapies
ayurveda, 269; biofeedback, 269; Chinese, 275; focusing, 270, 271; Hawaiian, 275, 276; hypnotherapy, 272; Japanese, 274; Native American, 274, 275; pet therapy, 272, 273, 274; polarity therapy, 270; reflexology, 270; subliminal tapes, 270

health care team
attitude of, 143, 144; and flare, preparing for, 131; and FMS support groups, 145, 146; and primary care physician choices, 144; and response to pain, 202

heart health and bodywork, 239

heartburn. *See* esophageal reflux

heat therapy, 25, 57, 72

hiatal hernia. *See* esophageal reflux

histamine, 35, 36, 53, 69, 72, 127

HIV, 43, 176

home life. *See also* family issues
bed-making, 297; clothing issues, 300, 301; coping with visitors, 295; educate guests, 296, 298; "house rules list," 295; household chores, 297, 301, 302; kitchen chores, 302, 303; physical comfort, 300; rules for surviving, 297, 298; setting limits, 298; tricks to make life easier, 299–303

HPA-axis
adrenal glands, function of, 140; disruption as cause of fatigue, 69, 70; and estrogen loss, 135; FMS disruption of, 108; hypothalamus, function of, 140; pituitary gland, function of, 140; and sympathetic nervous system, regulation of, 139

hypermobility
as coexisting condition, 44; as perpetuating factor, 56, 57; and rebound contraction danger, 256; and TrPs, 70

hyperpronation. *See* feet, pain

hypnogogic sleep stage, 114, 192

hypnopompic sleep stage, 114

hypnosis, 272

hypoglycemia
as coexisting condition, 44; defined, 44; and diabetes, 234; and family clusters, 234; "fasting," defined, 233; guaifenesin for, 234; and Irritable Bowel Syndrome, 124; reactive, as perpetuating factor, 52, 53, 221 and the "shakes," 73; symptoms of, 53

hypometabolic state, 191

hypometabolism
BT2 panel test for, 53; as coexisting condition, 44; defined, 44; as perpetuating factor, 52

hypothalamus, 69, 140. *See also* HPA-axis

I

ice
for nerve entrapment treatment, 25, 261; for guaifenesin-induced headache, 222; in spray and stretch massage, 249

immune (inflammatory) cascade, 232, 234

immune system
dysfunction of, 73; and pregnancy problems, 135; thymus gland, role in, 216; and yeast infections, 177

impotence, 93, 95, 292

infections, 52, 53, 73

insomnia. *See also* sleep disturbances
and alpha-delta sleep anomaly, 115; drugs for, 203, 204, 205, 206; forms of, 115–116; nicotine, role in, 116; and stress, 115; as depression symptom, 180, 183

insulin, 228, 233

intestinal cramps, 91, 92

irritable bladder, 92, 94,

Irritable Bowel Syndrome
aggravating factors in, 122, 123; and TrPs, 124, 125; causes of, 122; ileocaecal valve, role in, 124, 125; medications for, 123, 124; peppermint oil for, 124, 216; as symptom of FMS/MPS Complex, 92, 94; symptoms of, 121

"irritable everything syndrome." *See* sensitivity amplification syndrome

itchiness, 71, 80, 203

J

jaw pain, 98. *See also* Temporomandibular Joint Syndrome

journal keeping
as coping behavior, 162; and family dynamics, 288; and fibrofog, 173; getting started, 169–170; goals for, 168; to identify fears, 184; for medication records, 164, 211; and negative emotions, 164; and pain, 67; to prevent flare, 129; requirements for, 165–166; rereading, 164; rules for, absence of, 166; and self-esteem, 163; for self-help with Irritable Bowel Syndrome, 123; and sleep disturbances, 119; suggestions for, 167–168; and TrPs, 166

K

knee problems. *See* buckling knee

L

latent TrPs
  activated by bodywork, 239; defined, 25; and tennis- ball acupressure, 55
laughter, 160, 161, 175, 322
Leaky Gut Syndrome
  causes of, 123; food and chemical intolerance in, 123; and inflammatory cascade, 232; and seratonin formation, 233; small intestine functioning, 232, 233; vitamins for, 215, 231
leg cramps, 98, 118
ligaments, 19
light therapy. *See* Seasonal Affective Disorder (SAD)
low-back pain, 26, 92, 93, 95, 136
lupus, 9, 41, 44, 182
lymph, 36

M

massage therapy
  Alexander Technique, 247, 260, 261; Bowen therapy, 247, 248; craniosacral release, 248; Feldenkreis method, 248, 361; Jin Shin Do acupressure, 248; proprioceptor neuromuscular facilitation, 249; and rebound contraction, 247; Reiki, 249; spray and stretch, 249; strain-counterstrain, 250; and toxic wastes, 246, 247
mast cells, 36, 37
medications (general). *See also* medications (specific); nonprescription medications
  addiction and dependency, 111, 202, 361; analgesics, 203, 205, 206; anti-inflammatory, 206; antidepressants, 204, 205, 206; antifungal, 204; antihistamines, 203, 204, 205, 206; and breast milk, 136; for chronic pain, 109–111, 202, 203, 361; and dreams, 119; for FMS/MPS Complex conditions, 203–206; for gout, 220; guaifenesin therapy, 219–225; guidelines for use, 209–211; and jet lag changes, 348; and lactose intolerance, 203; NSAIDs. 123; and nerve receptor sites, 109; and neurotransmitters, 108; and pregnancy, 133; psychoactive, 203; record keeping, 164, 213–214; side effects, 212, 213; for sleep disturbances, 204, 205, 206; specific serotonin re-uptake inhibitors (SSRIs) 108, 119, 205, 206, 207; unusual reactions to, 72, 209
medications (specific). *See also* medications (general)
  Ambien, 203; Atarax, 203; Benadryl, 203, 204; BuSpar, 204; Desyrel, 204; Diflucan, 47, 177, 204; Effexor, 204; Elavil, 74, 204; EMLA 204; Flexeril, 204; Fluori- Methane, 204; Guaifenesin, 219–225; Hismanal, 204; Imitrex, 204, 205; Inderal, 205; Klonopin, 74, 205; Librax, 205; Lidocain, 116; Pamelor, 205; Paxil, 205; Potaba, 20, 205; Procain, 38, 205; Prozac, 205, 206;
  Quotane, 206; Relafen, 206: Sinequan, 206; Soma, 206; Tagamet, 206; Ultram, 206; Wellbutrin, 207; Xanax, 207; Zoloft, 207
meditation
  on berry picking, 196; connection, 198; defined, 191, 192; on a fence, 196, 197; focusing, 271; guided imagery, 193–196; and hypometabolic state, 191; procedure for, 192–193; and sensory overload, 191; and sleep disturbances, 119; types of, 193–196; walking, 193, 194
melatonin
  and depression, 215; and light sensitivity, 74; and SAD, 215, 216; and sleep, 120, 215, 216
menstrual problems, 93
meralgia paresthetica, 103
Merkel's discs, 71
metabolic waste
  and bodywork, 239; and GMS/ultrasound treatment, 252; guaifenesin therapy for, 221, 222, 223, 224; and Leaky Gut Syndrome, 232; in myofascia, 20; and TrPs, 24, 37, 52
microstim, defined, 252
migraine
  as FMS symptom, 83; prescription drugs for, 204, 205
mindfulness. *See also* meditation
  defined, 197; distraction, value of, 199; focusing exercise for, 197
mitral valve prolapse, 44, 45, 91, 239
molds, 70, 125
Morton's foot, **60, 61**, 96, 102
Morton's neuroma, 62, 102
MPS. *See* Myofascial Pain Syndrome
MPS patients
  gender distribution in, 31; misdiagnosed as multiple sclerosis, 45; misdiagnosed as osteoarthritis, 45
mucus secretions, 79, 220, 221, 222
multiple chemical sensitivities, 45, 69,123
multiple sclerosis, 45
  action of, 20; contractures of, 21; electrical loading of, 118; of inner eye, **81**; "jumpy," 74; and neurotransmitters, 13; and oxygen supply, 253; rebound contractures of, 240; stretching, 255, 256; sustained contraction, effect on, 36; and wastes, 20, 24
muscle fibers, 18, 19
muscles. *See* metabolic waste; myofascia; trigger points (specific);
muscle twitches. *See* fasciculation
musculoskeletal imbalance, 24
music, as stress reducer, 162
myelin, 45, 238
myofascia. *See also* metabolic waste
  adhesions and scar tissue, 19, 20; and circulation, 20; contractures of 21; defined, 17; as elastic framework, for muscles, 238; functions of, 37; and ground substance, 18; and ligaments, 19; and mitral valve prolapse, 239; and nerves, 20,

21; splint formation, 36, 118; structure of, 18, 19; and TrPs, 19; and wastes, 20, 24, 221

Myofascial Pain Syndrome. *See also* chronic MPS; FMS/MPS Complex; MPS patients; symptoms of MPS; trigger points (general)

    diagnosis of 32, 33; difference between FMS and, 31–32; FMS as perpetuating factor, 33; motor coordination problems as symptom of, 76; as neuromuscular condition, 30; not inflammatory condition, 203; not progressive illness, 26, 30; physical therapies for, 244; specific pain of, 31; trigger points as cause of, 26, 29; water temperature requirement, 254

N

narcotics, for nonmalignant chronic pain, 202, 203, 361. *See also* drug addiction

nausea, 92, 135, 239

neck congestion, 30–31, 91, 245

negative emotions

    cognitive therapy for, 184; distractions for, 199; identifying fears and, 184; journal keeping and, 164; minimizing, 155, 156, 158

nerve cells, number of, 113

nerve conduction, loss of, 21, 75, 116

nerve entrapment

    chiropractic medicine for, 245; defined, 25; of femoral cutaneous nerve, 103; heat therapy for, 261; ice therapy for, 261; and impotence, 292; and Morton's neuroma, 62; in neck, 91; pudendal, 93, 95; and sleep; problems, 116; and writing, 85

nerve function, 75

nerve receptors

    and endorphins, 108; "fight or flight" response, 13, 20; and neurotransmitters, 108; and sensitivity amplification, 13

nervous system

    communications in, 238; dorsal column in, 238; and glial cells, 174, 238; parasympathetic, defined, 139; prescription drugs for calming, 206; and spinal cord, 128; spinalthalamic sensations, 238; and stress, 140; sympathetic, defined, 139

neuroma, defined, 62

neurons, function of, 238 .

neuropraxia. *See* nerve conduction

neurotransmitters. *See also* growth hormone; histamine: melatonin; seratonin

    calcification effects on, 18; decreased blood flow to brain effects on, 173; defined, 13, 17; electromagnetic sensitivity and, 75; and HPA-axis, 140; and medications, 108; in muscle communication, 13; and nicotine, 116; and noise, 326; and numbness and tingling, 75; and oxygen depletion, 146; and psychoactive drugs, 203; receptor sites of, 108, 109; and sleep disturbances, 116; and substance P, 68, 69; and systemic dysregulation, 31

nonprescription medications

Calme Forte, 216; chromium picolinate, 215; coenzyme Q10, 215; L-threonine, 216; melatonin, 215; peppermint oil, 216; Phaxyme, 217; raw thymus, 216; salt water, 217; value of, 215; vitamin C, 215

NSAIDs, 203, 233

numbness and tingling, 25, 75, 103

nutrition. *See also* food allergies and sensitivities

    carbohydrate, fat, and protein ratios, 229, 230; diet for reactive hypoglycemia, 234; eating wisely, 231, 232; and electrolytes, 228, 229; excess carbohydrate consumption, symptoms of, 228; types of nutrients, 227

O

obstructive sleep apnea, 71, 117

orthotics, 102. *See also* shoes

osteoarthritis, as coexisting condition, 45

P

pain. *See also* chronic pain

    and blood pressure, 107; and bodywork, 238; as chief symptom of FMS, 9; children's perceptions of, 352,353; and depression, 10, 13; difference between FMS and MPS, 31–32; heat therapy for, 261; ice therapy for, 25, 242, 249, 261; and immune system suppression, 107; medications for, 202, 203; menstrual, 353; of phantom limb, 100; psychogenic, 202; quitting smoking, effect on, 50; and sensitivity amplification, 13; and sexual intercourse, 291, 292; spasticity, 21; terms used to describe, 112; time lag between stimulus and sensation, 238; tolerance for, 202; TrP pain compared to tender point, 26

Parkinson's Disease, as coexisting condition, 45

past issues

    avoidance of, 318, 319; counseling for, 317; as crime victim, 316; examination of, 315, 316; and natural disasters, 316; and poverty, 317; validation, 318; and war, 317

peer counseling, 151, 312, 313

peristalsis, 122

perpetuating factors

    air pollution, 50; allergies, 53; anemia, 53; behavioral factors in, 49–52; biochemical factors in, 52–56; body asymmetry, 23, 56; cancer, 54; chronic sleep deprivation, 50, 113; computer or typewriter use, 57; constipation, 55; Crohn's Disease, 54; defined, 49; depression/anxiety as, 50, 51; electrolytic balance, 52; "good sport syndrome," 50; fallen arches, 60; FMS for MPS, 33, 36; FMS/MPS foot, 60; foot deformities, 103; furniture, 25, 57; hemorrhoids, 56; ill-fitting shoes, 58; immobility, 57, 58; infections, 52, 53; intrinsic foot TrPs, 59; mechanical factors in, 56–62; Morton's foot, **60, 61**; Morton's neuroma, 62; MPS for FMS, 36; muscle abuse, 51; nutritional inadequacies, 52; obesity, 50; poor posture, 51; prolonged sitting, 58; reactive hypoglycemia, 221; repetitive motion, 51; smoking, 50; tryptophan, lack of, 52; vitamin inadequacies, 52

pet therapy, 272–274

phantom limb pain, 100

pharmacists, 211, 212

physical comfort, suggestions for, 300

physical therapy. *See* bodywork

physician. *See* doctors; primary care physician

pituitary gland, defined, 140

post-nasal drip, 30–31, 69, 76, 77

post-polio muscular atrophy. *See* post-polio syndrome

post-polio syndrome, as coexisting condition, 45, 46

post-traumatic hyperirritability syndrome (PTHS), 30

prayer
healing power of, 198; of the Tibetan Physician, 243

pregnancy
gestation length, 135, 136; heat intolerance, 136; hormone fluctuations in, 135; increase of MPS symptoms during, 134; joint pain in, 134; low-back pain, 136; morning sickness, 135; nonprescription sleep aids for, 203; post-partum depression, 135; remission of FMS during, 133, 134; unsafe medications during, 133

premenstrual syndrome (PMS), 291, 353

primary care physician. *See also* doctors
bringing a "handler" to, 330; checklist for initial visit, 358, 359; choosing, 355–356; cost of, 363; and diagnostic issues, 361; "Good Doctor Checklist," 357; guidelines for good relationship with, 363; initial visit to, 358; letter to, 362; and medication issues, 361; negative attitudes of, 360, 361; records, obtaining, 359; repeat visits to, 359, 360; tape recording, 360; test results, copies of, 359; worksheet for interviewing, 356, 357

progressive illness, defined, 26

Q

Qi Gong. *See* Chi kung

R

Raynaud's phenomenon, 10, 44, 46, 74, 86

reactive hypoglycemia. *See also* hypoglycemia
and carbohydrate metabolism, 233–235; diets for, 227, 234; glucose tolerance test, not good for, 234

referred pain patterns of TrPs, similarity of, 23, 26

Reflex Sympathetic Dystrophy Syndrome, as coexisting condition, 46

relinquishment exercise for family and friends, 290

remission of FMS
actions to take during, 146, 147; with guaifenesin therapy, 222, 223; during pregnancy, 133

repetitive motions
and eyes, 52; as perpetuating factor, 51; and work, 322

repetitive strain injury, 255, 256

Restless Leg Syndrome, 103, 118, 135, 216

rheumatoid arthritis, 12, 41, 46, 141, 142

ropy bands. *See* trigger points (general)

S

sacroiliac joint dysfunction, 62, 134

salicylates, 221, 224

salt, 228, 229

satellite TrPs, 25, 29, 30, 31

scar tissue, 19, 20, 71, 206. *See also* myofascia

sciatica, 95, 96, 134

Seasonal Affective Disorder (SAD)
and depression, 181; melatonin for, 215, 216; as symptom of FMS, 74; therapies for, 181, 182

secondary TrPs, 25, 29, 30, 31

self-administered bodywork
breathing exercises, 259, 260; callanetics, 258; contract for bodywork routine, 262, 263; doorway exercise, 252; guidelines for walking, 257, 258; heat therapy, 261; hypermobility, warning, 256; ice therapy, 261; limits for, 253; "Native American Lope," 257; posture and body mechanics, 260; Qi Gong, 263; repetitive motion, danger of, 255; rocking-chair exercise, 257; self-massage, 254; stretching, 255, 256, 258, 324, 345; Tai Chi Chuan, 263; tennis ball acupressure, 261, 262; water aerobics, 254; yoga, 263

self-advocacy
communication skills for, 281; guidelines for, 282, 283; know your rights, 280; letter writing as, 283, 284; persistence, necessity of, 282; and self-esteem, 279, 280; steps toward, 279, 280; and support, 281

self-empowerment. *See also* self-esteem
actions to take during remissions, 146, 147; choosing a primary care physician, 144; defined, 143; and depression, 180; goal setting, 146; and letter writing, 148; physical examination for, 144, 145; raising, 149–150; and smoking, 146; sources of, 148; support network for, 145, 146

self-esteem
abuse issues, 149, 319; affirmations for, 150; and chronic pain, 141, 142, 148; and journal keeping, 163; and negativity, 149, 150; raising, 149–153; and self-advocacy, 279, 280; and self-image, 151; sources of, 148, 149; subliminal tapes for, 153; techniques for improving, 151, 152

sensitivity amplification syndrome, 13

sensory overload, medication for, 206

seratonin
carbohydrate craving, 70; functions of, 108; and immune dysfunction, 73; and Irritable Bowel Syndrome, 122; and Leaky Gut Syndrome, 233; and migraines, 83; receptor sites for, 108; and SAD, 181; and sleep problems, 37, 118; and weather sensitivity, 267, 268

sexual intercourse, 93, 291, 292

shoes. *See also* clothing; feet; Morton's foot
    flexible for balance, 103; ill-fitting, as perpetuating factor, 58, 59; inserts for, 58, **61**; for walking exercise, 258

side effects, 212, 213

sinus infection, 31, 76, 118. *See also* post-nasal drip

skin
    blotches, 12, 69, 70, 71; hypersensitive, 20, 72, tests unreliable for FMS/MPS Complex, 69

sleep
    and bodywork, 239; and depression, 183; NREM sleep, 114; REM sleep, 114, 118, 119; and sex, 183; stages of, 114; and weight loss diets, 183

sleep deprivation, 115, 116. *See also* sleep disturbances

sleep disturbances
    apnea, 71, 117; bruxism, 118; cervical pillows for, 294; and chronic fatigue, 70, 294; in FMS, 13, 37; hypnic jerk, 118; insomnia, 114–116; melatonin for, 74; nocturnal cramps, 118; and obesity, 118; as perpetuating factor, 51; during pregnancy, 134, 135; Restless Leg Syndrome, 118; sinus problems, 118; sleep- inducing methods for, 119, 120; and TrPs, 113, 114, 116

sleep patterns in FMS/MPS Complex, 116, 117

small intestine, 232, 233

smoking, 50, 146

Social Security Administration (SSA), 333, 334, 335, 336, 337, 338. *See also* disability

Social Security Disability (SSD), 333. *See also* disability

Social Security Income (SSI), 333. *See also* disability

spasticity, 12, 21, 76

specific serotonin re-uptake inhibitor (SSRI), 108, 119, 205

SPECT scan, 173

spinal cord. *See* nervous system

spine manipulation, 245, 246

stress
    as cause of TrPs, 24, 140; and chronic pain, 109; and Irritable Bowel Syndrome, 122; music to relieve, 162; and self-esteem, 149; and sex, 291; and sleep, 115; as triggering event for FMS, 116

subliminal tapes, 153, 270

substance P, 68, 69

suicide, prevention of, 311

supporters
    avoiding burnout, 309; coworkers as, 307; finding, 306, 307; and flare, 308; meetings for, 309; working with, 307, 308

support groups
    and active listening, 306; and community activities, 307; confidentiality of, 311; delegating responsibility, 308, 309; and depression, 311; finding 306, 307; newcomer's packet, 312; number of people needed, 305, 306; and peer counseling, 312–314; personal stories of, 305; and social isolation, 310; starting your own, 310, 311, 312; strengthening, 308, 309; and suicide prevention, 311; women's support network, 330

symptoms of FMS. *See also* symptoms of FMS/MPS Complex; tender points

achiness, 68; carbohydrate craving, 70; dizziness, 75; electromagnetic sensitivity, 75; fibrofog, 171; fingernail ridges, 12; fluctuating, 8; heartburn, 86; hiatal hernia, 86; light sensitivity, 74; low-grade fever, 9; menstrual problems, 93; migraines, 83; numbness or tingling, 75; pain, 9, 12; pelvic pain, 8; SAD, 74; the "shakes," 73; skin mottling, 12, 69, 70, 71; sleep apnea, 71; spasticity, 12, 21; stiffness, 12; susceptibility to infection, 73; sweat problems, 72; tender points, 10, 11; urine, foul-smelling, 93; vomiting, 86; water retention, 203

symptoms of FMS/MPS Complex. *See also* symptoms of FMS; symptoms of MPS
    allergies, 69; big toe pain, 98; blackfly and mosquito attraction, 68; bodywide achiness, 68, 69; breast pain, 87; bruxism, 74, 80; buckling knee, 100; burning or redness of inner thigh, 103; chest tightness, 91; chronic dry cough, 78; clumsiness, 76; compulsive urination insomnia, 115, 116; dark specks in vision, 81, 82; dermographia, 72; difficulty climbing stairs, 101; dizziness, 84; dry mucus membranes, 79; electromagnetic sensitivity, 75; esophageal reflux, 86; fatigue, 69, 70; fibrofog, 171; fluctuating blood pressure, 79; fluctuating body weight, 79; FMS/MPS foot, 102; foot pain, 102, 103; foot slap, 98; frozen shoulder, 42, 87; frustration, 72; growing pains, 68; hair loss, 70, 71; hamstring pain, 102, 103; heat and cold sensitivity, 72; hiatal hernia, 91; impotence, 93, 95; intestinal cramps, 91, 92; irritable bladder or bowel, 87, 92, 94; itchiness, 71; jaw problems, 79; "jumpy" muscles, 74; low-back pain, 93, 95; lumbago, 95; mid-shoulder pain, 85; mitral valve prolapse, 91; muscle cramps, 100; nausea, 92; night driving difficulties, 73; outer thigh sensitivity, 103; overgrowing connective tissue, 71; pain when writing, 85; painful intercourse, 92; rapid heartbeat, 91; Restless Leg Syndrome, 103; ringing in ears, 78; roof- of-the-mouth itch, 70; runny nose, 76, 77; sciatica, 95, 96; shin splints, 98; shortness of breath, 87; stiff necks, 83, 84; "stitch in the side," 87; swallowing difficulties, 77, 78; thick mucus secretions, 72; weak ankles, 96; weak hand grip, 87, 88; yeast infections, 70

symptoms of MPS. *See also* symptoms of FMS/MPS Complex
    balance problems, 103; bruxism, 80; ear pain, 81, 82; eye pain, 81, 82; growing pains, 68; headache, 82; motor coordination problems, 76; unexplained toothaches, 81

syndrome, defined, 8, 9

T

teeth grinding. *See* bruxism

Temporomandibular Joint Syndrome
    as coexisiting condition, 46; as symptom of FMS/MPS Complex, 79, 80; and toothaches, 81

tender points
    changing into TrPs, 36; clusters of, 12; and the Copenhagen official definition of FMS, 10;

defined, 10; distribution in traumatically
caused FMS, 32; examining for, 10; locations of,
10–12; painful areas outside of, 31; pairs of, 10,
11; symmetrical distribution of 10, **11**; and TrPs,
28

tendons, 18, 19

tennis-ball acupressure
to compress TrPs, 261; to decrease water retention,
54; instructions for, 262; and Irritable Bowel
Syndrome, 125; and visualization, 262

thymus extract, 73, 216

thyroid deficiency. *See* hypometabolism

toothaches, 81

travel
checklist for, 348–349; and decompression time ,
345; "evergreen hotel rooms," 348; and jet lag,
348; limited mobility hotel accommodations,
346; and medications, 347, 348, 349; as
perpetuating factor, 57; resources for, 347, 348;
stretching on auto trips, 345; tips, 346–347

triggering events, 13, 14, 116

trigger point cascade, defined, 31

trigger point injections, 38, 39, 205

trigger points (general). *See also* latent TrPs; satellite TrPs;
secondary TrPs; trigger points (specific)
balance problems, 103; bloating, 91, 92; bodywork
for, 240; and breathing, 259; causes of, 19, 24–25;
chest tightness, 91; constipation, 54, 55; defined,
23, 25; distribution in MPS, 32; dizziness, 75, 84;
ear pain, 77; electronic stimulation for, 244; eye
problems, 76, 79, 81, 82; facial, 47; foot
problems, 98, 102; frozen shoulder, 42, 87;
galvanic muscle stimulation for, 250, 251, 252;
and growing pains, 68; and guaifenesin, 221;
hand grip, 25, 87, 91, 92; head rolls, danger of,
197; headaches, 82, 83; hypermobility, 70;
hypoglycemia, 53; and ill-fitting shoes, 58, 59;
immobility as activator, 255; and impotence, 93,
95; inappropriate therapies for, 244; initiating
events of, 30, 32; intestinal cramps, 91, 92;
irritable bladder or bowel, 92, 124, 125; leg
problems, 96, 98; low-back pain, 95; mapping
of, 33; menstrual cramps, 91, 92; motor
coordination, 75; muscle cramps, 100; muscle
strength, 25; neck problems, 30–31, 83, 84;
numbness and tingling, 75; painful sexual
intercourse, 93; perpetuating factors, 49, 54, 55;
post-nasal drip, 30; rebound contraction, 240,
246, 261; referred pain patterns of, 23, 25, 26;
and repetitive motion, 51, 255, 322; ropy bands,
25; shortness of breath, 87; swallowing
problems, 79; symptoms of, 27–28; and tender
points, 25, 28; tennis-ball acupressure for, 261;
toothaches, 81; types of pain caused by, 26;
ultrasound treatment for, 250, 251, 252;
variability of, 28; work-related, identifying, 322

trigger points (specific)
abdominal oblique: and hiatal hernia, **87**, 91; and
irritable bladder or bowel, **87**, 92
adductor longus: and buckling knee, 100, **101**
adductor magnus: and hamstring pain, 103; and
menstrual problems, 93
adductor pollicis: and pain when writing, **85**, 86

brachioradialus: and thumb pain and tingling, **84**,
85, 86
coccygeus: and menstrual problems, 93
digastric: and rhinitis, **77**; and swallowing
problems, 77; and toothaches, 81
dorsal interosseus: and foot deformities, 59
external oblique: and esophagael reflux, **87**; and
irritable bladder or bowel, 87, 92
gastrocnemius: and hamstring pain, **99**, 102; and
leg cramps, 98, 99; and Restless Leg Syndrome,
103
gluteus maximus, 55: and growing pains, 68, 351
gluteus minimus: and pregnancy, 134; and sciatica,
95, **96**
gluteus medius: and pregnancy, 134
gracilis: and burning or redness of inner thigh, 103
hamstrings: and phantom limb pain, 100; and
sciatica, 96, **97**
iliocostalis: and appendicitis-like pain, 92, **94**; and
menstrual pain, 93, **94**
iliopsoas: as perpetuating factor, **54**, 55; and
low-back pain, 95; and hamstring pain, **54**, 102
internal oblique: and irritable bladder or bowel, 94
intrinsic foot: 59, **60**, 103
levator scapulae: and stiff necks, **83**, 84
long flexor: 103
masseter: and bruxism, **80**; and ear problems, 78,
80; and jaw problems, 79, 80; toothaches, 81
McBurney's Point: and appendicitis-like pain, 92,
95
medial pterygoid: and ear pain, 77, **78**
multifidi: and irritable bladder or bowel, **92**, 93;
and nausea, 92, 93
opponens pollicis: and pain when writing, **85**, 86
orbicularis oculi: and eye problems, **82**
pectoralis: and chest tightness, **89**, 91; and
hypersensitive nipples, 87, 89; and rapid
heartbeat, 89, 91
peroneal: and ill-fitting shoes, 58, **59**; and shin
splints, 98; and weak ankles, 96, **97**
piriformis: and appendicitis-like pain, 92; and
impotence, 93; as perpetuating factor, 54, **55**;
and pain with intercourse, 93, and sciatica, 96
platysma: and prickling "electric" face, **79**
posterior cervicle: and headaches, 82, **83**; and stiff
necks, 84
psoas: during pregnancy, 134
pyramidalis: and irritable bladder or bowel, 92;
and menstrual problems, 93
quadratus lumborum: and low-back pain, 95
quadriceps: and buckling knee, 100, **102**; and
difficulty climbing stairs, 101, 102: and
hamstring pain, 102, 103; and myalgia
paresthetica, 103
rectus abdominis: and appendicitis-like pain, 92;
and irritable bladder or bowel, 94; and
menstrual problems, 93
sartorius: and difficulty climbing stairs, 99, 101;
and leg cramps, 98, 99; and myalgia
paresthetica, 103
scaleni: pain referral pattern of, 25, **26**; splinting of,
77; and spinal nerve entrapment, 91; and weak
hand grip, 91
serratus anterior: and shortness of breath, 87, **88**,
260

soleus: and circulation, **100**; and foot pain, 100, 102; and leg cramps, 98, 100; as "second" heart, 98, 256;

splenius capitis: cause of sore spot on head, **84**

splenius cervici: and eye problems, 81, **82**; and migraines, 83

sternalis: and breast pain, 87, **90**; and rapid heart beat 90, 91

subscapularis: and frozen shoulder, **42**, 43, 87; restricting rotating arm movement, 51

sternocleidomastoid (SCM): and balance problems, **27**; and eye problems, 27; cascade effect of, 31; and chest tightness, 91; and chronic dry cough, 78; and dizziness, 84; and headaches, 82, 83; and hypoglycemia, 53; and motor coordination, 75; splinting of, 77; and pregnancy, 134

temporalis: and eye problems, 81; and migraines, 83; and TMJ, **80**

thorocolumbar: and sciatica, 96, 101

tibialis: and foot problems, **98**, 102; and weak ankles, 96, 98

trapezius: and eye problems, 81; and migraine, 83; and stiff neck, 84; and TMJ, **80**

vastus lateralis: and myalgia paresthetica, 103

vastus medialis: and buckling knee, 100, **101**; and difficulty climbing stairs,100

TrPs. See trigger points (general); trigger points (specific)

tryptophan, 37, 52

U

ultrasound therapy , 224, 250, 251, 252

urination
compulsive urination insomnia, 115, 116; foul-smelling, 93; frequent, as symptom of FMS/MPS Complex, 92,; and phosphoric acid, 220

V

vaginal discharge, 172, 222

vapocoolant spray, 91, 204, 249

vision problems. *See* eye problems

visualization, 151, 193–196, 262

vitamins, 157

vocational rehabilitation, 328, 330

vomiting, 92. *See also* esophageal reflux

vulvar vestibular syndrome, 176

W

wastes. *See* metabolic waste

water
and heated pools, 182; retention caused by medications, 203; therapy, 161; and yeast, 173

weight
and flare, 129; fluctuations as symptom of FMS/MPS Complex, 74; gain or loss as symptom, 180; perception of and spills, 76

workplace issues. *See also* workstation
Americans With Disabilities Act of 1992 (ADA), 326; clothing, 323; company disability plan, 322; coworkers, 326, 327; education and training, 330, 331; employers, 326; environmental issues, 326; evaluating a job, 327, 328; National Rehabilitation Information Center, 326; Office of Economic Development, 329; Office of Equal Opportunity, 326; physical risks, 321; Plan to Achieve Self-Sufficiency, 328, 329; Project on Women and Disability, 330; repetitious movements, 322; SCORE (Service Corps of Retired Executives), 329; self- employment, 328; Small Business Development Centers, 329; supervisors and medical conditions, 323; vocational rehabilitation, 328; women's support networks, 330

workstation
computer screen distance, 324; keyboard and mouse issues, 324, 325; lighting, 326; optimizing tips for, 323–326; proper chair, 324; stretching at, importance of, 324; wrist rests, 325

Y

yeast problems
acidophilus for, 176; antibiotics for, 176; antibody test for infection, 70, 125; antifungal medication for, 204; and birth control pills, 176; and bladder complaints, 176; and diabetes, 176; "die-off," 47, 128, 177; diet for, 177; and fibrofog, 173, 175, 176–177; and flares, 128; as FMS/MPS Complex symptom, 70; and HIV, 176; infection as coexisting condition, 46; overgrowth, 47; prescription drugs for, 205

Name Index

Anderson, Bob, 256, 258
Anderson, Craig, 251
August, Lynne, 216, 228
Balfour, William, 7
Bourne, Edmund, 182
Butler, Sharon, 18, 19, 256
Campbell, John, W., Jr., 305
Carneiro, Norton Maritz, 268
Chopra, Deepak, 143, 164, 286
Clauw, Jay, 173
Freidman, Neil, 271
Gendlin, Eugene, 271
Goldstein, Jay, 173
Grad, Marcia, 234
Hanh, Thich Nhat, 142, 191
Johnston, Lynn, 160

Karni, Avi, 119
Kennedy, John F., 257
London, Wayne, 173, 177
Mason, John, 340
Moldofsky, Harvey, 117
Morton, Dudley, 60
Murray, Michael T., 124
Nye, David, 117, 178
Osler, Sir William, 155, 268
Phillips, Wendell, 334
Polter, Joseph, 335
Potter, Claudia, 221
Radnor, Alan T., 335
Travell, Williard, 250
Warfield, Carol, 109

Other New Harbinger Self-Help Titles

The Daily Relaxer, $12.95
Living with Angina, $12.95
The Power of Two, $12.95
Living with ADD, $17.95
The Body Image Workbook, $17.95
Taking the Anxiety Out of Taking Tests, $12.95
The Taking Charge of Menopause Workbook, $17.95
It's Not OK Anymore, $13.95
PMS: Women Tell Women How to Control Premenstrual Syndrome, $13.95
Five Weeks to Healing Stress: The Wellness Option, $17.95
Choosing to Live: How to Defeat Suicide Through Cognitive Therapy, $12.95
Why Children Misbehave and What to Do About It, $14.95
Illuminating the Heart, $13.95
When Anger Hurts Your Kids, $12.95
The Addiction Workbook, $17.95
The Mother's Survival Guide to Recovery, $12.95
The Chronic Pain Control Workbook, Second Edition, $17.95
Fibromyalgia & Chronic Myofascial Pain Syndrome, $19.95
Diagnosis and Treatment of Sociopaths, $44.95
Flying Without Fear, $12.95
Kid Cooperation: How to Stop Yelling, Nagging & Pleading and Get Kids to Cooperate, $12.95
The Stop Smoking Workbook: Your Guide to Healthy Quitting, $17.95
Conquering Carpal Tunnel Syndrome and Other Repetitive Strain Injuries, $17.95
The Tao of Conversation, $12.95
Wellness at Work: Building Resilience for Job Stress, $17.95
What Your Doctor Can't Tell You About Cosmetic Surgery, $13.95
An End to Panic: Breakthrough Techniques for Overcoming Panic Disorder, $17.95
On the Clients Path: A Manual for the Practice of Solution-Focused Therapy, $39.95
Living Without Procrastination: How to Stop Postponing Your Life, $12.95
Goodbye Mother, Hello Woman: Reweaving the Daughter Mother Relationship, $14.95
Letting Go of Anger: The 10 Most Common Anger Styles and What to Do About Them, $12.95
Messages: The Communication Skills Workbook, Second Edition, $13.95
Coping With Chronic Fatigue Syndrome: Nine Things You Can Do, $12.95
The Anxiety & Phobia Workbook, Second Edition, $17.95
Thueson's Guide to Over-the-Counter Drugs, $13.95
Natural Women's Health: A Guide to Healthy Living for Women of Any Age, $13.95
I'd Rather Be Married: Finding Your Future Spouse, $13.95
The Relaxation & Stress Reduction Workbook, Fourth Edition, $17.95
Living Without Depression & Manic Depression: A Workbook for Maintaining Mood Stability, $17.95
Belonging: A Guide to Overcoming Loneliness, $13.95
Coping With Schizophrenia: A Guide For Families, $13.95
Visualization for Change, Second Edition, $13.95
Postpartum Survival Guide, $13.95
Angry All the Time: An Emergency Guide to Anger Control, $12.95
Couple Skills: Making Your Relationship Work, $13.95
Handbook of Clinical Psychopharmacology for Therapists, $39.95
Weight Loss Through Persistence, $13.95
Post-Traumatic Stress Disorder: A Complete Treatment Guide, $39.95
Stepfamily Realities: How to Overcome Difficulties and Have a Happy Family, $13.95
The Chemotherapy Survival Guide, $11.95
Your Family/Your Self: How to Analyze Your Family System, $12.95
Being a Man: A Guide to the New Masculinity, $12.95
The Deadly Diet, Second Edition: Recovering from Anorexia & Bulimia, $13.95
Last Touch: Preparing for a Parent's Death, $11.95
Self-Esteem, Second Edition, $13.95
I Can't Get Over It, A Handbook for Trauma Survivors, Second Edition, $13.95
Concerned Intervention, When Your Loved One Won't Quit Alcohol or Drugs, $12.95
Dying of Embarrassment: Help for Social Anxiety and Social Phobia, $12.95
The Depression Workbook: Living With Depression and Manic Depression, $17.95
Focal Group Psychotherapy: For Mental Health Professionals, $44.95
Prisoners of Belief: Exposing & Changing Beliefs that Control Your Life, $12.95
Men & Grief: A Guide for Men Surviving the Death of a Loved One, $13.95
When the Bough Breaks: A Helping Guide for Parents of Sexually Abused Children, $11.95
When Once Is Not Enough: Help for Obsessive Compulsives, $13.95
The Three Minute Meditator, Third Edition, $12.95
Beyond Grief: A Guide for Recovering from the Death of a Loved One, $13.95
Leader's Guide to the Relaxation & Stress Reduction Workbook, Fourth Edition, $19.95
The Divorce Book, $13.95
Hypnosis for Change: A Manual of Proven Techniques, Third Edition, $13.95
When Anger Hurts, $13.95
Lifetime Weight Control, $12.95

Call **toll free, 1-800-748-6273,** to order. Have your Visa or Mastercard number ready. Or send a check for the titles you want to New Harbinger Publications, Inc., 5674 Shattuck Ave., Oakland, CA 94609. Include $3.80 for the first book and 75¢ for each additional book, to cover shipping and handling. (California residents please include appropriate sales tax.) Allow four to six weeks for delivery.

Prices subject to change without notice.